TREATING WOMEN
WITH SUBSTANCE USE DISORDERS
The Women's Recovery Group Manual

Also by Shelly F. Greenfield

Women and Addiction: A Comprehensive Handbook
*Edited by Kathleen T. Brady, Sudie E. Back,
and Shelly F. Greenfield*

Treating Women
with Substance Use Disorders

THE WOMEN'S RECOVERY GROUP MANUAL

Shelly F. Greenfield

THE GUILFORD PRESS
New York   London

© 2016 The Guilford Press
A Division of Guilford Publications, Inc.
370 Seventh Avenue, Suite 1200, New York, NY 10001
www.guilford.com

Printed in the United States of America

This book is printed on acid-free paper.

Last digit is print number: 9 8 7 6 5 4 3 2 1

The author has checked with sources believed to be reliable in her efforts to provide information
that is complete and generally in accord with the standards of practice that are accepted at the
time of publication. However, in view of the possibility of human error or changes in behavioral,
mental health, or medical sciences, neither the author, nor the editor and publisher, nor any other
party who has been involved in the preparation or publication of this work warrants that the
information contained herein is in every respect accurate or complete, and they are not responsible
for any errors or omissions or the results obtained from the use of such information. Readers are
encouraged to confirm the information contained in this book with other sources.

Library of Congress Cataloging-in-Publication Data

Names: Greenfield, Shelly F., author.
Title: Treating women with substance use disorders : the women's recovery
    group manual / Shelly F. Greenfield.
Description: New York : The Guilford Press, [2016] | Includes bibliographical
    references and index.
Identifiers: LCCN 2016013925 | ISBN 9781462525768 (paperback : acid-free
    paper)
Subjects: LCSH: Women—Substance use. | Substance abuse—Treatment. |
    Women—Mental health. | BISAC: PSYCHOLOGY / Psychopathology / Addiction. |
    MEDICAL / Psychiatry / General. | SOCIAL SCIENCE / Social Work. |
    PSYCHOLOGY / Psychotherapy / Group. | MEDICAL / Nursing / Psychiatric.
Classification: LCC RC564.5.W65 G74 2016 | DDC 362.29082—dc23
LC record available at *http://lccn.loc.gov/2016013925*

For Allan, Danny, and Jacob—
who provide great support, love, humor,
and inspiration

About the Author

Shelly F. Greenfield, MD, MPH, is Professor of Psychiatry at Harvard Medical School and Chief Academic Officer at McLean Hospital, where she also serves as Chief of the Division of Women's Mental Health and Director of Clinical and Health Services Research and Education in the Alcohol and Drug Abuse Treatment Program. The Women's Recovery Group grew out of her extensive research and clinical work in the field of substance use disorders, with a particular focus on women and addiction. Dr. Greenfield has authored more than 125 articles and book chapters. She is Chair of the National Institute on Drug Abuse Clinical Trials Network gender special interest group and past Chair of the American Psychiatric Association's Council on Addiction Psychiatry, and serves on the Board of Directors of the American Academy of Addiction Psychiatry and on the Advisory Committee on Services for Women of the U.S. Substance Abuse and Mental Health Services Administration. A member of the American College of Psychiatrists and a Distinguished Fellow of the American Psychiatric Association, Dr. Greenfield is a recipient of the R. Brinkley Smithers Distinguished Scientist Award from the American Society of Addiction Medicine and the A. Clifford Barger Award for Excellence in Mentoring from Harvard Medical School.

Preface

This book is designed for therapists who treat women with alcohol and drug use disorders. It presents the Women's Recovery Group (WRG), an evidence-based group therapy for women with substance use disorders (SUDs) who are heterogeneous with respect to their alcohol or drug use disorders, presence of co-occurring psychiatric disorders, and ages and stages of life. The WRG was designed as a gender-responsive, single-gender group therapy that can be implemented in a variety of practice settings in both a semi-open or open enrollment (i.e., rolling) group format. It emphasizes both women-focused content and the mutual support gained from an all-women group composition. It is a relapse prevention, cognitive-behaviorally oriented group therapy that emphasizes self-care and developing skills for relapse prevention and recovery. The WRG can therefore be implemented as a component of treatment in a mixed-gender treatment setting, providing a gender-responsive group therapy for women with SUDs, or it can be provided in a single-gender women's treatment program as a component of gender-responsive care.

Alcohol and drug use disorders are a growing health problem among women, but significant barriers impede women's access to addiction treatment that is responsive to their needs. Obstacles to recovery for women with alcohol and drug use disorders include stigma, lack of support from partners and family, and competing responsibilities between recovery, work, and the needs of children and other family members. In addition, many women with SUDs also have co-occurring disorders such as depression, anxiety disorders, and eating disorders. These co-occurring conditions can affect recovery but are often not addressed in group therapy for alcohol and drug use disorders. The WRG was developed to provide a gender-responsive group therapy for women to address many of these clinical characteristics and other issues that are common for women with alcohol and drug use disorders.

This treatment was developed and tested in two clinical trials that demonstrated its efficacy, participant and therapist satisfaction with the group, and the feasibility of implementing the group in real-world clinical settings. This book provides the therapist with background information on women and addiction as well as the empirical evidence supporting the WRG.

It comprises a complete manual on how to conduct each session and also includes the informational handouts and skills practices for participants, check-in and check-out sheets, and bulletin board materials to be posted at each session. It is my hope that this book will make the WRG widely available so that it can assist many more women in their recovery from alcohol and drug problems.

Acknowledgments

There are many individuals and institutions that have contributed to the development of this treatment. I would like to gratefully acknowledge the National Institute on Drug Abuse and its support for the Stage I and Stage II trials of the Women's Recovery Group (WRG) through Grant Nos. R01 DA 015434 and K24 DA019855. In addition, the contributions of collaborators, co-investigators, consultants, research assistants, and study therapists were essential in developing this treatment. Among the co-investigators and consultants who were key individuals in the development of the treatment are Genie Bailey, MD, Kathleen Brady, MD, PhD, Hilary Connery, MD, PhD, Dennis Daley, PhD, Garrett Fitzmaurice, ScD, Hadine Joffe, MD, Grace Hennessy, MD, Robert Gallop, PhD, Roger Weiss, MD, Mike Robbins, PhD, John Rodolico, PhD, Aaron Hogue, PhD, and Mirka Koro-Ljungberg, PhD. I would also like to acknowledge the key role of the studies' group therapists, Crystal Cote, LMHC, Patty Diaferio, LICSW, Judy Faberman, LICSW, Heather Harley, LICSW, Monika Kolodziej, PhD, Marjorie Joseph, LICSW, Sue O'Donnell, MA, Barbara Raymond, LICSW, Ruth Reibstein, EdD, Laura Ruegg, LICSW, and Bronwen Wirta, LICSW. Lynn Carlson, LICSW, provided additional feedback on clinical implementation outside of the research setting. Each of the studies relied on the excellent help of a talented research study staff including Michele Crisafulli, MA, Amanda Cummings, PhD, Cathryn Freid, PhD, Julia Kaufman, BA, Laura Kuper, BA, Brittany Iles, BA, Melissa Lincoln, BA, Kate McHugh, PhD, Rebecca Popuch, BA, Michelle Rapoza, CAC, Katie Schlebecker, BA, BS, Dawn Sugarman, PhD, Elisa Trucco, PhD, and Sara Wigderson, BA. Finally, the Stage I and Stage II trials were conducted at the Alcohol and Drug Abuse Treatment Program, Division of Alcohol and Drug Abuse, of McLean Hospital in Belmont, Massachusetts, and Stanley Street Addiction and Recovery (SSTAR) in Fall River, Massachusetts. I wish to thank Michele Crisafulli, MA, Sara Wigderson, BA, and Brittany Iles, BA, for their careful attention to preparation of several versions of the manuscript. I would also like to thank Jim Nageotte, Senior Editor at The Guilford Press, whose guidance no doubt contributed to a much better and more helpful book. There are numerous individuals throughout both of these treatment programs who supported the studies through patient referrals and in other significant ways, and I would like to acknowledge their contributions, without which we could not have learned about the WRG. McLean Hospital has supported my development as a clinician and researcher and has provided the essential resources and environment for the development of this treatment. Finally, I would like to thank the many patients who participated in the studies that helped develop the WRG. I hope that the WRG will be a helpful resource for women who struggle with addiction and will provide insights, support, and tools for their healthy recovery.

Contents

Purchasers of this book can download and print the materials
in Appendices A and B at *www.guilford.com/greenfield-forms*
for personal use or use with clients.

PART I

Introduction to
the Women's Recovery Group

In this section of the book, we first review information about women and substance use disorders and then provide detailed information about how to conduct the Women's Recovery Group (WRG). Chapter 1 reviews the prevalence of alcohol and drug problems in women, the effects of substance use disorders on women's health, and the rationale for providing group therapy in women-only treatment groups. We then present an overview of the WRG. In Chapter 2 we first describe all of the key elements of the WRG, including therapist style, group content and process, WRG theme and central recovery rule, and participant characteristics. Then we will present the details of the format of the WRG, including implementation in open- versus closed-group format, setting up the group room, and conducting the pre-group meeting. Detailed information is then provided on the structure of the group sessions, including check-in, review of skills practices, presentation of session topic, open discussion, wrap-up and reading of take-home messages, distribution of skills practice, and check-out. This chapter concludes with tips for managing common clinical situations as well as adapting the WRG to individual therapy.

CHAPTER 1

Treating Women
with Substance Use Disorders

Substance use disorders (SUDs) are a growing health problem among women (Brady, Back, & Greenfield, 2009). However, compared with men, women are less likely to receive treatment for substance use disorders in the course of their lifetimes (Dawson, 1996; Mojtabai, 2005; Wu & Ringwalt, 2004). Specific barriers and obstacles to receiving care for women include stigma, lack of child care for those who are parenting, lack of support from partners and family, and insufficient financial resources, among others (Greenfield, Trucco, McHugh, Lincoln, & Gallop, 2007b; Greenfield, Brooks, Gordon, Green, Kropp, et al., 2007a). In addition, women often report a preference for women-only treatment, perceiving that such care provides a greater sense of comfort and safety for its members; however, lack of access to such treatment poses a barrier for many of them.

Women with SUDs differ from men in a number of characteristics, including the prevalence of co-occurring psychiatric disorders, medical problems, barriers to care, and reasons for relapse (Greenfield et al., 2007a). There is evidence that some of these issues may not be adequately addressed in mixed-gender substance abuse treatment groups (Kauffman, Dore, & Nelson-Zlupko, 1995; Nelson-Zlupko, Dore, Kauffman, & Kaltenbach, 1996). Since the mid-1990s, several group therapies for a number of subgroups of women with SUDs have been developed and empirically tested. For example, some group therapies have focused on treating women who are pregnant and parenting (Luthar & Suchman, 2000; Mackie-Ramos & Rice, 1988), or who have a specific co-occurring disorder (such as posttraumatic stress disorder) (Hien, Cohen, Miele, Litt, & Capstick, 2004; Najavits, Weiss, Shaw, & Muenz, 1998). However, in many clinical settings and practices, treatment-seeking women with SUDs are quite heterogeneous with respect to the type of substance they use, their age, their background (e.g., with or without a trauma history, children, partner), whether they have co-occurring psychiatric disorders (e.g., mood, anxiety, posttraumatic stress, eating disorders), and, if so, which disorders they may have.

In light of this, we recognized that there was no evidence-based recovery group therapy for treatment-seeking women who are heterogeneous with respect to their abuse or dependence on a range of substances (e.g., opioids, alcohol, cocaine), a variety of other psychiatric disorders (e.g., depression, anxiety, eating disorders), as well as different ages and stages of life (e.g., pregnant, parenting, widowed). We, therefore designed the Women's Recovery Group (WRG) to fill this gap.

How This Book Is Organized

The balance of this chapter provides background on SUDs in women, followed by an overview of the WRG and the current evidence for the WRG treatment. The chapter also includes quick reference tables, therapist examples, and discussion points in text boxes that provide concise summaries of the material presented as well as clinical illustrations relevant to running the WRG. Chapter 2 provides specific information on how to conduct the WRG treatment and includes therapist examples. Part II of this book provides a detailed therapist guide to conducting each of the 14 topic-oriented sessions as well as an individual pre-group meeting. Appendix A and Appendix B contain all the supporting materials for conducting the treatment, including a therapist self-assessment tool and materials to copy and post on a bulletin board during sessions, check-in and check-out sheets that are passed among participants, and session-specific participant educational sheets and skill practices for distribution. A section with references to research on the WRG as well as additional reading for each session topic is also provided in Appendix B.

Prevalence and Course of SUDs in Women

Gender differences in the rates of SUDs have been observed in both the general population and in treatment seekers, with a greater prevalence of SUDs in men than women (Lopez-Quintero et al., 2011). However, in the last two decades it has become clear that the gender gap in the prevalence of alcohol and drug use is narrowing (Centers for Disease Control and Prevention, 2013; Substance Abuse and Mental Health Services Administration, 2012). For alcohol use disorders, good evidence indicates that this is accounted for by the rising prevalence of these disorders among girls and women in recent birth cohorts, with rates in boys and men remaining fairly steady (Grucza, Bucholz, Rice, & Bierut, 2008). Until the 1980s, alcohol use disorders were thought to be five times as common among men as among women (Robins & Regier, 1991); however, by the 1990s, it had become clear that these rates had changed, with men being only 2 to 2.5 times as likely to have an alcohol problem as women in the course of their lifetime. Drug use disorders are approximately twice as likely in men as women, and in some instances, depending on the substance, these rates are even closer (Greenfield et al., 2007a).

In recent decades, girls have been initiating their use of alcohol, tobacco, and other drugs at approximately the same age as their male counterparts (Centers for Disease Control and Prevention, 2013; Greenfield et al., 2007a; McHugh, Wigderson, & Greenfield, 2014; Substance Abuse and Mental Health Services Administration, 2012). This is of clinical and public health concern because compared with men, women have increased vulnerability to the physical and medical adverse consequences of alcohol and other drugs. In particular, women can experience a so-called telescoping course of their addiction, which means shorter average intervals than men between first use and first problem use, between first problem use and dependence, and between dependence and treatment (Piazza, Vrbka, & Yeager, 1989; Randall et al., 1999). The telescoping course means that, even with fewer years at lower doses than men, women experience on average more medical, psychiatric, and social consequences of their addiction. A number of clinical studies demonstrate that with fewer years of use, women experience more psychological distress, mood and anxiety disorders, exposure to childhood and adult trauma and associated symptoms, greater mental health problems, and more family and employment problems (Grella, 2008; McKay, Lynch, Pettinati, & Shepard, 2003; Stewart, Gossop, Marsden, Kidd, & Treacy, 2003; Wechsberg, Craddock, & Hubbard, 1998). There is also evidence that women who use substances such as alcohol, nicotine, or stimulants may experience more rapid dependence on these substances (Hernandez-Avila, Rounsaville, & Kranzler, 2004; Sugarman, Brezing, & Greenfield, 2013).

Women with SUDs are more likely than men to have co-occurring psychiatric disorders, such as depression, anxiety disorders, and eating disorders (Cohen et al., 2010; Greenfield et al., 2007a). These mental health problems can complicate treatment of SUDs (Brown, 2000; Compton, Cottler, Jacobs, Ben-Abdallah, & Spitznagel, 2003; Greenfield et al., 1998; Kranzler & Tinsley, 2004; Sinha & Rounsaville, 2002). In addition, women with SUDs are more likely to have a history of childhood and adult trauma than men with SUDs (Hien, Cohen, & Campbell, 2005). Some studies have found that histories of trauma can be associated with poorer SUD treatment outcomes (Brown, 2000; Comfort, Sockloff, Loverro, & Kaltenbach, 2003; Green, Polen, Lynch, Dickinson, & Bennett, 2004; Greenfield et al., 2002; Sugarman, Kaufman, Trucco, Brown, & Greenfield, 2014). In spite of the increasing prevalence of alcohol and drug use disorders, the earlier ages of initiation of use, and the telescoping course of SUDs in women, women are less likely than men to seek or receive treatment for their addiction (Dawson, 1996; Greenfield et al., 2007a; Wu & Ringwalt, 2004). While women may seek treatment for other co-occurring psychiatric disorders, such as anxiety and depression in mental health settings, they may not discuss their co-occurring problems with alcohol or drugs and their alcohol and drug use may therefore remain undetected and untreated (Weisner, 1993; Weisner & Schmidt, 1992).

Outcomes of Treatment of SUDs in Women

Once in treatment, a convergence of evidence demonstrates that there are few gender differences in success rates of treatment for women and men (Greenfield et al., 2007a), but recovery trajectories may differ longitudinally. One study of long-term outcomes for older women and men with alcohol dependence demonstrated that women were twice as likely as men to be abstinent at the 7-year follow-up, and the strongest predictor of outcomes for both men and women was the length of the initial treatment episode (Satre, Blow, Chi, & Weisner, 2007). Another study demonstrated more self-help use among women with alcohol dependence at the 16-year follow-up and that self-help engagement had greater association with drinking reductions for women than for men (Timko, DeBenedetti, Moos, & Moos, 2006). A longitudinal study of outcome showed that at 36 months there were no gender differences in drug and alcohol use but that women reported more psychological distress while men had more criminal justice involvement (Grella, Scott, & Foss, 2005).

While a convergence of evidence shows that gender itself does not predict treatment outcomes, studies have demonstrated a number of gender-specific prognostic factors that affect treatment outcomes (Greenfield et al., 2007a). For example, a co-occurring diagnosis of depression, anxiety, or PTSD may adversely affect SUD treatment outcomes for men and for women (Brown, 2000; Cohen et al., 2010; Compton et al., 2003; Greenfield et al., 2007a; Greenfield et al., 1998; Kranzler & Tinsley, 2004; Sinha & Rounsaville, 2002). Because these disorders are more prevalent among women than men, they may disproportionately affect women's recovery. The same is true for histories of trauma and other characteristics. There is evidence that treatment that addresses these and other gender-specific factors in recovery can enhance SUD treatment outcomes for women (Greenfield et al., 2007a). For example, programs for pregnant and parenting women with substance use disorders that provide child care and prenatal care can have improved treatment outcomes for women (Ashley, Marsden, & Brady, 2003; Orwin, Francisco, & Bernichon, 2001). In addition, several longitudinal studies have demonstrated different pathways to recovery for women and men (Grella, 2008).

A Rationale for Women-Only Treatment Groups

Few randomized trials have compared all-women's treatment to mixed-gender treatment for SUDs. Several studies that have compared women's residential treatment programs with mixed-gender treatment programs have not found superior outcomes for women-only residential compared with mixed-gender treatment (Bride, 2001; Kaskutas, Zhang, French, & Witbrodt, 2005). However, a number of studies have found that programs that provide enhanced services for women that focus on women's specific needs have higher rates of treatment completion and improved outcomes (Claus et al., 2007; Orwin et al., 2001; Smith & Marsh, 2002), and a systematic review of multiple studies provides convergent evidence on enhanced treatment outcomes for women in women's programming tailored to women's specific treatment needs (Grella, 2008). Such gender-responsive treatment for women is strengths-based, stresses the importance of relationships, and is trauma-informed (Covington, 2003; Grella, 2008).

There are therefore several rationales for single-gender SUD treatment groups for women. These include patient preference; the opportunity to enhance comfort, support, and cohesion within treatment groups; and the opportunity to present women-focused content (Greenfield, Cummings, Kuper, Wigderson, & Koro-Ljungberg, 2013a). In several qualitative studies, women report decreased sex-role stereotyping and feeling safer in a single-gender substance abuse treatment group (Kauffman et al., 1995; Nelson-Zlupko et al., 1996). A preference for single-gender groups may exist for a wide range of reasons such as dissatisfaction with treatment or self-help groups that are mixed-gender or predominantly male; a positive experience with an all-women's recovery or self-help group in the past; and a history of trauma or abuse such that an all-women's treatment format feels safer and more comfortable. Patient preference in a variety of medical and psychiatric treatments is often a factor in satisfaction and provides one rationale for a single-gender format for treatment of SUDs. For example, in one study comparing single-versus mixed-gender programs, lesbian women, women with dependent children, and women with trauma histories were less likely to drop out of a single-gender than mixed-gender SUD treatment program (Copeland & Hall, 1992).

Women report feeling an enhanced sense of comfort and support in an all-women's treatment setting. They report feeling that there is a sense of easy communication within a group of women and that because of this shared understanding and communication, they can move more rapidly to discuss difficult issues that are often obstacles to recovery (Greenfield et al., 2013a). Some of these issues focus on sexuality, male or female partners, and histories of abuse, among others. Discussion of these difficult issues and the effect they have on addiction and recovery is often critical for many women, but may not be possible in a mixed-gender context. In one qualitative study of the WRG, women reported feeling nonjudgmental support on the part of other women in the group and a sense of validation of their own experience that is helpful in recovery from alcohol and drug addiction (Greenfield et al., 2013a).

Finally, a single-gender SUD group therapy format provides the context for women-focused content. For example, in the WRG, the topics provide information and education about the antecedents and consequences of alcohol and drug problems that are especially pertinent to women. Specific topics include the effects on recovery of women and caretaking; women and their partners; the effect of substance problems on women's health; substance problems through a woman's life cycle; substance use and women's reproductive health; mood, anxiety, and eating disorders and SUDs; and violence and abuse.

Studies of the effectiveness of gender-specific treatment for women with SUDs have increased in number since 2000, but nevertheless remain relatively few (Greenfield et al., 2007a). Studies of women's treatment programs (e.g., residential or day hospital programs) that may or may not be compared with mixed-gender treatment, have produced mixed results depending on the population studied, the outcomes evaluated, and the comparison groups chosen. Nevertheless, evidence is accumulating that treatment that focuses on women's specific needs and services can provide enhanced outcomes for women (Greenfield et al., 2007a; Greenfield & Grella, 2009; Grella, 2008). Ongoing research in this area holds promise in expanding our understanding about the characteristics of women who might benefit the most from women-focused treatment and how to maximize the effectiveness of these clinical services.

Overview of the WRG

The WRG is a relapse prevention group therapy that utilizes a cognitive-behavioral approach for women who are heterogeneous with respect to their age, stage of life, specific substance used, and the presence or absence of co-occurring psychiatric disorders.

Goals of the Group

The major goals of the group are (1) to promote abstinence from all substances including alcohol; (2) to improve understanding of specific aspects of substance use disorders, recovery, and relapse that are relevant to women; and (3) to help participants develop skills and strategies that will be useful in preventing relapse and promoting recovery.

The WRG uses a 90-minute, structured relapse prevention group therapy session with a cognitive-behavioral focus that includes session topics based on gender-specific antecedents, consequences, and treatment outcomes for SUDs. There are 14 specific session topics (see Table 1.1) that can be flexibly chosen in any order for a 12-week sequence of groups, or all 14 topics can be used for a 14-week sequence.

Each session is structured with a brief check-in, review of the previous week's skill practice, presentation of that day's session topic, an open discussion, the reading of the take-home messages, distribution of the skill practice sheet for the upcoming week, and a check-out.

The group makes use of visual aids (in the form of bulletin board materials) and session-specific educational sheets and skill practices for participants. Bulletin board materials stating the group theme "Recovery Means Taking Care of Yourself," the central recovery rule "Recovery = Relapse Prevention + Repair Work," and the symptoms of substance problems are posted weekly (see Table 1.2). Summary points and take-home messages from the day's topic change weekly and are also posted.

The group theme—"Recovery Means Taking Care of Yourself"—emphasizes self-care and the idea that recovery is both a major part of self-care and that self-care activities will also enhance recovery. Therapists should refer back to this group theme throughout the treatment by encouraging self-care activities and routines that enhance recovery. The central recovery rule—"Recovery = Relapse Prevention + Repair Work"—emphasizes that recovery must encompass both relapse prevention and repair work (see Table 1.3). Repair work includes repairing the damage to self and relationships due to substances and learning how to enjoy your life substance-free.

The WRG sessions that focus mainly on relapse prevention include Sessions 2, 3, 6, and 8 (see Table 1.3), which encourage identifying triggers to using and building alternative skills and coping to prevent substance use. Other sessions, such as Sessions 11, 13, and 14, focus on other domains of life including disclosure, achieving a balance, and having fun without using

TABLE 1.1. WRG Session Topics

- Session 1. The Effect of Drugs and Alcohol on Women's Health
- Session 2. How to Manage Triggers and High-Risk Situations
- Session 3. Overcoming Obstacles to Recovery
- Session 4. Managing Mood, Anxiety, and Eating Problems without Using Substances
- Session 5. Women and Their Partners: The Effect on Recovery
- Session 6. Coping with Stress
- Session 7. Women as Caretakers: Can You Take Care of Yourself While You Are Taking Care of Others?
- Session 8. Using Self-Help Groups to Help Yourself
- Session 9. Women's Use of Substances through the Life Cycle
- Session 10. Violence and Abuse: Getting Help
- Session 11. The Issue of Disclosure: To Tell or Not to Tell?
- Session 12. Substance Use and Women's Reproductive Health
- Session 13. Can You Have Fun without Using Drugs or Alcohol?
- Session 14. Achieving a Balance in Your Life

TABLE 1.2. Central Recovery Rule and Group Theme

Central Recovery Rule: Recovery = Relapse Prevention + Repair Work

Group Theme: Recovery Means Taking Care of Yourself

substances. These are part of "repair work." Certain sessions have elements of both relapse prevention and repair work including those focused on partners, the caretaking role, and violence and abuse. Both relapse prevention and repair work are central to recovery.

The WRG also emphasizes the message that while differences might exist between individuals in the group, all participants are united in seeking treatment for their problems with substances.

Therapists can refer to the common symptoms of substance problems that are posted on the bulletin board weekly (see Table 1.4) in order to highlight a key point for participants: that while they may differ in the specific substance they use, symptoms of co-occurring disorders, and family and social circumstances, they share with one another at least some of the symptoms of substance problems posted on the board. They also share a desire to recover.

TABLE 1.3. The WRG Central Recovery Rule: Recovery = Relapse Prevention + Repair Work

Relapse prevention

- Identify triggers and high-risk situations.
- Plan to avoid high-risk situations and develop coping skills to deal with unavoidable situations.
- Create a "trigger-free" environment.
- Get treatment.

Repair work

- Repair damaged relationships and damage to self.
- Learn to enjoy life substance-free.

WRG sessions include both relapse prevention and repair work.

Sessions focusing on relapse prevention and/or repair work

Relapse prevention

1. Effects of drugs on health
2. Managing high-risk situations
3. Obstacles to seeking treatment
4. Managing mood, anxiety, eating disorders
6. Using self-help to help yourself
8. Coping with stress

Repair work

11. Issue of disclosure
13. Can you have fun?
14. Achieving a balance

Elements of both

5. Women and their partners
7. Women as caretakers
9. Women's use of substances through the life cycle
10. Violence and abuse
12. Reproductive health

Therapist Examples: Discussing the Central Recovery Rule

Example 1

THERAPIST: I think to just keep in mind that there is a timeline to recovery. The first part is relapse prevention and not using drugs and alcohol, and the second is the repair work you can do to work on the circumstances in your life and come to a better place with those things. And it takes time and it's so hard to work on the relapse prevention part, especially when life is feeling that bad to you.

Example 2

THERAPIST: This sort of brings home to me—we were talking about the repair work that happens after we sort of, you know, there is the relapse prevention and there is the repair work piece of it—that some of the repair work piece of it has to do with learning how to interact with families in a way that's helpful.

PARTICIPANT: Right.

THERAPIST: And it's also relapse prevention work, and it's kind of both together. So in some ways, working on relationships so they're not triggering, working on relationships so that they're helpful, and working on relationships so that they're good all around—I can see that all as being part of the relapse prevention, repair work continuum.

Table 1.4 lists symptoms that are common to individuals experiencing substance-related problems. Individuals with these symptoms may or may not qualify for a diagnosis of a substance related disorder. For example, the American Psychiatric Association's (2013, p. 483) *Diagnostic and Statistical Manual of Mental Disorders*, fifth edition (DSM-5), specifies 11 symptoms that are common to SUDs. DSM-5 notes that SUDs can be further specified as mild, moderate, or severe based on the number of these symptoms that the patient experiences. Generally patients having two or fewer symptoms have a mild disorder, those with three to five symptoms qualify for moderate severity, and those with six or more are considered to have a severe disorder. For information related to assessment of SUDs and psychiatric disorders as well as standard criteria

TABLE 1.4. Common Symptoms of Substance Problems

- Increasing the amount of the substance(s) used over time.
- Trying unsuccessfully to cut down or stop using substances.
- Spending an increasing amount of time using substances, often leading to decreasing time spent in other activities related to work, school, relationships, or recreation.
- Having craving for the substance(s) when you are not using.
- Continuing to use substances even knowing they cause or worsen problems with work, family, school, relationships, or other activities.
- Using substances even when knowing they cause physical or mental health problems or when they may be physically dangerous to use.
- Developing tolerance to the substance over time (i.e., developing a need for more of the substance in order to achieve the desired or usual effect).
- Experiencing withdrawal symptoms when substance use stops or is reduced.

TABLE 1.5. Four Levels of Participation

- Attendance every week
- Active listening
- Sharing and responding
- Doing the skill practices between sessions

for the diagnosis of substance-related disorders according to the World Health Organization's *International Classification of Diseases*, version 10 (ICD-10), or the American Psychiatric Association's DSM-5, the reader is referred to standard texts (Stevens & Dennis, pp. 107–116, and Woody & Cacciola, pp. 117–122, in Ruiz & Strain, 2011; World Health Organization, 1992; Greenfield & Hennessy, 2015; American Psychiatric Association, 2013).

The WRG encourages an environment of mutual support and social connectedness. Throughout the group women are encouraged to participate in four different ways (stressing that women assess their own comfort with each level of participation): attending the group, active listening, sharing and responding, and doing the skill practices between sessions. The WRG recognizes that not everyone will be able to participate at all four levels; however, everyone is encouraged to participate as much as she is able at all four levels as best outcomes may be achieved through full participation (see Table 1.5).

The WRG was designed to include two main components of group therapy that are posited to be key effective components of the treatment: (1) the all-women group composition and (2) women-focused topics to provide education about the antecedents and consequences of addiction in women, as well as women-focused recovery topics (see Table 1.6). The WRG was designed to include both components in order that the all-women group composition would enhance comfort and support for participants, facilitate group cohesion, and promote communication. The women-focused topics would provide education specific to the women participants.

The effect of patient–therapist gender matching in individual therapy has been the subject of studies and has produced mixed results (Fiorentine & Hillhouse, 1999; Sterling, Gottheil, Weinstein, & Serota, 1998, 2001). Because patient–therapist gender matching may affect treatment outcomes, in the studies comparing the WRG to mixed-gender group therapy, all therapists conducting either the WRG or mixed-gender group therapy were women. It is therefore not known what effect a male therapist would have on the outcomes of the WRG and we currently recommend that the group be led by a woman therapist.

TABLE 1.6. Key Components of the WRG

All-women group composition
- Enhances group cohesiveness; sense of safety, comfort, and support.

Women-focused topics
- Provides education on gender-specific antecedents and consequences of SUDs for women.

The Distinction between the WRG and Other Group Approaches

The WRG is a cognitive-behaviorally oriented relapse prevention treatment that focuses on understanding internal and external triggers to substance use and works on developing strategies to manage these triggers, rather than using substances. The WRG focuses on thoughts, feelings, and environmental cues that may make the person more vulnerable to drug craving. It stresses identification of the individual's own triggers, learning skills that foster one's own recovery, discussion of ambivalence about the recovery process, and thinking through practical problems that might be obstacles to staying abstinent and in recovery. The WRG utilizes cognitive-behavioral methods such as a focus on an individual's cognitions and feelings that might trigger craving to use and helps develop alternative ways to manage these thoughts and feelings. The WRG also provides "skills practices" to be completed between sessions. However, the WRG differs from standard cognitive-behavioral therapy (CBT) groups in that it does not exclusively focus on identifying and changing cognitions and feelings that might be triggers to substance use, nor does it set the expectation that doing the "skills practice" between sessions is a required part of the group. Rather, the WRG uses this approach (e.g., identifying thoughts and feelings that may provide triggers to substance use), and provides skills practices as an element of the treatment, but other key elements of treatment are utilized as well. These other key elements of treatment include the mutual support of the other women participants and group cohesiveness that are achieved through both the single-gender group composition, the dedicated session time for open discussion of recovery-oriented concerns as a standard part of each group session, the supportive atmosphere established by the therapist (e.g., nonconfrontational and emphasizing commonalities rather than differences among participants), and education about antecedents and consequences of SUDs in women. These WRG-specific elements are not standard components of CBT groups.

The WRG is not a psychodynamically oriented group. While the WRG does have time in the session dedicated to open discussion of recovery concerns, it focuses on the present and the future but does not explore the past and the effect of early relationships on current problems. The WRG might explore an individual's past relapses insofar as this helps illuminate the patient's triggers and alternate ways that she might cope with those triggers.

The WRG is more directive than motivational interviewing or motivational enhancement insofar as the therapist and patient are clear that the goal of the WRG is abstinence from all drugs and alcohol. On the other hand, women in the WRG are heterogeneous with respect to substance used and treatment history. Like motivational interviewing or motivational enhancement, the WRG adopts a nonjudgmental, nonconfrontational stance and encourages participants to explore ambivalence as part of their risk for relapse. In addition, women report any use, slips, or lapses they might have had during the weekly check-in. Often these circumstances are explored during the open discussion. Women in the group may be abstinent from one substance (e.g., alcohol) but struggling with ambivalence regarding cessation of another drug (e.g., marijuana). They may also be engaged in a first treatment or may have recently relapsed after a period of sobriety.

The WRG encourages individuals to make use of self-help groups, but the WRG is not a 12-step group, nor is it a 12-step facilitation group. The WRG does not include the directive that all participants must use self-help or attend a self-help group in the course of the WRG treatment. Instead, Session 8, "Using Self-Help Groups to Help Yourself," discusses the pros and cons of many self-help groups and encourages participants to discuss their own experiences. It also explores issues pertaining to women utilizing self-help and examines women-only versus mixed-gender self-help groups.

Because the WRG is not a 12-step group, the therapist should not ask participants to identify themselves as "an alcoholic and/or an addict," to review specific steps from the 12-step model, or to say the Serenity Prayer. Similarly, because the WRG is not a psychodynamic group, the therapist will not focus on transference or interpersonal issues within the group and how they might relate to their own families of origin, or ask participants to explore early relationships and how they have bearing on the participant's current situation. Rather, in the WRG participants are asked to identify high-risk situations and internal and external triggers, and to assess what they have been able to do to facilitate their own abstinence or what actions have made them feel more vulnerable. They are asked to identify alternative strategies to managing triggers rather than using substances. In the course of the therapy, the WRG provides a variety of approaches and resources for women who are trying to prevent relapse and recover from their SUD. These approaches include learning to identify individual triggers and alternative strategies to cope and manage them; education about alcohol and drug's adverse consequences on women's health, as well as antecedents and consequences of alcohol and drug use disorders that are specific to women; skill practices designed to reinforce the session topics; education about self-help; open discussion of recovery related issues; and mutual support from other women participants in a nonconfrontational group that emphasizes self-care, preventing relapse, and focusing on repairing domains of life (e.g., family relationships, feelings of shame) that have been harmed through the process of addiction.

What Is Different about the WRG?

There have been other substance use disorder recovery groups for women, and some have been manual-based. However, to our knowledge, the WRG is the first recovery group for women who are heterogeneous with respect to the type of substance used, age and stage of life, and presence or absence of co-occurring psychiatric disorders. The manual-based WRG has been tested empirically in Stage I and Stage II behavioral treatment development trials and tested in comparison with an effective, manual-based, mixed-gender group treatment for SUDs. While there have been other group treatments for women, these have generally focused on a specific group of women, such as women offenders, women with co-occurring trauma and SUDs, pregnant and parenting women, among other specific groups. Some of these group therapies have been studied for their efficacy and effectiveness in randomized trials and others have not; some are now supported by evidence but others are not. In many clinical practices and programs, clinicians need to treat a heterogeneous group of treatment-seeking women with SUDs, but prior to the WRG there were no manual-based, empirically supported, women-focused recovery groups that would fit this clinical need. The WRG is empirically supported and utilizes a cognitive-behavioral, relapse prevention approach with a structured group format, an all-women group composition, and women-focused group content. The investigators hypothesized that the all-women group composition and the women-focused group content synergize to produce improved outcomes for women participants.

Outcomes Research on the WRG

The WRG was initially developed and tested in a small randomized controlled Stage I behavioral development trial funded through the National Institute on Drug Abuse (NIDA). The goal of the WRG Stage I pilot study was to develop a manual-based, 12-session WRG and to pilot-test this new treatment in a randomized controlled trial against mixed-gender group drug counseling (GDC). GDC is an effective manual-based treatment for SUDs delivered in a mixed-gender format. GDC was chosen because it approximates standard group treatment delivered in community-based SUD treatment programs. The format of GDC is similar to the WRG in that it can be delivered as 12 weekly 90-minute sessions, each focusing on a specific topic. The goals of GDC are to facilitate abstinence, encourage mutual support, and teach new ways to cope with substance-related problems. GDC is delivered in a mixed-gender group composition and does not address gender-specific themes for men or for women (Greenfield et al., 2007b).

After the initial development of the WRG manual, two 12-session WRG groups were conducted in sequence with a total of 13 women participants in order to determine the group's feasibility, as well as patient and therapist satisfaction with the group treatment. Minor modifications to the manual were made in response to feedback from patients, therapists, and experts who reviewed the manual. Then, in the pilot stage, women were randomly assigned either to the WRG or mixed-gender GDC, with a total of 16 women assigned to the WRG and seven women and 10 men assigned to the control group, GDC. The groups were run in a semi-open format. Groups started with four participants, and participants were added until there were a total of eight in each group. Each participant continued in the group for the entire 12-week sequence until completion. Because randomization in this Stage I trial took place with a single GDC group in which half the participants were men, there were about half as many women assigned to GDC as to the WRG.

In this Stage I trial, participants were predominantly white and well educated, with more than 90% having some college or a graduate education. Forty-one percent of the women participants were married. Overall, there were no demographic differences between women assigned to the WRG and those assigned to GDC, except that the women assigned to the WRG were younger on average (mean age 45 years) than those assigned to GDC (mean age 58 years). Because of this statistically significant difference, all outcome analyses for the pilot study controlled for age differences between groups.

The study was open to women with any current substance dependence (in addition to any nicotine dependence). Eighty-six percent of the women enrolled in the study had current alcohol dependence as their primary substance dependence. In addition, approximately 7% had current cannabis dependence, 3% had current cocaine dependence, and 3% had other current stimulant dependence. Although alcohol dependence was the current substance dependence for the majority of the women, almost 70% of these women also had lifetime histories of other SUDs, including cannabis, cocaine, other stimulants, opioids, sedatives, and hallucinogens (Greenfield et al., 2007b).

In many respects, participants had rates of co-occurring psychiatric disorders that were similar to what would be expected in an outpatient population of women seeking treatment for SUDs. For example, more than one-third had a current mood disorder and 75% had a history of mood disorder in their lifetime. Thirty-one percent had a current anxiety disorder and 44%

had a history of anxiety disorder in their lifetime. Approximately one-third of enrolled women met criteria for a personality disorder. It is important to note that women who met criteria for current, active PTSD, bipolar disorder, and psychotic disorders were excluded from the Stage I study. There were no significant differences in the prevalence of psychiatric disorders between women enrolled in the WRG and GDC groups.

Feasibility and assessment of patient satisfaction with the WRG were major goals of the Stage I trial. In the prepilot phase, 100% of participants enrolled completed the treatment and the follow-up assessments. In the pilot phase, 81% of women randomized completed treatment. Satisfaction with groups was assessed using the Client Satisfaction Questionnaire (Nguyen, Attkisson, & Stegner, 1983). While satisfaction with both the WRG and the GDC groups was high, women were significantly more satisfied with WRG than GDC. Subsequent research not included in the original paper demonstrated that greater satisfaction with the WRG group was attributable to a number of perceptions and experiences of the women participants. These included women's perception that there was enhanced comfort, support, and feelings of safety in the WRG group, as well as greater ease of communication among the women. Women appreciated the focus on educational topics related to women's recovery as well as the open discussion that allowed for immediate connection and support. Women participants stated that they shared the intimate details of their addiction and recovery in the all-women's format, which would not have been possible for them in a mixed-gender setting, and that this had been a key ingredient in their satisfaction with the group and their recovery (Greenfield et al., 2013a).

The Stage I pilot study also assessed outcomes at the end of treatment and 6 months posttreatment. The main outcomes assessed were the decrease in days per month of any substance use compared with use at baseline (i.e., 60-day period before entering the study) and for those who used alcohol, the decrease compared with baseline of the average number of drinking days per month, drinks per drinking day, and changes in the alcohol severity composite scores. The Time Line Follow Back (Sobell & Sobell, 1992) and the Addiction Severity Index (McLellan et al., 1992) were used to ascertain frequency and quantity of substances used, as well as severity. At the end of the 12-week group treatment, on average women in both the WRG and GDC reduced their days of any substance use and days of alcohol use; there were no significant differences in these substance use outcomes between the WRG and GDC. However, during the 6-month posttreatment follow-up, the WRG participants demonstrated a pattern of continued reductions in substance use while women in GDC did not. In addition, women in the WRG pilot with alcohol dependence had significantly greater reductions in average drinks per drinking day and improvement on the alcohol composite scale than women in the mixed-gender GDC group at 6 months following treatment completion.

The Stage I trial concluded that the newly developed 12-session, women-focused WRG was feasible with high satisfaction among participants. It was as effective as mixed-gender GDC in reducing substance use during the 12-week in-treatment phase *and* produced significantly greater reductions in drug and alcohol use in the 6 months following treatment than did mixed-gender GDC. In spite of the small size of the sample of women enrolled in the Stage I trial, these results were promising. The investigators therefore pursued several additional analyses of the initial data from the trial in order to ascertain if there were certain characteristics of women who might have had different outcomes depending on whether they were assigned to the WRG or GDC.

For example, analysis of the Stage I data examined baseline self-efficacy and substance use outcomes among women assigned to the WRG and GDC. Self-efficacy is generally defined as the belief that an individual has the ability to cope effectively with a particular high-risk situation, and abstinence self-efficacy is known to play a role in SUD treatment outcomes (Trucco, Connery, Griffin, & Greenfield, 2007). Generally, high self-efficacy is associated with better treatment outcomes than low self-efficacy. Nonetheless, in the Stage I trial, women with low self-efficacy who were assigned to the WRG had the greatest decrease in days per month of substance use during the 12-week treatment and in the 6 months after treatment, while the women with low self-efficacy enrolled in the GDC increased their days of use both during the treatment and in the 6-month follow-up period. There were no significant differences in reduction of days of substance use between women with high self-efficacy who were assigned to the WRG or GDC during treatment or in the 6-month follow-up period. However, women with low self-efficacy assigned to the WRG exceeded women with high self-efficacy in either group in the magnitude of reductions in days of substance use each month (Cummings, Greenfield, & Gallop, 2010).

Changes in coping were assessed using a standard measure administered at baseline and at the end of the 12-week treatment during the Stage I trial. This analysis showed that there were no significant differences in coping-change scores between groups but that the relationship of certain types of coping changes with treatment outcomes varied by treatment group. For example, increases in problem-focused coping were associated with decreased drinking days in the WRG but with increased drinking days in GDC. For both groups wishful thinking was associated with increases in substance use, and increases in social support coping were associated with decreases in use in both groups (Kuper, Gallop, & Greenfield, 2010).

More than one-third of women in both the WRG and GDC groups had co-occurring depression and anxiety disorders. The 36 women enrolled in the Stage I trial were administered self-report and clinician-rated measures of anxiety (Beck Anxiety Inventory [BAI]; Beck, Brown, Epstein, & Steer, 1988); depression (Beck Depression Inventory [BDI]; Beck & Steer, 1987), and general psychiatric symptoms (Addiction Severity Index [ASI]; McLellan et al., 1992). An analysis of changes in these symptoms throughout the trial showed that women in both groups demonstrated significant improvement in depression, anxiety, and general psychiatric symptoms that were not related to changes in their substance use (McHugh & Greenfield, 2010). Symptom reductions were especially notable among women with greater psychiatric symptom severity at baseline.

In order to understand women's experiences in the WRG compared with the mixed-gender GDC, semistructured interviews with 28 women study participants were conducted and transcripts were analyzed for themes. Compared to GDC, women in the WRG more frequently endorsed feeling safe; embracing all aspects of one's self; having their needs met; and feeling intimacy, empathy, and honesty. In addition, women endorsed the theme that group cohesion and support allowed them to focus on gender-relevant topics supporting their recovery (Greenfield et al., 2013a).

Given the preferences women often articulate for the safety and comfort of single-gender group treatment (Greenfield et al., 2013a; Nelson-Zlupko et al., 1996), the underlying theory of the WRG is that the all-women group composition would be a key effective component in the treatment and would enhance supportive and empathic affiliation among group members compared with mixed-gender group treatment. In order to examine affiliative statements made in the WRG and GDC groups, 28 group therapy tapes were coded and compared for five types of affiliative statements. This study found that in the WRG, there were more frequent statements that were coded as "affiliative" compared with GDC. In the mixed-gender GDC, women were more likely to give than to receive an "affiliative" statement (Greenfield, Kuper, Cummings, Robbins, & Gallop, 2013b). This study demonstrated that an element of the enhanced support and safety that women endorsed in the WRG (Greenfield et al., 2013a) may be the greater frequency of supportive and affiliative statements exchanged by the group members in the single-gender WRG compared with the mixed-gender GDC.

Because of the small sample size and the relative homogeneity of the sample in the Stage I trial, the next phase of the study was to assess the effectiveness of the WRG relative to GDC in a Stage II randomized controlled trial using a larger group of women who were heterogeneous with respect to the substances they used, presence of co-occurring psychiatric disorders, trauma histories, and age and stage of life (e.g., pregnant, parenting, or neither; with or without a partner). The Stage I trial was implemented in a semi-open enrollment format. However, group therapy is most often implemented in clinical settings in an open (e.g., rolling) enrollment format in which participants can enter at any time in the group sequence and exit the group after 12 weeks are completed (Morgan-Lopez & Fals-Stewart, 2006; Washton, 2005) rather than starting and ending with a cohort of other participants. Therefore, a second aim of the Stage II trial was to demonstrate the feasibility of implementing the WRG in an open-enrollment group format at two outpatient clinical sites.

In the Stage II trial, participants were included if they were substance-dependent and had used substances within the past 60 days. Fifty-two women were randomized to the WRG and 48 to GDC. Substance use outcomes were assessed at months 1–6 and month 9. The Stage II trial was implemented at two clinical sites in an open enrollment format with groups continuously "rolling" for 24 months. Among women participants enrolled in the trial, current substance dependence diagnoses included 88% alcohol, 17% opioid, 15% cocaine, 9% cannabis, and 9% sedatives. Co-occurring psychiatric disorders among women participants included major depressive disorder (61%), anxiety disorders (22%), and posttraumatic stress disorder (20%). Seventy-five percent of the women had an Axis I disorder and 17% had an Axis II disorder (according to DSM-IV-TR criteria; American Psychiatric Association, 2000), with avoidant personality disorder accounting for the majority of the Axis II disorders (76.5%). The mean age of women participants was 47 years, with a range of 23–79 years; 95% were white; 32% were married, 35% divorced or separated, and 25% were never married (Greenfield et al., 2014b).

The Stage II trial found that women in both the WRG and GDC had reductions in mean number of substance use days during treatment (12.7- vs. 13.7-day reductions for the WRG and GDC, respectively) and 6 months posttreatment (10.3- vs. 12.7-day reductions), but there were no significant differences between groups. Overall, women in both the WRG and GDC groups had significant ($p < .0001$) reductions from baseline in mean number of alcohol use days during treatment (9.9- and 12.4-day reductions for the WRG and GDC, respectively) and at 6 months posttreatment (8.3- and 12.2-day reductions). Similarly, women in both the WRG and GDC groups had significant ($p < .05$) reductions in mean number of drug use days during treatment (3.0- and 1.5-day reductions for WRG and GDC, respectively); however, at 6 months posttreatment, the reductions were significant for the WRG (2.8-day reduction; $p < .05$) but not for GDC (1.6-day reduction; $p > 0.1$). In addition, women in both the WRG and GDC groups had significant ($p < .0001$) reductions in mean number of heavy drinking days during treatment

(8.6- and 12.1-day reductions for the WRG and GDC, respectively) and at 6 months posttreatment (8.0- and 11.8-day reductions).

In the Stage II trial, the WRG demonstrated comparable effectiveness to standard mixed-gender treatment (i.e., GDC) and was feasibly delivered in an open-group format typical of community treatment. The investigators concluded that the study demonstrated that the WRG is an effective manual-based group therapy with women-focused content that can be implemented in an open-enrollment format in a variety of clinical settings for women who are heterogeneous with respect to their substance of abuse, co-occurring psychiatric disorders, and life stage (Greenfield et al., 2014b).

In summary, the WRG was developed and tested in a small pilot study in the context of a Stage I trial. In this study, on average, reductions in days of substance use and drinking days per month for women in the WRG were equivalent to reductions for women in a standard mixed-gender GDC group during the 12-week treatment trial. However, on average, women assigned to the WRG continued to improve and decrease their alcohol and other substance use in the 6 months following treatment, while those assigned to GDC continued at the same level or increased their substance use during that same time period. Importantly, the WRG was feasible to conduct in a semi-open format and received ratings of high satisfaction from its participants. From the additional analyses of the Stage I trial data it appears that the effect of changes of coping on treatment outcome varied with the group treatment and those with improved problem-focused coping assigned to the WRG had improved treatment outcomes. In addition, the evidence from the pilot study showed that women with low self-efficacy were best served by the women-focused WRG. Symptoms of anxiety and depression decreased in the course of treatment, especially among those with greater symptom severity at baseline. Women in the WRG had high satisfaction with the group treatment and endorsed feeling safe and having their needs met. There is evidence that the WRG group process has a greater frequency of affiliative statements between group members providing support and empathy. These findings suggest that women who have low self-efficacy and may be considered especially vulnerable because of these characteristics may do especially well in the WRG. When the WRG was administered in the semi-open enrollment groups in the Stage I trial, the 6-month posttreatment outcomes were better than GDC. The groups in the Stage I trial had a more stable group membership due to the semi-open enrollment compared with the larger Stage II trial that was implemented in two sites in an open-enrollment format characteristic of clinical settings in the community. In this Stage II trial, women participants were heterogeneous with respect to their substance disorder, trauma histories, presence of co-occurring psychiatric disorders, and life stage, and had within-treatment reductions in days of substance use that were sustained at 6-months posttreatment and were comparable to mixed-gender GDC (Greenfield et al., 2014b). Taken together, the findings of the Stage I and Stage II trials demonstrate that the WRG is an effective group treatment for women with substance use disorders who are heterogeneous with respect to the substance used as well as co-occurring psychiatric disorders that can be implemented in an open-enrollment format typical of community treatment settings. The next chapter will provide detailed information on how to conduct the WRG.

CHAPTER 2

Conducting the Women's Recovery Group

Conducting any group therapy calls for special skills on the part of the group therapist, including attention to the setting and group membership. Conducting the WRG requires attention to group membership, the choice of whether to run the group in an open or a closed format, attention to the group room setup including bulletin board materials as well as participant educational sheets, and the selection of group topics and their sequence.

This chapter discusses in detail how to conduct the WRG. The chapter first presents therapist characteristics and the style of conducting the group. Next there is a section on participant characteristics, who is appropriate for the group, and the use of other concurrent treatments. The chapter then provides information on the different possible methods of group enrollment (i.e., open vs. semi-open and closed groups) and a discussion on choosing the number of group sessions and topics. The chapter then provides information on setting up the group room. This is followed by a guide to conducting the pre-group meeting and then a detailed description of conducting the group sessions. The chapter concludes with tips for managing common clinical situations such as participant emergencies, slips and relapses, and missed sessions, as well as suggestions for how to conduct the WRG as an individual session with a single participant.

Therapist Characteristics and Style

The therapy is designed for a woman therapist and an all-women group. The therapist's work should be characterized by warmth, openness, acceptance, and friendliness without violating boundaries. The WRG therapists in our studies included counselors, social workers, psychologists, and psychiatrists. They had varied clinical backgrounds in SUD treatment and different theoretical orientations. The WRG is designed to be a relapse-prevention, cognitive-behaviorally focused intervention; this treatment manual should provide the guidance that allows therapists

> ### Who Is the Best Type of Therapist to Run the WRG?
>
> The Stage I and Stage II trials had women therapists as the WRG therapists. The WRG has not been conducted in any of our studies with a male therapist, and the all-women group composition (which does include a woman therapist) is an important element of the WRG. I therefore recommend that the WRG be conducted by a female therapist. The WRG therapists in our studies have had different backgrounds, including counselors, social workers, psychologists, and psychiatrists. They have also had varied clinical backgrounds in treating SUDs and different theoretical orientations. The WRG is designed to be a relapse-prevention, cognitive-behavioral intervention; the manual should provide guidance that allows therapists of varied backgrounds and orientations to learn to conduct the WRG with women with SUDs. Most research on effective therapists indicates that the patient's perception of the therapist's level of empathy and genuine interest in the patient are the most significant effective characteristics of therapists, and this is likely to hold for the WRG as well.

of varied backgrounds and orientations to learn to conduct the WRG with women with SUD. The therapist should be able to keep the group on-task. The therapist should not be judgmental, harsh, confrontational, or condescending toward the participants.

Key Elements of the WRG

Several key elements of the WRG are important to highlight and may distinguish it from other group therapies. These include gender-specific group content, a group process that emphasizes similarities rather than differences in addiction and recovery among women participants, a group theme promoting self-care, and the group's central recovery rule that specifies both relapse prevention and repair work. In addition, the WRG specifies four levels of participation that allow each woman to engage based on her own sense of comfort but provides encouragement to engage at all levels. The WRG also balances the presentation of thematic material with group discussion. This section provides details of each of these elements of the WRG.

Group Content

For those who use substances, there are important gender differences in social factors, co-occurring psychiatric disorders, histories of sexual and physical assault, biological responses and medical consequences, reproductive health, use of substances through the life cycle, triggers, and coping strategies. Many of these issues may not be as effectively addressed for women in a mixed-gender recovery group as in an all-women recovery group. The specific topics in each session of the WRG are meant to cover 14 of these issues. In each session, a specific topic is addressed by the group leader using a participant educational sheet that is distributed and a bulletin board display of the essential points made in the participant informational sheet as well as the session's take-home messages. The topic is meant to educate the participants about an area that relates to women with SUDs who are trying to recover. The topic is also meant to generate discussion and additional ideas among the participants.

Group Process

As discussed earlier, there is evidence that women in all-women groups experience a greater sense of freedom to express direct concerns about personal and interpersonal issues than they might in a mixed-gender group. The all-women composition also enhances group cohesion and affiliation, and this may be an important factor in promoting the success of the group, as well as the effectiveness of the group for the individuals who participate.

The relationships among the group members and between the group members and the therapist also affect the character of the group. For example, group members often find that the responses from other members who have been in situations similar to theirs can be quite beneficial. Other aspects of the group process can also interfere with or impede group progress. For instance, if one member of the group is having a particularly difficult time, her difficulties may begin to absorb the attention of all of the members or may provoke feelings of discouragement. This process within the group may need to be commented upon in order to refocus the group on their common task. In addition, if members begin to focus on differences among themselves (e.g., one member uses self-help and another does not; one member is sober and another is still struggling; one member is committed to abstinence and another member is still dealing with ambivalent feelings), it is important for the therapist to remind members of the group that they are all there for common reasons: (1) they all have substance problems and (2) they are all trying to help themselves in recovery. In the group therapy room, in addition to the bulletin board postings of the central recovery rule, group theme, take-home messages, and discussion topic summary points, there will always be a list of symptoms of substance problems that are common for people with SUDs. At moments when group members are highlighting their differences, the therapist can point out that all of them were enrolled in the group because they likely have several of these symptoms listed on the board, and this is what is common to all of them. In spite of their differences, each person has symptoms of substance problems and each wants to recover. This approach emphasizes commonality among participants and deemphasizes differences, thus helping to promote mutual support, affiliation, and group cohesion (one of the hypothesized key effective ingredients of the WRG).

As I mentioned earlier, the WRG is primarily a cognitive-behaviorally oriented, relapse-prevention group. However, group process and interpersonal relationships can play a role in two ways. Group process and interpersonal relationships among members can become a focal point for the therapist when they are interfering with the group's focus on the primary task (i.e., recovery and relapse prevention). On the other hand, increased comfort and familiarity within the context of an all-women's group can promote a feeling of safety among group members. This feeling, in turn, can enhance group cohesion and affiliation and is likely therefore to be a positive therapeutic ingredient of the WRG.

Group Theme and Central Recovery Rule

The major group theme of the WRG is "Recovery Means Taking Care of Yourself," as I stressed in Chapter 1. Many of the themes of the group sessions return to the principle that women in the group need to increase their self-care. This means paying attention to their triggers, urges, and cravings; planning to avoid high-risk situations; making time for recovery activities; asking for help; figuring out ways to take care of themselves even as they care for others; and taking care of their physical and mental health. This theme is a thread through all of the group sessions. It is helpful to have the theme "Recovery Means Taking Care of Yourself" posted on the bulletin board throughout all of the sessions (included in Appendix B materials).

The central recovery rule of the WRG is "Recovery = Relapse Prevention + Repair Work." This central recovery rule encompasses the skills and behaviors that are addressed throughout the WRG treatment. For example, relapse prevention includes identifying triggers and high-risk situations, planning to avoid such situations, and developing coping skills to manage situations that can't be avoided. It also involves making your environment as "trigger-free" as possible and getting treatment. Repair work includes repairing the damage to self and relationships due to substance related problems and learning how to enjoy your life substance-free. The sessions in the WRG address both relapse prevention and repair work. The central recovery rule is posted on the bulletin board throughout the sessions (included in Appendix B). The group therapist should refer to the central theme and the central recovery rule throughout the group sequence.

The Four Levels of Participation in the WRG

One key principle of the WRG is that it provides a safe, supportive, and respectful group environment. In providing this environment, the WRG emphasizes the approach that each member's participation in the group is important but that each person in the group participates at the level at which she feels most comfortable. The WRG specifies four levels of participation that are reviewed during the pre-group meeting. The first level of participation is *coming to group*. The importance of group attendance is reinforced during the pre-group meeting and at each session as an important principle of the group. Participants need to attend groups to help themselves but there is also a responsibility toward other group members. The second level of participating is *actively listening* to other group members while in group. The WRG emphasizes that even when a person may not be comfortable sharing or responding to another's contributions in the group, actively listening to other members is important for her own learning and also in supporting other group members in recovery. The third level of participation is *sharing and responding*. Insofar as the participant is comfortable, she should share her own experiences. The therapist asks the participant to share within her own "comfort zone." The fourth level is *doing the skill practices* between the sessions. Skill practices help the participant reinforce the learning in each group session and to personalize that learning for her own recovery. The WRG emphasizes that the more each participant can participate in each of these four ways, the more helpful the group will be for her recovery.

Starting and Stopping the Group on Time

It is important to start and stop sessions on time, no matter how many participants are there at the specified time for the start of the group. If by the end of the group there are missing participants, it is common for group members who are present to express their disappointment or anger that other participants are missing the group while they themselves have made the effort to attend. They may also express concern or worry about why another group member missed a session. In this instance, it is helpful for the group therapist to express understanding of the group members' feelings, saying something like, "It is understandable to feel concerned about Ms. X." It may then be helpful to say something like, "As you know, whenever anyone misses group, I always call to check in and make sure she is all right." These sorts of statements help promote a feeling of safety within the group.

The Balance between Presenting Material and Group Discussion

The group is designed to provide both specific didactic information and time for group discussion. In order to provide both, each group lasts 90 minutes. However, the therapist will have to judge how much time to devote to topic presentation versus discussion. This will depend to some extent on the number of participants in the group at any one time and the degree to which the participants are willing and able to engage in discussion. For example, a group with 10 participants will need to provide less time for each individual participant to speak than a group with four participants. Some groups will have strong group cohesion and participants who are capable of empathic listening and supportive interpersonal interactions. Although the therapist will wish to encourage these attributes and skills, groups will vary in the participants' abilities in this regard. Therefore, the group therapist will have some latitude in structuring the sessions.

What Is the Ideal WRG Group Size?

We have run groups with as few as two participants (e.g., when there were absences of other group members) and as many as 10 participants. Generally, the group works best when there are at least four and no more than eight participants. The group could run with 10–12 participants but the therapist would need to adjust the time allotted for the different group components. For example, in order to accommodate this group size, the therapist would likely need to shorten one or more parts of the session such as a shorter check-in and check-out period, shorter topic presentation, or shorter open discussion.

Patient Characteristics: Who Is Appropriate for the WRG?

This treatment is designed for a group of women who are heterogeneous with respect to age and background, drug and alcohol use disorders, co-occurring psychiatric disorders, and trauma histories, but whose main common characteristics are that they have substance-related disorders of varying severity and are willing to work toward the goal of abstinence. In our studies of the WRG, all participants qualified for a DSM-IV diagnosis of SUD; however, they varied in severity, with some women engaging in a first treatment and others having had numerous previous treatments, and some women having more severe symptoms and consequences of their substance use than others. It may not be necessary for participants to meet DSM-IV or DSM-5 or ICD-9 or ICD-10 criteria for substance-related disorders; however, women are most likely to benefit from the WRG if they are concerned about their substance use and wish to remain abstinent. The group is designed to encompass adult women age 18 and older. Women may have problems with more than one substance or dependence on a single drug, including alcohol. However, the studies of the WRG excluded women with current intravenous drug use, who are likely to benefit from a more comprehensive program. The group could be used as a component of care in a treatment program for women with intravenous drug use but the group was not specifically designed for this population. The group is also designed to be used by women with co-occurring psychiatric disorders such as anxiety, depression, eating disorders, and other disorders that will not generally impair their attention and focus in a group. WRG would not be indicated for women suffering from psychotic disorders or for women with bipolar disorder; there are group therapies specifically designed for such patients, such as Integrated Group Therapy (IGT) (Graham et al., 2003; Weiss & Connery, 2011). The Stage II trial of the WRG included women with posttraumatic stress disorder (PTSD) and a range of personality disorders. However, if PTSD is the main focus of treatment, a specific group treatment, Seeking Safety (Najavits et al., 1998), for women with SUDs and co-occurring PTSD is available, or another treatment such as COPE (Back et al., 2012) may be useful. Patients for whom co-occurring borderline personality disorder is a major treatment focus may best be served by a dialectical behavior therapy group (Linehan et al., 1999). The Stage II trial included women with PTSD and borderline personality disorder as well as several women with bipolar II disorder. These co-occurring disorders were stable and were being addressed in concurrent treatment.

There will likely be heterogeneity among the women participants in the duration and severity of their substance disorder. For some women, this may be their first treatment, and for others their 5th, or 10th. Some women may have had problems with substances for decades, while for others onset and progression may be more recent. Even though these differences exist, the therapist can help the group focus on the commonality among all members: that they have

---

Who Is Appropriate for the WRG?

Can Women with Both Alcohol and Drug Problems Be in This Same Group?

The WRG was designed for women with SUDs who are heterogeneous with respect to the primary substance used. All of the WRG groups in the studies had women with both alcohol and drug dependence (in addition to any nicotine dependence). The WRG stresses the symptoms of substance problems that are common for all the women in the group and lists these symptoms on the bulletin board every week to underscore what is common to everyone in the group no matter what other characteristics may differ among them (e.g., type of substance used, age, other psychiatric disorders).

Is It Possible to Have Very Young Adult Women and Much Older Women in the Same Group?

Yes. The WRG was designed for women who are heterogeneous with respect to age. In the studies of the WRG, the mean age of group members was in the mid-40s; however, groups were conducted with women ranging in age from their early 20s through their late 70s. Observation of group process during the studies indicated that this multigenerational approach was generally a significant strength of the group. Younger women benefited from learning from the experiences of some of the older women in the group, and older women similarly found it helpful to learn about the younger women's experiences. It is also true that age does not correlate with severity of substance problems or with progress in recovery. In the studies of the WRG, we observed that sometimes younger women had moved forward to stable recovery while older women in the group were still struggling. These older women learned from their younger group members and also provided the younger members with support and praise for being motivated toward their recovery at an early stage of their lives.

substance problems and are trying to learn how to remain abstinent and recover from their SUD. This provides a group environment that allows members to be supportive of one another in spite of differences in duration or type of substance problem.

Is There Any Type of Patient Who Is Not Appropriate for the WRG?

The Stage I trial of the WRG excluded women with current, active PTSD, bipolar disorder I and II, and psychotic disorders. The Stage II trial excluded patients with bipolar I and psychotic disorders but included women with stable PTSD and bipolar II disorder. PTSD was excluded in the Stage I trial in order to test the hypothesis that women other than those with current PTSD could benefit from a women-focused group therapy for SUDs; however, patients with stable PTSD and bipolar II disorder were included in the Stage II trial. Patients with bipolar I and psychotic disorders were excluded because there is evidence that there are specific treatments for patients with these disorders and co-occurring substance use disorders that are effective (Drake, Mueser, Brunette, & McHugo, 2004; Weiss & Connery, 2011). Generally, such effective group therapies integrate treatment targeted at both disorders simultaneously.

In general, the WRG will not be appropriate for women who have other psychiatric disorders with symptoms that are very unstable or are not being adequately treated. For example, a woman with severe depression may need to have treatment for her depression in order to fully participate in the group. Likewise, a woman with active PTSD may need to be in concurrent treatment for the PTSD if she is to be able to benefit from the WRG. Women who are actively self-destructive or who have active suicidal ideation are not generally appropriate for the WRG, as these other symptoms and behaviors often need specific, intensive treatment that is not provided by the WRG. On the other hand, the WRG can be an adjunctive treatment for women with SUDs who are in appropriate treatment targeted at another psychiatric disorder (e.g., in an eating disorders treatment program, trauma program).

The Stage I and Stage II trials did not include women who were currently administering drugs intravenously (though they may have had a past history of IV use). We decided to exclude these individuals from the studies because evidence suggests that individuals with active IV drug use would benefit most from a more intensive program than a weekly outpatient recovery group. That said, while the WRG would not be an ideal stand-alone treatment for women trying to become abstinent and prevent relapse to intravenous drugs, in clinical practice, it would be possible to use the WRG as one component of a comprehensive program treating women with IV opioid dependence.

When Should a Participant Be Removed from the WRG?

In our studies of the WRG, it was rare that we removed a participant from the group. Circumstances that might lead to removing a participant from the WRG might be if a participant is dangerous to herself or others (for example, through self-destructive behaviors, assault or threatened assault of others, or selling of drugs or inviting other group members to drink or use drugs with them). In such an instance, this member's continuation in the group would generally not be advisable, and clinically appropriate referrals would be made. We have had participants in the WRG who had a significant relapse such that referral to a more intensive level of care (e.g., inpatient medical detoxification, intensive outpatient, or residential programming) was required (for substance use or for a co-occurring psychiatric disorder). Generally, those participants returned to the group when their conditions were stabilized.

Concurrent Treatments

The WRG was designed as an outpatient, weekly, relapse-prevention group, and participants may be in some other treatments concurrent with the WRG. Participants may be in individual therapy, individual pharmacotherapy, couple or family therapy, and self-help groups. In the studies of the WRG, women were not able to be in another group therapy for SUD concurrently with WRG. They were able to be in another group therapy with a different focus (e.g., anger management group, trauma group, bereavement group). However, in clinical practice, this same restriction would not apply. Some women may be in another effective group treatment for SUD and wish to add a women-focused recovery group. Such combined treatments should be utilized when clinically appropriate.

Conducting the WRG in Open versus Closed Group Format

The group is designed to function as a "closed," "semi-open," or "open" enrollment group, depending on the treatment context and needs. There are advantages and disadvantages to each of these strategies. In a closed group, the entire group of six to eight individuals begins the first session together, and no one else is enrolled once the group begins. In a semi-open group, new members are entered only up to a specific number of group sessions (e.g., up to the third group session), and then enrollment is closed. In an "open" (or rolling) group format, the group begins with a specified number of people (e.g., four participants), and then enrollment continues as new participants who are appropriate for the group become available. A closed format has the advantage that the group begins and ends together, and this is likely to promote greater group cohesion and affiliation. On the other hand, the closed format has the limitation of needing to wait for the complete number of participants before starting the group, which often necessitates making some participants wait to get started. A semi-open format has the advantage of limiting the wait time of participants who are ready to begin immediately, but may delay the process of group cohesion (Greenfield, Crisafulli, Kaufman, Freid, Bailey, et al., 2014a). In addition, new members who start after the first session may feel less "a part of the group" than the "old" members or that they missed something. In the semi-open format, sessions are added at the end of the sequence to cover the earlier, "missed" sessions that members who entered after the first group did not attend. All members should be encouraged to attend these because repeating the topics can also be helpful. The "open format" (or rolling group format) is the most common format in community practice. This means that the sessions continue to go in sequence and then repeat as soon as one sequence is completed. In this format, new participants are added continuously, which may be advantageous and particularly appropriate if the group were adopted as part of an SUD treatment clinic setting, residential, or day treatment program. The main disadvantage is that group coherence and affiliation are likely to be diminished as members come and go.

Formats for Conducting the WRG

Should I Run the WRG in a Semi-Open or Closed Group Format?

We have run the WRG in both semi-open and open formats. The Stage I trial of the WRG used a semi-open format. The advantage to this approach is that the group can begin with fewer than the total number of participants (e.g., four participants) and add additional members (e.g., another four) in the first few weeks. Then the group can close to new admissions until the sequence is completed. In this format, the later entrants to the group will finish up with a smaller number of individuals if the first four group members choose to complete the group after 12 sessions. On the other hand, these four members could be invited to stay until the end and repeat several sessions. The advantage of the semi-open format is that the therapist does not need to wait to collect the total number of participants to begin. Sometimes when waiting for eight members to be ready to join, the initial members recruited for the group must wait in a holding pattern for a number of weeks. Depending on the clinical needs of the patients such a wait time can be too long. The semi-open format also allows for the eight participants to participate for the majority of groups together. Such a stable membership lets the women get to know one another fairly well and facilitates group cohesion, social bonding, and social support. All of these factors are advantageous for the WRG model and have been rated as highly important by women who have participated in the WRG in the past.

Should I Run the WRG in an Open-Enrollment Group (e.g., Rolling) Format?

An alternative to the closed or semi-open format is to run the WRG group in an ongoing, open-enrollment format and to continue to add participants weekly as patients who are clinically appropriate are available to join. There are many advantages to this format and a few disadvantages. One advantage is that many clinical settings run groups continuously on a weekly or twice-weekly basis and receive participants into these groups as they are admitted to the clinical program. The WRG is designed to be effective in this type of setting, and the Stage II trial was conducted in precisely this format for this reason. In this format, when the therapist is first getting started, the group can begin with as few as three or four women, and then the therapist can continue to add new participants as they are available. Thus, this approach conforms to the reality of many practice settings and allows patients who are clinically appropriate to be added when they are ready so that they do not need to wait. The disadvantage to this format is that group attendance changes, and the group may be less cohesive. A stable group attendance (e.g., the same core group of women) may only overlap with one another for four to six sessions and may need to adapt to a new member each week that they are attending. This can decrease group cohesion and group affiliation, thereby diminishing the type of social support that is one hypothesized mechanism of action of the WRG. The reality of the design of the WRG is that it was shown to be effective in both open and semi-open formats and it is flexible so that it can be adapted for either format.

Choosing the Number of Group Sessions and Topics

Although the manual is designed as a 12-week relapse prevention group, there is some flexibility in this design, allowing it to be tailored to specific treatment settings, patient populations, and enrollment approaches. The manual contains 14 sessions, each with a specific topic. For some groups of women, all topics may be appropriate; for other groups, some of the topics may be less useful or even unnecessary. For example, the session on violence and abuse may be less appropriate in a treatment setting where many of the patients are also in a "trauma" group, or if the group is conducted in a trauma treatment program as a gender-responsive SUD treatment group, and the therapist may elect to exclude this session topic. Thus, the group leader may decide to cover 12 topics in 12 weeks or 14 topics in 14 weeks. Another possibility is that the group therapist may spread discussion of certain topics over two full group sessions. So, for example, a group therapist might choose to spend two sessions on triggers and two sessions on coping strategies, and then devote subsequent sessions to each of the 12 other topics. (This particular sequence would have a duration of 16 weeks.)

Numbers and Topics of Group Sessions

Can I Do the WRG for 14 Weeks and Use All Session Topics?

It is absolutely fine to run the WRG for 14 weeks and to use all 14 topics. In the initial Stage I prepilot study, all 14 topics were used and assessed for their acceptability and participant satisfaction. If you opt to use only 12 topics over a 12-week sequence, it is also reasonable to hand out the additional material for the two sessions you will not be presenting.

Are There Other Frequency of Sessions and Duration of the WRG That Are Possible?

In the Stage I and Stage II trials, the WRG was run as a once weekly group. However, the WRG format is designed to be flexible so that it can adapt to a number of different types of clinical settings. For example, to run a total of 12 sessions, the WRG could be run twice weekly for 6 weeks or three times weekly for 4 weeks. In a residential setting, sessions could be conducted on a daily basis for 2 weeks, thereby covering all 14 topics. There are other examples of frequency and duration of sessions that would be possible depending on the clinical program and needs of the patients.

Can Participants Stay for Longer Than the 12-Week Sequence?

Yes. It is fine for participants to continue in the group for as long as it is helpful. If the group is run continuously in an open, rolling format, a participant could elect to repeat the entire sequence. For some women, working through the sessions and skill practices more than once, as well as gaining the ongoing support from other women in the group, will be helpful for their recovery.

Can I Present the Topics in a Different Order?

Yes. In our studies of the WRG, we did adhere to a specific order so that all of the group sequences would be consistent across study groups. However, the WRG is designed so that the sessions can be presented in the order that makes the most sense for the individual group members. For a closed group or at the start of the semi-open or open format it is suggested that the therapist begin with "The Effect of Drugs and Alcohol on Women's Health," as we did in the Stage I trial. However, experience in our studies with the semi-open and open format demonstrated that women successfully entered the group with any session topic, and the sequence of topics did not seem to matter. Therefore, the therapist has discretion over the order of topics. One potential clinical advantage to this flexibility is that specific topics might come up during a session (e.g., women might discuss their problems with depression during open discussion), and the therapist might elect a session topic (e.g., "Managing Mood, Anxiety, and Eating Problems without Using Substances") for the following week that specifically addresses this issue. It is also fine for the therapist to conduct the WRG using the session sequence as it is written in this book. In sum, the topic order is flexible and allows the therapist to adapt the sequence to what is most clinically appropriate in the setting where she is conducting the group therapy.

The enrollment strategy will also influence total duration of the group therapy. A closed group that covers all 14 topics will last 14 weeks, whereas a semi-open group that enrolls through group #3 and chooses all 14 topics will last 16 weeks. In an open enrollment (rolling admissions) group, members enter the group at any time and continue along ideally for the entire sequence. This is the typical delivery format for most outpatient SUD treatment programs and the Stage II trial delivered the WRG treatment in this format in order to test its feasibility, effectiveness, and acceptability in the format most typical of treatment programs. In this approach there is no start or finish to the sequence. **It is important to note that there is no definitive order in which the groups must be conducted, and topics are meant to be used in a continuous loop if that is most appropriate to the participants or to the treatment setting.** In the case of an open, rolling group, it will be important to spend a few minutes at the beginning of each session for group members and the therapist to introduce themselves. For example, the therapist will say at the introduction of each group and before the welcome: "Welcome. Today we have a new group member. Can we all go around the room and say our names? I am Susan, the group therapist. . . . " During the group discussion, the therapist may also need to explain references to another specific session topic to which she may refer, so that everyone in the group understands the reference.

Setting Up the Group Room and Checklist of Materials Needed Each Week

The WRG uses a number of materials to help women learn about recovery from SUDs and self-care. These consist of visual aids posted in the group room each week as well as patient hand-outs and skill practices for each of the 14 sessions. The bulletin board materials that should be posted at every session as well as the take-home messages specific to each session are included in Appendix B. Therefore, before you begin each week's group, you should post the materials listed in Table 2.1.

Materials Needed to Conduct the WRG

You should also have the check-in and check-out sheets, the session-specific therapist overview, and the three patient handouts for each session's topic. Some therapists will put copies of the participant's session-specific informational sheets in a file folder and make these available at every group in case a participant missed the previous week's group and would like the partici-pant sheets. Alternatively, some participants may have done the skill practice but left their sheets at home and would like a copy to use during the beginning of the group session when the skills practice is reviewed. Table 2.2 is a checklist of the materials needed for conducting the WRG.

TABLE 2.1. Materials to Be Posted in the Group Room Each Week

- Central recovery rule of the WRG: *Recovery = Relapse Prevention + Repair Work*.
- WRG theme: *Recovery Means Taking Care of Yourself*.
- Common symptoms of substance problems.
- Session-specific bulletin board outline.
- Session-specific take-home messages.

TABLE 2.2. Checklist of Materials to Conduct the WRG

- Pre-Group Meeting Information (Participant Sheet PG.1): To be used in 30-minute pre-group meeting.

- List of Sessions and Topics (Participant Sheet PG.2): This list of sessions will be distributed during the pre-group meeting.

- Readings and Resources for Recovery (Participant Sheet PG.3): This is a list of resources for participants to be given out during the pre-group meeting.

- Check-In Sheet and Check-Out Sheet: These can be printed on opposite sides of the same paper. Laminating this sheet will help maintain longevity.

- Three session-specific participant sheets for each of the 14 sessions:
  ○ Participant overview of session topic
  ○ Take-home messages for the session
  ○ Session-specific skills practice

- Bulletin board materials posted at every session: Central Recovery Rule, Group Theme, Common Symptoms of Substance Problems.

- Bulletin board materials specific for sessions: Bulletin board outline and take-home messages for Sessions 1–14. These should be posted in the group room for each session.

- Three-ring binders or folders (optional): Providing binders or folders is optional but binders or folders can help participants file their session-specific sheets and skill practice sheets; the therapist can encourage participants to bring the binders or folders every week.

Conducting the Pre-Group Meeting

The WRG is designed for women who are heterogeneous with regard to age and other characteristics, drug and alcohol use disorders, and co-occurring psychiatric disorders. We assume that depending on the clinical setting (e.g., outpatient, partial hospital, residential, intensive outpatient, inpatient), the participant has had a complete psychiatric and substance use evaluation, and has now been referred to the WRG. Information regarding the assessment of participants with SUDs and other psychiatric disorders is beyond the scope of this book but is summarized in a number of textbooks and other sources (e.g., Greenfield & Hennessy, 2008, 2015; Ruiz & Strain, 2011; American Pyschiatric Association, 2013).

Once the participant has been assessed and referred to the WRG, before she enters the group, it is important for the therapist to conduct one individual 30-minute pre-group meeting with her. It is helpful to have this meeting within a week of when the participant will begin group. The pre-group meeting will allow the therapist and the participant to become acquainted with one another and for the therapist to establish rapport with the individual participant. It also allows the participant to ask specific questions about the group. The pre-group meeting enables the therapist to review with the participant the group ground rules and expectations, as well as tips for how the participant can help herself in recovery. During this session, the therapist should stress the need for weekly attendance. She can emphasize the differences between individual therapy and group treatment and how the group works best when all members attend. Finally, the participant can express any particular concerns about herself including things that she does not wish to share with the group.

The participant and therapist review together Participant Sheet PG.1 (Pre-Group Meeting Information, included in Appendix A). The therapist can print two copies of this form. At the end of the pre-group meeting, the therapist and the participant sign the form to signify her commitment to the group and each can keep a copy. The participant can use the form as a reference for the basic principles and ground rules of the group and the therapist can include the form in her records. The therapist may also choose to present the participant with a three-ring binder or folder at the pre-group meeting so that the participant can keep all of the group informational sheets and skill practices sheets organized. The signed pre-group meeting sheet can be the first sheet for the participant to place in the binder or folder. The therapist should also provide the patient participant with two additional informational sheets: the List of Session Topics (Participant Sheet PG.2), and Readings and Resources for Recovery (Participant Sheet PG.3). The therapist can tailor the list of Session Topics and cross out any sessions that will not be covered. Participant Sheet PG.2 also has a space at the bottom for the therapist's name and contact number and for additional contacts (e.g., other clinician, emergency, or clinic contact information) that the therapist might want the participant to have.

Because one of the most important aspects of the pre-group meeting is establishing rapport with the participant, the therapist should begin the meeting with an open, warm, nonconfrontational tone and express enthusiasm for the group and the changes that individual group members may be able to accomplish in the course of the group therapy. The therapist should begin by introducing herself and asking what led the participant to seek out this particular group. Hopefully, this will lead to a discussion of the participant's substance disorder and her current motivation for treatment and abstinence.

In addition to establishing rapport with the participant, another important task that the pre-group meeting can accomplish is emphasizing the need for attendance. Here the therapist can explain to the participant that individual and group therapy are different from each other. In individual therapy, there is a one-to-one relationship with the therapist. If the participant misses the treatment, she is the one who is missing out. In group therapy, on the other hand, there is a relationship with other members of the group. The commitment the participant makes is not only to herself and the therapist, but also to the other group members. Just as she will benefit from and count on the presence and participation of the other group members, they will count on her. Thus, in order for the treatment to be helpful, the participant must attend, and this is true for her as well as for the other group members. It is important here to stress that *everyone* feels ambivalent about coming to treatment at some time, no matter who she is and no matter what treatment it is. No matter how ambivalent one is, though, it is important to come anyway. The only exception to this rule is if the participant is intoxicated or using on the day of the group; this would be the one reason the therapist would ask the participant *not* to come. That said, the therapist would want and expect the participant to attend the following week. Although the goal of the group is abstinence, slips and relapses are not uncommon, and the purpose of the group is to help participants learn from mistakes and get the support they need to figure out alternative and more effective ways of coping.

In the context of this discussion it is important for the therapist to emphasize that participants can be tempted to drop out of group treatment either because they are doing well or because they are doing poorly. It is normal for participants to have these thoughts but it is very important not to act on them. Encourage the participant to speak to you if she notes that she is having problems with the group and is tempted to drop out.

The next step in the pre-group meeting is to present to the participant a balanced view of the group and what can be gained from the WRG. It is helpful here to ask the participant if she has specific concerns or questions that she might wish to ask the therapist. The therapist can then answer the participant's questions about the group. Specific points that the therapist should cover during the pre-group meeting include the following:

1. *Explain the length and duration of the groups* (e.g., 90 minutes weekly for 12 weeks). Give the participant the List of Session Topics (Participant Sheet PG.2) with the therapist and/or contact name and number to call with questions or concerns.

2. *Review Pre-Group Meeting Information* (Participant Sheet PG.1). After reviewing each of the points on this sheet have the patient sign and the therapist countersign the two sheets. Keep one for the therapist's records and give the other to the participant. The participant can place this in her three-ring binder or folder if provided.

3. *Provide the participant with Readings and Resources for Recovery* (Participant Sheet PG.3).

4. Ask the participant if there are things that she would like the therapist to know about her before the group starts.

5. Ask the participant if there are things she would *not* wish to share with other group members during the group.

6. Explain to the participant issues of confidentiality including the need to break confidentiality if there is imminent risk of harm to self or others, as well as any mandated reporter laws in the therapist's state (e.g., mandated reporting for suspicion of childhood abuse, elder abuse). At this time, it is reasonable to ask the participant to sign a release of information for the therapist to communicate with other clinicians should a clinical situation arise that the therapist feels ought to be communicated with the participant's therapist, psychiatrist, or other clinicians involved in her care.

7. Review the group rules with the participant as follows:
   - The participant should attend group weekly.
   - However, the participant should not come to the group if she is intoxicated. If she does come intoxicated she will not be permitted to join the group, but her safety will be considered and appropriate steps for safety and clinical care will be taken (e.g., sending her home with a family member, not letting her drive, taking her car keys, calling an ambulance).
   - It is important that the participant take part in the group. There are several levels of participation, and the participant is encouraged to participate at all of the levels as she feels comfortable to do so. The first level of participation is *coming to group*. The second level is *actively listening* to other group members while in group. The third level is *sharing and responding*. Insofar as the participant is comfortable, she should share her own experiences. The therapist asks the participant to share within her own "comfort zone." The fourth level is *doing the skill practices* between the sessions. Emphasize that the more the participant can take part in each of these levels, the more helpful the group will be for her recovery.
   - Emphasize that not every aspect of every group will be helpful to every individual, but that overall there should be many aspects that are helpful to each participant.
   - Emphasize that safety is very important, both physically and emotionally, within the group. The group therapist will be attentive to making sure that the group is safe for all participants, which will lead the group therapist to call individuals who miss

groups to ensure follow-up. It will also necessitate that members who are intoxicated do not attend the group but are helped to be safe themselves. It may lead the therapist to intervene in discussions within the group that might cause some members to feel unsafe. Respecting confidentiality of other members is expected. Whatever is said in the group, remains in the group.

- Participants ought to call the therapist (and/or another contact person if there is one) with questions or concerns.

After this discussion, the therapist should ask the participant again if she has any final questions and answer them. Finally, the therapist should end the meeting on an upbeat note by telling the participant that she is looking forward to seeing her at the first group and letting her know again the time and place of the group. If it is possible for the therapist to call participants with a reminder the day before the group, this helps ensure optimal attendance. If the therapist (or another office or program staff person) will be providing reminder calls, she should let the participant know she will get a reminder call the day before the group, as this is normal procedure for the group.

Conducting the Group Sessions

Before starting the WRG, it will be important for the therapist to review the structure of each WRG session and learn the elements of conducting each session. Each group session includes the check-in and introductions, the review of the previous week's skill practice and reminder of the last week's group, the presentation of the topic, open discussion, the wrap-up and reading of the session's take-home messages, distribution and description of the skill practice for the coming week, and the check-out. This section describes each of these components of the group session. On a weekly basis, the therapist will need to review the background and content of each individual session (presented in Part II of this book) in order to be prepared to present the material relevant to that specific group session.

Structure of Group Sessions

The WRG consists of several core components that should each be covered in every session. The core components, along with general time guidelines, are listed in Table 2.3.

The core components listed in Table 2.3 should be delivered at each session and in the order specified. The proportion of time spent on each component should approximate what is specified later. However, the suggested duration for each component may vary to some extent from one group to the next depending on the number of group members, their level of active participation, or the specific session topic. The therapist may choose to vary the time allotted to each component depending on what seems most appropriate for a particular session and with a specific group of participants. For some groups, more time will be spent on the check-in, with discussion and comments from other group members. For other groups, the individuals may be less talkative and more focused on the therapist presentations. In this case, the group therapist may make the check-in component shorter and the presentation and discussion of material longer. For example, with more group members, the therapist may spend more time

TABLE 2.3. Core Components of Each WRG Session

- Introduction (5 minutes).
  In the first group (and for every group with new members if using an open, rolling format) before check-in, the therapist should go around the group and have each participant state her first name. The therapist should then emphasize:
  - Safety and confidentiality.
  - Group session's 90-minute duration will start/stop on time.
  - Coming to group no matter what, even if struggling to be sober (except if intoxicated or using on day of group).
  - Orientation to the bulletin board materials.
- Check-in (15 minutes).
  - 2 minutes per person (e.g., for an eight-person group, 16 minutes; for a five-person group, 10 minutes).
- Review of last week's skill practice and topic (5 minutes).
- Presentation of this week's topic and distribution of topic overview (25 minutes).
- Open discussion (30 minutes).
- Wrap-up and reading of take-home messages (2 minutes).
- Distribution and description of this week's skill practice (3 minutes).
- Check-out (5 minutes).

on the check-in component (e.g., 20 minutes) and less time on the open discussion (e.g., 20–25 minutes).

In addition, *there will be varying levels of reading ability and health literacy among group members.* If the participant sheets that summarize each session's topic information are presented at a reading grade level that exceeds those of group members, the therapist can refer to, and emphasize, the "bulletin board" take-home messages for each session. These take-home messages are distributed to group members as participant sheets and are available in Appendix A along with the session overview and skill practice.

A detailed discussion of each of the core components of the WRG sessions is described below.

Introduction (5 Minutes) and Check-In (15 Minutes)

The check-in is a critical part of each group. If the session is a semi-open or open enrollment format, the new members should be introduced at the beginning of the group by saying something like, "Today we have a new group member. Before we begin, can everyone introduce herself." If a regular member returns after an absence or a missed group, it is helpful to welcome that person back and for the therapist to say she is glad the group member has returned. Group members can go quickly around the room and state their first names.

The therapist can proceed with the formal check-in. She should say something such as "Let's start with the check-in" and pass the check-in sheet to a participant to get the check-in started.

The check-in establishes the tone for the group. If everyone is doing well, the tone is more likely to be optimistic. If everyone is having great difficulty the group may feel discouraged. If one or two people are having a rough time, other group members may participate during open discussion and be solicitous and supportive.

In some instances, the check-in may run a little longer than the time allotted, as each person reflects on the stressors and triggers of the past week, her level of craving, the way she managed this, which coping strategies she used that were helpful, other ways she may have coped with a situation, and anything significant she thought or did related to the skill practice. It is nevertheless important to adhere to the 2- to 3-minute time limit per person during the check-in and to defer longer discussions to the discussion portion of the group. The therapist can facilitate moving through the check-in by saying in response to a difficult week or an individual's distress, "Thank you for bringing that up in your check-in. I know we will have time to return to discuss this more when we have open discussion."

The check-in sheet helps group members adhere to the structure and time limit of the check-in. Each group member answers the check-in questions on the sheet and then passes the sheet to the next group member. The Check-In sheet and Check-Out sheet are provided in Appendix B. These two sheets can be laminated to diminish wear and tear and can be copied double-sided so that check-in and check-out questions are on reverse sides of the same sheet. It is important to spend approximately the same amount of time on each person's check-in. A brief comment on a theme that may have come up after each check-in can be useful. On the other hand, a simple "thank you" can be sufficient if there is no specific comment the therapist wishes to say. It is helpful to listen to the check-in reports and note any particular reports that relate to the topic of the day so that the therapist can bring this information into the discussion later. It

---

Therapist Examples

Orienting Group Members to the Bulletin Board Materials

THERAPIST: So I'm going to orient you to the things that are up there on the wall. The green sheets stay up every week because those are the fundamental things about this group. And we will go back over these WRG themes and recovery rules and refer to them throughout the sessions. So the WRG group theme is that "recovery means taking care of yourself." The central recovery rule is that "recovery = relapse prevention + repair work" and we will learn more about the specifics of that throughout our sessions. And then the commonality of what brings everyone here—the central thread that brought everyone into the WRG group—are the common symptoms of substance problems. It doesn't mean that you have experienced all of these symptoms, but some of these should look familiar to you and that's what brings everyone here today. That and the desire to recover from substance problems. . . .

Creating a Positive Atmosphere

THERAPIST: (*talking at first to a participant who wasn't feeling completely well*) It's good to see you here, and just do the best you can. I appreciate your effort. The other part of participation other than attendance is listening, so we're all here and respectful to one another, and talk one at a time, and listen to one another, participating in the group at your own comfort level. So people add to the discussion as they see fit. None of that is forced, we ask people at their own comfort level to contribute if you have thoughts about what people are talking about or on the topic.

is important to bring themes from the check-in into the open discussion later during the group rather than focusing on them during the check-in.

On the other hand, a patient's check-in may relate to other topics that have been previously discussed in the group and may not be relevant to the topic of the day. So, for example, a patient's check-in may center on her continued ambivalence about her sobriety. If this occurs on a week when the topic is Women's Use of Substances through the Life Cycle, it may be difficult to relate this patient's check-in to the topic of the day. So, in this instance, the therapist may choose to comment by saying, "These feelings of ambivalence you are bringing up today are very important. We have discussed in some other sessions how it is possible to have strong feelings of wanting to stay sober and wanting to use at the same time. I wonder if you have some thoughts about how to help yourself with this?" The patient may then spend another minute discussing this issue, and then the therapist can move onto the next patient for check-in. If the subject requires more than a minute for comment, the therapist might say, "These feelings of ambivalence you are bringing up today are very important. We have discussed in some other sessions how it is possible to have strong feelings of wanting to stay sober and wanting to use at the same time. I think this is important and want to make sure we return to this topic during our open discussion later in the session."

If, during the check-in, a patient participant brings up an emergency or crisis situation that warrants individual attention, the therapist may say in front of the group, "I would like to discuss that with you individually for a few minutes after the group." This statement allows the group members to know that the therapist intends to help the individual (see additional discussion in "Dealing with Emergencies," pp. 42–43). If the issue does not warrant individual attention, the therapist can mention that this would be good to discuss more during the discussion portion of the group and then try to bring the issue back up at that time. For example, if a participant says she is distressed by a marital crisis that happened in the previous week, the therapist might say something like, "This seems like a very difficult situation and, as we have discussed here, intimate relationships have a very important role in women's recovery. I would like to make sure we discuss this further when we come to open discussion. OK?"

After all the participants have checked in, it is good to try to pull together a common theme if possible and relate this theme to the day's topic. If several people have discussed losses and the topic is "How to Manage Triggers and High-Risk Situations," the therapist might say something like, "A number of people have discussed losses today, and that is one possible type of trigger that can make women vulnerable to using substances. Today we are going to discuss a range of triggers including some that are typical for anyone with a substance problem but some of which may be more typical or more powerful for women. . . ." Another therapist response might be, "It sounds like a number of you faced some difficult challenges but were able in many instances to come up with excellent strategies and ways of coping so that you didn't use substances. It is very helpful to hear about some of these ways of coping with tough situations that you have used. . . . Today, after we review the skill practice, we will be discussing. . . ."

Review of Last Week's Skill Practice and Topic (5 Minutes)

The next component of the WRG is a brief review of the previous week's skill practice (unless this is the first group). The therapist should say something like, "Last week's skill practice asked you to write down at least one trigger that you confronted during the week and three ideas for alternate coping strategies. Can anyone share her answers?" The review of last week's session and skill practice should be brief. The therapist can remind group members that the skill practices are designed to be helpful and are important to do between sessions. If a participant says she has forgotten to do it, the therapist can also say that the skill practice is there as a resource and that even if she misses doing it one week, it still may be helpful to try it in the coming week. If there are group members who may have a pattern of not doing the skill practice, the therapist might say "I know it is hard for some of you to complete these skill practices in advance. I wonder if we could talk about what things get in the way and have people brainstorm about solutions." For a group member who is present and missed the previous week's group, the therapist can hand out the previous week's skill practice so the participant will have it as a resource.

Another aspect of reviewing the skill practice is that this also serves to remind group members of the previous week's topic, which accomplishes two additional goals. First, for those who attended the previous week, it establishes some common thread from week to week. Second, for those who missed the group, or for new members of the group, it helps fill them in on what took place the week before.

Presentation of This Week's Session Topic and Distribution of Topic Overview (25 Minutes)

The next component of the session is the presentation of the session topic. It is helpful to make the transition to this portion of the group by relating the session-specific topic to themes from the day's check-in (or perhaps to past check-ins). Before beginning to discuss the topic, the therapist should pass out the session-specific informational sheet that is included for each session-specific topic (see Appendix A). The session-specific sheets included in Appendix A represent a concise outline of the information that is provided in greater detail for the therapist in the session-specific background information that is part of each session plan in Part II of this book. In the Stage I and II trials of the WRG, more detailed background information was routinely provided to women participants as session-specific informational sheets. The goal of this book is to make the WRG flexible for implementation in diverse settings serving women who are heterogeneous with respect to educational attainment and health literacy, and to decrease the time burden for therapists preparing materials for each session. Therapists may therefore elect to refer participants interested in more detailed information on a particular topic to the additional resources provided in Participant Handout PG.3 in Appendix A. This model allows therapists to assess the level of detail that would be most helpful to the women participants in their specific group and setting.

It is helpful to provide a three-ring binder or folder to each group member as she joins the group (see Table 2.2 on materials needed to run the group). Participants can be encouraged to keep their session-specific sheets and skill practices sheets in the three-ring binder or folder, bring them to each group, and keep for their own future reference.

In some instances, the therapist may choose to begin the topic presentation with the *take-home messages* posted on the bulletin board. For example, the therapist can say, "Today we will review several of the most important points of today's topic and review the take-home messages first." These take-home messages highlight at the outset of group the important points that participants should come away with, and they will be repeated at the end of the discussion. The depth with which the therapist presents material will depend on the needs of the group participants. In some instances, it will serve the needs of the group to keep the discussion simple and focused on the main points of the session-specific informational sheets and take-home messages. For other groups, the women will want more in-depth information. The participant sheets, bulletin board materials, and take-home messages are meant to bring a degree of flexibility to the session, so that it can be tailored to individual group members' needs including reading and health literacy grade levels that may vary among group members and between groups. Some women may ask for more detailed information, in which case they may be directed to Participant Sheet PG.3, Readings and Resources for Recovery, that was distributed during the pre-group meeting and provides websites and books for additional reading. For other group members, the session-specific informational sheets and take-home messages will provide sufficient written detail. The therapist can tailor this degree of information to the needs of the group members.

The topic presentation is meant to be *interactive* rather than in a lecture format. The therapist should use the outline in the "Therapist Overview" for each session (contained in Part II). The bulletin board session-specific outlines (contained in Appendix B) are one to three pages long and should be posted in each session along with the session-specific take-home messages (contained in Appendix B). These outlines can guide the therapist in presenting the material. The presentation of the session topic should take approximately 20–25 minutes and leave another 25–30 minutes for open discussion. The presentation by the therapist should move seamlessly into the open discussion. In total, the presentation and open discussion together should occupy anywhere from 45 to 50 minutes, depending on the length of the check-in and group size. For example, a group with fewer members will have a shorter check-in and may spend more time on the topic presentation and open discussion. The open discussion should end with approximately 10 minutes left in the 90-minute session to have adequate time to summarize the take-home messages, distribute and describe the skill practice for the following week, and do the check-out.

The session-specific bulletin board materials (i.e., the topic-specific outline and take-home messages) and the therapist's topic-specific overviews are meant to be guidelines and not specific scripts. The therapist should present the material in an interactive style. As long as the overall guiding principles of the group are followed and the main points of the topic are covered, it is more important to attend to group members' questions and thoughts about the material than to cover every detail. One way to *facilitate discussion* during the presentation of the topic is to present the first one to two points of the session material and then pause and ask something like, "Does anyone relate to this in the past or present?" or "Does this ring any bells for anyone?"

Because the group is likely to be heterogeneous with regard to members' backgrounds and levels of education, it is important to keep that in mind and gear the presentation accordingly. It is also sometimes helpful to remind people that there are some things that will be common to everyone and that there are other things that will be different for each group member. If necessary, the therapist can refer back to the bulletin board poster on the symptoms of substance problems to remind participants that while people differ in many ways, everyone in this group has in common at least some of these symptoms of alcohol and drug problems and a desire to be in recovery. It is most important to involve participants in a discussion of the topic and have them relate the material to their own experiences. In addition, the therapist can raise themes and experiences that have come up in the past or even during that group session that relate to the material. So, for example, in Session 11, "The Issue of Disclosure: To Tell or Not to Tell?," the therapist might say something like, "I know this is an issue that many of you have brought up over time and has been an area of concern. For some of you, there has been a feeling of needing to keep your recovery secret, and for others you have felt good about telling certain people in your life and getting their support. Some of you have also experienced having someone else disclose your recovery without your permission, and we have talked about the feelings that has caused. So, today's session will really focus on the pros and cons of disclosing your substance problem and your recovery. . . ."

It is helpful to emphasize that it is normal for people in early recovery to be struggling with the urge to use and the desire to recover. The therapist can emphasize that it is excellent when a group member is able to discuss this struggle openly and honestly with the group and gain group support. The therapist can also say something like, "I know that it is really feeling like a struggle right now. I wonder if you can think of ways to help yourself move in the direction you seem, on balance, to want to go in . . . and that is to be able to manage these difficult parts of your life without relying on substances. . . ." Such statements and questions like these on the part of the therapist emphasize the group's solid rule of abstinence from substances but also maintain an empathic stance regarding the individual participant's struggle to achieve this goal. In this way, the therapist should proceed through the session topic outline covering the main points in an interactive format.

It is also helpful to try to bring everyone into the discussion while also observing the overall group rule that people discuss things when they feel safe to do so, and that verbal participation is voluntary. The therapist might say things like, "I wonder if anyone else has had this experience or might wish to comment on this. . . ." These invitations to participate may be a way to engage participants who may be more peripherally involved in the discussion.

Open Discussion (30 Minutes)

The topic presentation and open discussion components should encompass 50–55 minutes of the 90-minute session. Open discussion is a very important component of the WRG. The purpose of the open discussion is for participants to speak about recovery-related concerns. These concerns may include ongoing discussion about the session's topic. However, open discussion may also focus on other areas such as something that came up in the check-in earlier in the session, a difficult situation that a member encountered in the past week, or another recovery concern. When the group is working optimally, participants will often interact with one another with minimal intervention from the therapist. On the other hand, the therapist may need to summarize themes she is hearing from group members, relate participants' discussion to the session's topic or other WRG topics, or relate the content of the discussion to the WRG theme of self-care or the central recovery rule. Sometimes there is a seamless transition from the presentation of the topic into the open discussion part of the session. At other times, the therapist can facilitate transition from the presentation of the session topic to the open discussion in a variety of ways such as by stating any of the following, for example:

> "We can now move into the open discussion part of our session. . . ."
> "Are there other things on people's minds today?"
> "I know there were a number of concerns raised during check-in; we could talk about those now or anything else people would like to discuss."

**Therapist Example: Referring in Open Discussion to the Theme
of "Recovery Means Taking Care of Yourself"**

THERAPIST: It is sort of the challenge that we talked about last week, too—that is that when you're a caretaker and you're used to putting on a certain face, it's much harder to take care of yourself and to ask for help when you need it. And sometimes people can really hold themselves well, like you were saying that you do—we want to be able to hold ourselves like that.

PATIENT: Yes . . . I want to do that but sometimes I need to ask for help and that is taking some care of myself rather than trying to show I'm all right when I am not.

THERAPIST: I agree. It is challenging to ask for help and take care of yourself in the midst of all those responsibilities. . . .

It is important for the therapist to bear in mind that qualitative interviews and group overview questionnaires with participants after the Stage I trial demonstrated that participants valued *both* learning the topical information presented and having time for open discussion with other participants in the group and weighed these as *equally important* to their overall experience of the WRG. Open discussion often takes place with little interaction on the part of the therapist, with women providing mutual support for one another using empathic and affirming statements (Greenfield et al., 2013b). Participant discussion should take precedence over the therapist's voice in open discussion. However, the therapist can summarize themes and relate the content of participants' discussion to the group theme of self-care or to other session topics of the WRG. This is a good way to jump-start discussion either at the beginning of open discussion or at any time that the discussion lags. If there is a lag in the discussion, or a specific concern is raised that necessitates therapist interaction during the open discussion, the therapist can intervene by underscoring a significant issue that has been raised and how it relates to the WRG themes of self-care, relapse prevention, repair work, or one of the specific WRG session topics. For example, women may discuss some aspect of being overwhelmed by family responsibilities and triggers to using by feeling pressure from caretaking responsibilities. The therapist may point out that this concern relates to other WRG topics about women, caretaking, and triggers. The therapist can often encourage discussion by asking, "I wonder if anyone in the group has encountered similar situations or feelings . . . ?" In open discussion the therapist should allow supportive and empathic group member interactions to take precedence over the therapist's voice. However, restating WRG themes and session topics and relating them to content of the discussion is a good way to jump-start discussion either at the beginning of open discussion or at any time that the discussion lags. It is worth noting that during the Stage I and Stage II trials, as long as the group had adequate size (usually four or more members), little was required of the therapist to begin or maintain discussion during open discussion.

Wrap-Up and Reading of Take-Home Messages (2 Minutes)

The take-home messages should be posted on the wall of the group room (see Appendix B; they are also available in Appendix A as session-specific participant sheets for distribution). With about 10 minutes left to go, the therapist should distribute the patient copy of the session's take-home messages (the second participant sheet for each session found in Appendix A). If for any reason it is not possible to post the take-home messages on the wall of the group room, the take-home messages distributed to group members can be referred to during group. Generally, the therapist can transition to this part of the session by summarizing in a few sentences what was discussed, highlight any themes, and then proceed to the take-home messages. The therapist should ask participants to read the take-home messages. So, for example, if there are four bullet points in the take-home messages, group members can each read one in turn. Having members read each bullet point of the take-home messages in turn is another way to engage the group.

Distribute and Describe the Skill Practice (3 Minutes)

After the wrap-up and take-home messages, the therapist should hand out the skill practice sheet for the coming week (see Appendix A). She should then describe to the group what the skill practice asks them to do and remind them that the skill practice is an important component of the WRG and is there as a resource to help them through their week. She can also remind group members that women will do best if they are able to participate in each component of the group (e.g., attendance, active listening, participation, and weekly skill practices).

Check-Out (5 Minutes)

The therapist can transition to this part of the session by stating simply, "It is time to move to our check-out." The check-out sheet (see Appendix B) is then passed from one member to the next as each person responds to the check-out question. As each member holds the sheet she answers the check-out question: "What will you do in the coming week to support your recovery?" and then passes the sheet to the next person. Finally, the therapist can conclude the group by thanking everyone, wishing everyone a good week, and saying she looks forward to seeing them next week.

Tips for Managing Common Clinical Situations

There are a number of clinical situations that are common in SUD treatment including slips and relapses, patient emergencies, and missed sessions. This section discusses each of these and provides guidance for the WRG therapist for managing each of these in the course of conducting the WRG.

Dealing with Slips and Relapses

Although the group is abstinence-focused, it is common for participants to have slips or relapses during the course of the group. The response to such slips in the group should promote learning for the individual who slipped and for the group as a whole. The therapist should help the patient try to link the substance use to any specific trigger, and then to think about what she might do differently if confronted with a similar situation in the future. For example, the therapist can help the patient think about alternate coping strategies. In the WRG, the therapist helps facilitate supportive discussion and can ask group members if they have suggestions for other ways of coping. It is most useful in this group for the leader to adopt a nonconfrontational style and to encourage problem solving, improved identification of triggers to use, and development of alternative positive ways of coping and managing triggers, urges, and cravings. Facilitating members' support of one another within the group was demonstrated in the studies of the WRG to be effective in enhancing the peer support and safe and comfortable group process of the WRG.

Dealing with Emergencies

A patient in the group may have an emergency or a crisis that needs immediate attention. In this instance, the patient should be seen individually. There are a number of ways to handle this situation, depending on the nature of the emergency, the timing of it in the group, and other resources the therapist might have available to her.

If a patient discusses serious issues warranting intervention (such as suicidal ideation or other dangerous behaviors such as self-harming behaviors or placing herself in unsafe situations), the therapist can say something like, "It seems that you are having a great deal of difficulty and are in distress. I wonder if we might meet to discuss it at the end of the group." This allows the patient to know the therapist is going to address her difficulties, and also allows other group members to know the concern is taken seriously, and the individual will be cared for, which promotes a feeling of safety in the group.

Although the group rules ask the participants not to come to the group intoxicated, if a participant does enter the group intoxicated, it is important that the group leader handle the situation immediately. It is important to have a procedure in place for this situation before the start of the group. It is helpful to have one or several clinicians who can be reached via pager or phone, to "back up" the therapist when participants show up intoxicated. This back-up person can then meet with the participant separately, while the group therapist continues with the group. The group therapist might say something to the group like, "It is important that Ms. X be helped now. Dr. Y is going to talk to Ms. X and see what the best way is to help her." It may be useful to remind the group members that there is a rule against coming intoxicated to the group because it can be unsafe, but that when someone does come intoxicated it is important to take care of her. In the meantime, the back-up clinician can wait with the participant until she is no longer intoxicated, can call a friend or family member (with permission), or can take further emergency steps if they are needed (such as calling an ambulance).

Finally, if a participant in a weekly WRG outpatient group begins to have increasing difficulties, such as escalating substance use, exacerbation of another illness, or another crisis or problem, it may be necessary to consider helping her to find other treatments to supplement the group work. For example, if the therapist observes that a patient is becoming increasingly depressed over a number of weeks, it might be helpful to meet with her for a few moments before or after the group. In this meeting, the therapist can say she has noticed that the patient has been struggling, and inquire whether she notices symptoms of increasing depression. If the participant acknowledges these symptoms, the therapist can then ask if she would like a referral to be evaluated for these symptoms. If the therapist believes the symptoms warrant it, she should strongly recommend that the participant seek an evaluation. In another instance, a group member might reveal severe marital or family distress. It may be appropriate, again, to request a few moments of participant's time before or after group and discuss the possibility of referral for family or couple therapy. Another important instance would be if a woman reveals domestic abuse or interpersonal violence or other issues of personal safety in the course of the group. If this should take place, it is imperative that the therapist discuss the need to be safe and then ask to see the participant after the group or perhaps in an individual meeting. The therapist must then assess with the woman the possibility that she is in physical danger. If she is, the therapist needs to raise with her seeking shelter, calling the police, and securing alternative housing, among other options.

How to Handle Patients' Missed Sessions

When group members miss sessions, it can raise questions or concerns among the other members, and even disrupt the treatment. So it is important to take steps to increase the likelihood of every member's participation in every session. There are several ways to cut down on missed sessions. The first is to discuss the importance of attending every group in the pre-group meeting. The second is to call each patient the day before the group and leave a message reminding her that the group is meeting the next day and stating the time the group meets. It is important to let participants know in advance that this is a routine group procedure, obtain the most appropriate number to call, and advise them that each of them will get a call each week. It is also important to let group members know that if something unexpected occurs that would cause them to miss group, they should call in advance to let the group therapist know they will not be attending and the reason for the missed session. Each group member needs to know that if she misses a session unexpectedly, the therapist will be calling her to assess how she is doing and to encourage her to come to the next group.

Adapting the WRG to Individual Therapy

During the Stage II trial investigating the effectiveness of the WRG, the groups were run in an open, rolling group format. Occasionally, because of participant absences or temporary low enrollment in the study, a single participant would be available for the group. In the context of the study, the group was held with only one participant. Therefore, over the course of several years of the study, a number of therapists had the experience of conducting the group session with a single individual participant. Their experience was that the process was different in many ways from conducting the group session. Nevertheless, they thought that the session was helpful to the individual who participated. They also found that certain minor adaptations in the format and conduct of the session enhanced the degree to which the session was helpful to the participant. These adaptations are summarized below.

Format and Duration of Session

In general, the therapists found that reducing the length of the session from 90 minutes to 60 minutes worked best for an individual participant. The regular format and structure of the session can then be followed. The participant can check in and then review the previous week's skill practice with the therapist. Following this review, the therapist can pass out the session-specific participant informational sheet and present the session topic. As with the group, the presentation of material should be done in an interactive style. The check-in, review of skill practice, and presentation of the topic can take approximately 25–30 minutes. Following these elements, the therapist can engage in open discussion with the individual for 20–25 minutes. In the last 5–10 minutes, the participant can read the take-home messages, the therapist can give the participant the upcoming week's skill practice, and the participant can check out.

Open Discussion

One obvious key difference between the WRG conducted as a group and the adaptation of this group structure to an individual is that there are no other participants to provide feedback and support. During open discussion with multiple participants, the dialogue is interactive among the participants. However, when the session is being conducted with one participant, the therapist has to be more interactive during open discussion than would otherwise be the case in the group.

It is important to emphasize that studies of the WRG have only yielded data on the group therapy format and not on its application to individual treatment. When the WRG is run in an open format, there may be occasions when only a single individual is available for the group on a specific date. Depending on the setting of the group therapy (e.g., outpatient clinic, office-based treatment, residential treatment, intensive outpatient), the therapist may or may not decide to hold group with a single participant. Should the therapist decide that running the group session with a single participant is consistent with the clinical setting and clinical needs of the participant, the general guidelines presented above are meant to be helpful to the therapist in conducting the session.

Therapist Self-Assessment in Conducting the WRG

A Therapist Self-Assessment in Conducting the Women's Recovery Group is included in Appendix B. This self-assessment tool includes 23 questions that will help the therapist assess the extent to which she is following the basic guidelines of the WRG model and how extensively she engages in specific therapist behaviors that are consistent with the WRG style of delivering this treatment. For each question, the therapist scores herself on a 0–4 scale, rating herself as conducting the WRG or engaging in each WRG-specific behavior not at all (a score of 0), rarely (1), somewhat (2), frequently (3), or extensively (4). Especially when the therapist is learning to provide the WRG treatment, she may wish to use the self-assessment tool after each session until she is comfortable that she is conducting the WRG with a high level of fidelity to the treatment model. Once she is comfortable conducting the WRG, the therapist may also wish to complete a self-assessment at specified intervals (e.g., after every four to six sessions) to ascertain that she is continuing to stay on target and is continuing to conduct the WRG using the fundamental principles and with extensive adherence to the WRG model. Over time, without self-assessment, therapists may drift from any manualized treatment model and this can diminish the effectiveness of the treatment. Empirically supported, evidence-based treatments such as the WRG are most effective when they are delivered with close adherence to the treatment model as specified in the treatment manual.

PART II

Group Sessions

Introduction to Session-Specific Topics

The 14 session topics are presented in this section. Each group session follows the format described in Chapter 2. Every session will begin with an introduction, check-in, and review of the previous week's skill practice and topic. The therapist will then present the session-specific topic, the group will proceed to open discussion, the therapist will wrap up, and the group will read the take-home messages. The therapist hands out and reviews the upcoming week's skill practice and then the group ends with the check-out.

The session-specific information in this section of the book includes "Background Information" for the therapist on the topic covered in each session, along with a detailed outline of that topic. Therapists should read the "Background Information" as they prepare for each session, and then use the detailed outline in the "Therapist Overview" while presenting this material during the session. Also, note that the detailed "Therapist Overview" complements the bulletin board materials (e.g., the session outline and take-home messages) and the first session-specific participant sheet for each session. (Other participant sheets for each session include a set of take-home messages, and a skills practice exercise.)

As I indicated earlier, Appendix A contains all of the reproducible materials for participants (session outline, take-home messages, and skills practice), and Appendix B contains all of the reproducible materials for therapists (e.g., the check-in and check-out sheets, as well as bulletin board materials, including each session's outline and take-home messages). You can photocopy these items from the book, or you can download and print them from the publisher's website (see the box at the end of the table of contents). This book is meant to be adaptable to a broad spectrum of educational attainment and health literacy among women participants. Some participants might prefer additional, in-depth topic information. For these participants, therapists can refer them to the additional resource information that is provided in Participant Handout PG.3, Reading and Resources for Recovery, in Appendix A. In the Stage I and Stage II trials, participants received detailed information similar to the background information provided to therapists. Practice settings, resource availability, and participant interest and literacy are all factors in the therapist's decision regarding the detail the therapist presents in the session.

The check-in sheet is passed around by participants, who each briefly orally answer the three check-in questions. The therapist should pass out the session outline (i.e., the first participant session-specific sheet) when she begins to discuss the topic for that session. Some participants may find the session outline a convenient place on which to take notes during the session. The bulletin board session-specific outline can be a guide for the therapist when she is presenting the topic, and can help participants follow the course of the discussion. After the open discussion and the wrap-up, the therapist distributes the patient copy of the take-home messages (i.e., the second session-specific participant sheet). Next, group members read the take-home messages taking turns reading each bullet point. After the reading of the take-home messages, the therapist should distribute the session-specific skill practice sheet (i.e., the third session-specific participant sheet) and describe the skill practice. Finally, every session concludes with the check-out; the check-out sheet is passed around as each participant orally answers the single check-out question.

Each of the 14 session plans that follows here provides:

- Session-specific therapist background information (Part II).
- Session-specific therapist overview (Part II).
- Participant sheet: Topic outline (Appendix A).
- Participant sheet: Take-home messages (Appendix A).
- Participant sheet: Skill practice (Appendix A).
- Session-specific topic outline and take-home messages to be posted as bulletin board materials (Appendix B).

The Effect of Drugs and Alcohol on Women's Health

In the closed group format, this will usually be the first session of the group because it introduces the concept of SUDs and establishes the "common ground" for everyone in the group. It also discusses the negative physical and health consequences of SUDs in women and the need to get and stay healthy through abstinence from substances. If this is an open format group, this may be the first session for some participants but not all participants. Many participants will encounter this session sometime in the middle of their sequence and not as the first group session. In preparing for this session and all sessions, it is important that the therapist read the "Background Information" and "Therapist Overview" below, as well as the session-specific participant sheets. The "Background Information" section provides the therapist with detailed information on the topic of the session—in this case, the effects of specific drugs and alcohol on women's health. The "Therapist Overview" that follows serves as a guide for the therapist to use during the session, and as an aid in presenting this background information.

Background Information

Common Symptoms of Substance Problems

The common symptoms of substance problems are listed below. The same symptoms apply to both drugs and alcohol.

- Increasing the amount of the substance(s) used over time.
- Trying unsuccessfully to cut down or stop using substances.
- Spending an increasing amount of time using substances, often leading to decreasing time spent in other activities related to work, school, relationships, or recreation.

- Having craving for the substance(s) when not using.
- Continuing to use substances even knowing they cause or worsen problems with work, family, school, relationships, or other activities.
- Using substances even when knowing they cause physical or mental health problems or when they may be physically dangerous to use.
- Developing tolerance to the substance over time (i.e., developing a need for more of the substance in order to achieve the desired or usual effect).
- Experiencing withdrawal symptoms when substance use stops or is reduced.

These symptoms of substance problems and SUDs are common to both women and men. However, one major difference between women and men with substance problems is the *course of the illness* and the *severity of the health effects*. In general, compared with men who have SUDs, women with SUDs use smaller quantities of substances (i.e., alcohol and drugs including nonmedical use of prescription drugs), less frequently, and for shorter periods of time, but women will progress more rapidly from onset of substance use to first having a problem with substances, to the later stages of dependence with the associated severe medical consequences. This phenomenon of the more rapid advancement of SUDs in women than in men is called the *telescoping course* of illness. Because of this accelerated course, particularly worrisome is the fact that girls are now starting to use substances (including alcohol) at increasingly younger ages and now start using at the youngest ages (10–14 years) at the same rate as boys.

Given this telescoping course of illness in women, what are the effects of specific substances on women's health?

Alcohol

Alcohol is metabolized differently by men and women. Although most alcohol is metabolized in the liver by a specific enzyme (i.e., alcohol dehydrogenase), some of that enzyme is also located in the stomach lining (i.e., gastric mucosa). Women have less of this enzyme in their stomachs than do men. When men drink alcohol, a substantial amount is broken down in the stomach lining before being absorbed into the bloodstream; however, in women there is much less breakdown (i.e., metabolism) of alcohol in the stomach lining. Therefore, for women most of the alcohol consumed is absorbed as pure ethanol. Women also have less total body water than do men. There is, therefore, less body water in which to "dilute" the alcohol in a woman's system once it is absorbed. As such, ounce per ounce of alcohol consumed, women have a higher concentration of alcohol in their blood. This is one reason why, after drinking comparable amounts of alcohol, women are seen to have higher blood alcohol concentrations than men, even allowing for differences in size and body weight.

Women often suffer many of the adverse health effects of alcohol sooner than do men and after consuming smaller quantities of alcohol overall than men. These health effects include effects on women's heart, liver, lungs, and brain including conditions such as cirrhosis of the liver, a heart condition called cardiomyopathy, hypertension, cognitive impairment, and disruption in reproductive function (e.g., loss of periods, loss of ovulation, premenstrual dysphoria, risk of early menopause). Some research has also shown that even a moderate daily intake (e.g., one drink per day) of alcohol can increase circulating levels of the hormone estrogen and may increase women's risk for breast cancer (Cao, Willett, Rimm, Stampfer, & Giovannucci, 2015).

Cocaine

When compared with men, women who use cocaine demonstrate the telescoping course of earlier initial use, younger age at first treatment, and more rapid development of dependence. Women using cocaine or crack are often more likely than men to smoke cigarettes, to have physical problems such as headaches after smoking crack, and to go to emergency rooms after smoking crack because of physical symptoms. Cocaine is a stimulant and produces subjective feelings of excitation, restlessness, euphoria, decreased social inhibition, and increased energy and concentration. It also causes physical effects (e.g., constricted blood vessels; increased heart rate, blood pressure, and temperature; and dilated pupils) and puts users at risk for stroke and heart attacks. Cocaine has many other adverse effects on the heart, stomach, lungs, and brain. It is not yet clear in what ways men and women may differ in the physical effects of cocaine. However, cocaine-dependent women may have problems with their menstrual cycle function, including galactorrhea (production of milk in the breasts), loss of menstrual periods, and infertility.

Opiates (Heroin, Oxycodone, Hydromorphone, Morphine, Etc.)

The telescoping course of illness is apparent with opiates, as we have seen in alcohol and cocaine disorders. Women are also at greater risk of death from their heroin dependence (Gjersing & Brettville-Jensen, 2014). Individuals who are injecting drug users have a higher mortality rate than individuals who are nondrug users (Perucci, Davoli, Rapiti, Abeni, & Forastiere, 1991). A systematic review by the World Health Organization found that while people who inject drugs have greater mortality overall, this risk for women is even greater than for men (Mathers et al,, 2013). Drug overdoses have continuously accounted for the majority of deaths in heroin users, with AIDS, medical problems, and suicide being other leading causes (Huang & Lee, 2013; Quaglio et al., 2001). For women, rates of heroin use doubled from 2002 to 2013. Between 2011 and 2013, past year heroin use disorders increased in women (Jones, Logan, Gladden, & Bohm, 2015).

Effects of opiate use include drowsiness, fluctuating mood, mental clouding, apathy, slowed movements, and lowered rates of breathing. Opiates may also cause dilation of blood vessels with resulting low blood pressure. Other effects of opiates are constipation and urinary hesitancy.

Many of the health problems associated with opiate abuse come either from self-neglect or from the complications of intravenous injections. Shared needles promote infections such as HIV, hepatitis B and C, staphylococcus aureus, and other agents that cause endocarditis, an infection of the heart lining. Poor health and other infectious organisms also increase the prevalence of syphilis and tuberculosis among women with opioid use disorders. Increasing numbers of deaths of heroin-dependent people may be due in part to the combination of heroin with other substances, such as cocaine and alcohol, and to the prevalence of HIV and other infections associated with shared needles.

Women appear to have greater medical consequences associated with their opiate dependence than men. Women have more respiratory diseases and problems with their urinary tract and genital infections. In addition, significantly more women than men with opiate problems have medical problems for which they do not receive medical care.

Marijuana

The most commonly cited heath consequences of marijuana use are anxiety or panic attacks, psychotic symptoms (e.g., paranoia), and impaired memory following chronic marijuana use. More women than men report panic attacks after smoking marijuana. There are also longer term effects of marijuana on brain function (Crean, Crane, & Mason, 2011). Heavy marijuana use has been associated with impairment in certain skills, such as pencil tapping, time estimation, size estimation, reaction time, and speed and accuracy tests. Memory impairment and deficits in math skills and verbal expression are also associated with heavy marijuana use. Compared to men who were frequent marijuana users, women who were heavy marijuana smokers had worse memory on certain tests. Marijuana also has adverse effects on the respiratory system. Compared with tobacco smoking, marijuana smoking is associated with a larger puff volume, a greater depth on inhalation, and a fourfold increase in breath-holding time. The prolonged exposure to tar and other irritants in marijuana cigarettes can lead to inflammation of the airways and eventually result in changes in the cells that line the respiratory system. This inflammation in the lungs of marijuana smokers is no different than in the lungs of tobacco smokers and seems to be the same in women and men. There may be increased risk of cervical cancer in marijuana-smoking women compared with those who do not use marijuana. There may be an adverse effect on female reproductive hormones, though a period of abstinence may allow for hormone levels to return to normal levels. Marijuana use can lead to physical dependence with an abstinence syndrome (withdrawal) when use is discontinued, including symptoms such as anxiety, sleep disturbance, changes in appetite, and marijuana cravings.

Neglected Self-Care

In addition to the direct health effects of specific substances, another important way that substances affect women's health is that while women are using drugs, they often *neglect themselves physically and psychologically* in a number of ways. Women often neglect going to the doctor for regular checkups that all women need. This means they may neglect getting preventive care, such as mammograms; PAP smears; routine lab work to check cholesterol and triglycerides; blood pressure checks; and other essential health care. Women may also neglect getting treatment for symptoms of infections because of their drug use, and these infections may get worse and lead to other health complications. There are other types of self-neglect and destructive behaviors that cause women physical and mental health problems that are associated with drug use. For example, some women may find themselves trading sex for drugs, or may have unprotected sex while intoxicated, and this can increase the risk of certain infections such as HIV, hepatitis B and C, and others.

Therapist Overview

Goals of This Session

- To learn common symptoms of substance problems.
- To understand differences between women and men in the *course of illness* and the *severity of the health effects*.
- To teach group members about the telescoping course of substance problems in women.

- To understand that substance problems result in self-neglect and diminished self-care.
- To understand that staying healthy and being well requires self-care, and part of self-care is abstinence from drugs and alcohol.

Session 1 Outline

- **Introduction** (5 minutes) to the group (*if this is the first session, or there are new participants in open group*).
  - ○ Emphasize:
    - Safety and confidentiality.
    - Session duration.
    - Importance of attendance (except if intoxicated or using day of session).
    - Orientation to the bulletin board materials.
- **Check-In** (15 minutes): Pass around the three-question check-in sheet.
- **Review of Last Week's Skill Practice and Topic** (5 minutes): *This review will take place if the group is an open (rolling) format group and not if this is the first session of a new group.*
- **Presentation of This Week's Topic and Distribution of Topic Overview** (25 minutes): Provide Participant Sheet 1.1.
  - ○ Interactive presentation and discussion of topic.
    - Introduce this session's topic.
    - Review common symptoms of substance problems.
    - Explain telescoping course in women.
    - Review adverse health effects of:
      - □ Alcohol
      - □ Cocaine
      - □ Opiates
      - □ Marijuana
      - □ Neglected Self-Care
- **Open Discussion** (30 minutes): Topics may include ongoing discussion of today's specific topic; discussion of issues brought up in the check-in; and other recovery-related topics. Open discussion often takes place with little interaction on the part of the therapist so that women may provide mutual support for one another. Participant discussion should take precedence over the therapist's voice in open discussion. However, the therapist can summarize themes and relate the content of participants' discussion to the group theme of self-care or to other session topics of the WRG. This is a good way to jump-start discussion either at the beginning of open discussion or at any time when the discussion lags.
- **Wrap-Up:** In the final few minutes of the open discussion, recap any themes of the open discussion and relate them to any WRG themes and transition to reading of the session topic's take-home messages.
- **Take-Home Messages** (2 minutes): Provide Participant Sheet 1.2. Participants can take turns and each read one take-home message; alternatively, the therapist can read them if this is more clinically appropriate.

- **Distribution and Description of This Week's Skill Practice** (3 minutes): Provide Participant Sheet 1.3. Quickly read through the skill practice sheet and encourage participants to do it before the next group and bring it with them to review.

- **Check-Out** (5 minutes): Pass around the one-question check-out sheet. Thank the members for coming and tell them you look forward to seeing them next time. Remember, it is important to start and stop the group on time.

Session-Specific Materials Needed

- Bulletin Board Outline and Take-Home Messages for Session 1.
- Participant Sheet 1.1: The Effect of Drugs and Alcohol on Women's Health.
- Participant Sheet 1.2: Session 1 Take-Home Messages.
- Participant Sheet 1.3: Session 1 Skill Practice: The Effect of Drugs and Alcohol on Women's Health.

Introduction

For the first session of a closed group, or when there are new members in an open group, the therapist should welcome participants; go around the room and have everyone state their first names; emphasize the safety and confidentiality of the group; that the 90-minute duration of the group will start and end on time each week; and the importance of attending each session.

Check-In

If this is the first session for any participant or for the group as a whole, introduce the check-in procedure and the Check-In Sheet. Explain that at the start of each session you will pass around the check-in sheet, which lists three questions:

1. Did you have any urges or cravings to use?
2. Did you use? If not, how were you able to remain sober?
3. Did you do the skill practice? If so, what did you do or find helpful?

(*Question 3 applies if the group is an open [rolling] format group, but not if this is the first session of a new group.*)

Group members are asked to respond orally to each of the three questions in a few sentences.

Review of Last Week's Skill Practice and Topic

This review will take place if the group is an open (rolling) format group, but not if this is the first session of a new group.

Presentation of This Week's Topic
and Distribution of Topic Overview

The therapist should distribute Participant Sheet 1.1 and introduce the session topic as "The Effect of Drugs and Alcohol on Women's Health." She can start out by explaining that today's topic is important because it first defines why all the group members are here today and what they have in common. The therapist can distribute Participant Sheet 1.1, saying, "We are first going to look at the symptoms of substance problems that are listed on this sheet and are also up on the bulletin board. Everyone will recognize many or all of the symptoms listed as being part of having a SUD or substance-related problems. Second, the session topic describes the specific impact of substances on women's health and emphasizes that in order to stay healthy, women must learn how not to use substances."

The therapist can then proceed to say, "Let's review what we mean by the common symptoms of substance problems. Most of you are in this group because you were diagnosed with an alcohol or drug use disorder. I have listed here the most common symptoms of substance problems. These symptoms or behaviors are typical experiences for women with substance use disorders." The therapist might invite members to read from the bulletin board the list of symptoms going around the room, or the therapist can read through these herself. After the therapist and/or group members read the list of the symptoms and behaviors, she can ask the group if they recognize any of them. This will usually generate comments such as "Yes, I have had all of these" or "I recognize all of them except. . . ." The therapist can then emphasize that having a problem or an SUD (e.g., drug and/or alcohol use disorder) is the "shared ground" or "what all the group members have in common." She can say, "Although there may be differences in what substance you have had problems with, or how long you have had this problem, or the severity of the consequences, having some of these symptoms and behaviors in common is why everyone is here today in this group."

Explanation of the Telescoping Course of SUDs in Women

After this discussion, the therapist can move on to the second part of the session, which addresses the course of illness and the severity of health effects of substances in women. She can introduce this part by saying, "Although the symptoms and behaviors of substance problems and substance use disorders are the same for both men and women, the health consequences of substance use disorders can be different." This leads to the definition of the *telescoping course of substance use disorders in women*. The therapist can explain that, in general, the telescoping course refers to the fact that women may use less of a substance and less frequently over a shorter period of time than do men before they begin to have health and medical consequences. These adverse consequences appear after shorter times of use and less heavy use. Here the therapist can state that this accelerated course of use is well documented for alcohol use disorders, and that there is evidence of this telescoping for other substances as well. These symptoms of SUDs are common to both women and men with substance disorders. However, one major difference between women and men with substance disorders is the *course of the illness* and the *severity of the health effects*. Generally, compared with men with SUDs, women with substance disorders use smaller quantities of substances (the term "substances" includes alcohol, illicit drugs, and nonmedical use of prescription drugs), less frequently, and for shorter periods of time, but women will progress more rapidly from onset of first substance use to first having a problem with substances, to the late stages of dependence with the associated severe medical consequences. This phenomenon of the more rapid advancement of substance disorders in women than in men is called the *telescoping course* of illness. Because of this accelerated course, particularly worrisome is the fact that girls are now starting to use drugs (including alcohol) at increasingly younger ages in more recent birth cohorts compared with previous birth cohorts and may start using at the youngest ages (10–14 years) at the same rate as boys.

The therapist can explain that this means that usually women have been using substances for fewer years before they begin to have more severe consequences (e.g., effects on liver or stomach, blackouts, increasing tolerance and need for greater quantity to achieve the same effect) than men. It is important to stop and ask if anyone has any thoughts about this issue or recognizes any of this in their own lives. The therapist might also point out that since substance problems run in families, sometimes women have had male relatives (e.g., fathers, grandfathers, uncles) with substance problems for several decades before they had severe adverse consequences or got help. Sometimes women think that this same time course will apply to them. However, because of the *telescoping course*, this may not be the case for women. The therapist can pause here to listen to group members' responses to this information.

Review of the Health Effects of SUDs

Given this telescoping course of illness in women, what are the effects of specific drugs on women's health? The therapist can highlight some specific points for each substance.

Alcohol

- Alcohol is metabolized differently by men and by women.
- Although most alcohol is metabolized in the liver by a specific enzyme (alcohol dehydrogenase), some of that enzyme is also located in the stomach lining (i.e., gastric mucosa).
- Women have less of this enzyme in the gastric mucosa (i.e., stomach lining) than do men.
- When men drink alcohol, a substantial amount is broken down (i.e., metabolized) in the stomach lining before being absorbed into the bloodstream.
- However, in women there is very little breakdown of alcohol in the stomach lining.
- Therefore, most of the alcohol consumed is absorbed as pure ethanol.
- Women also have less total body water than do men.
- There is less body water in which to "dilute" the alcohol in a woman's system once it is absorbed.
- As such, ounce per ounce of alcohol consumed, women have more concentrated alcohol in their bloodstream (i.e., higher blood alcohol concentrations).
- This is one reason why, after drinking comparable amounts of alcohol, women are seen to have higher blood alcohol concentrations than men, even allowing for differences in size and body weight.
- Women often suffer many of the adverse health effects of alcohol sooner than do men and after consuming smaller quantities of alcohol overall than men. These health effects include cirrhosis of the liver, a heart condition called cardiomyopathy, hypertension,

cognitive impairment, and disruption in reproductive function (e.g., loss of periods, loss of ovulation, premenstrual distress, risk of early menopause).
- Some research has also shown that even moderate daily intake of alcohol can increase circulating levels of the hormone estrogen and may increase women's risk for breast cancer.

Cocaine

- When compared with men, women who use cocaine demonstrate the telescoping course of earlier initial use, younger age at first treatment, and more rapid development of dependence.
- Women using cocaine or crack are often more likely than men to smoke cigarettes, to have physical problems such as headaches after smoking crack, and to go to emergency rooms after smoking crack because of physical symptoms.
- Cocaine also causes physical effects (e.g., constricted blood vessels; increased heart rate, blood pressure, and temperature; and dilated pupils).
- These effects put users at risk for stroke and heart attacks.
- Cocaine has many other adverse effects on the heart, stomach, lungs, and brain. It is not yet clear in what ways men and women may differ in the physical effects of cocaine.
- Cocaine-dependent women may have problems with their menstrual cycle function, including galactorrhea (production of milk in the breasts), loss of menstrual periods, and infertility.

Opiates (Heroin, Oxycodone, Morphine, Etc.)

- The *telescoping course of illness* is apparent with opiates, as we have seen in alcohol disorders.
- Women are likely to have a more rapid progression to addiction to opioids than men.
- Women are also at greater risk of death from their heroin dependence. A man with heroin dependence was found to be four times more likely to die than a man without heroin dependence; a woman with heroin dependence was found to be seven times more likely to die in any given year than a non-heroin-dependent woman.
- Drug overdoses have continuously accounted for the majority of deaths in heroin users, with AIDS, medical problems, and suicide being other leading causes (Huang & Lee, 2013; Quaglio et al., 2001).
- Most health problems associated with opiate use disorders come either from self-neglect or from the complications of intravenous injections.
- Shared needles promote infections such as HIV, hepatitis B and C, staphylococcus aureus, and other agents that cause endocarditis, an infection of the heart lining.
- Increasing numbers of deaths of heroin-dependent people may be related to overdose deaths, the combination of heroin with other substances such as cocaine and alcohol, and to HIV transmission and related illness.
- Significantly more women than men with opiate problems have medical problems for which they do not receive medical care.

Marijuana

- Most commonly cited heath consequences of marijuana are anxiety or panic attacks, psychotic symptoms (e.g., paranoia), and memory loss following more chronic marijuana use.
- More women than men report panic attacks after smoking marijuana.
- There are longer term effects of marijuana on brain function.
- Memory impairment and deficits in math skills and verbal expression are associated with heavy marijuana use.
- Marijuana also has adverse effects on the respiratory system.
- The prolonged exposure to tar and other irritants in marijuana cigarettes can lead to inflammation of the airways and eventually result in changes in the cells that line the respiratory system. This inflammation in the lungs of marijuana smokers is no different than in the lungs of tobacco smokers and seems to be the same in women and men.
- There may be increased risk of cervical cancer in marijuana-smoking women and an effect on female reproductive hormones, though a period of abstinence may allow for hormone levels to return to normal levels.
- Marijuana use can lead to physical dependence with an abstinence syndrome (withdrawal) when use is discontinued, including symptoms such as anxiety, sleep disturbance, changes in appetite, and marijuana cravings.

Neglected Self-Care

In addition to the direct health effects of specific substances, another important way that substances affect women's health is that while women are using drugs, they often *neglect themselves physically and psychologically* in a number of ways. Women often neglect going to the doctor for regular checkups that all women need. This means that they may neglect getting preventive care, such as mammograms; PAP smears; routine lab work to check cholesterol and triglycerides; blood pressure checks; and other essential health care. Women may also neglect to get treated for symptoms of infections because of their drug use, and these infections may get worse and lead to other health complications. When women neglect themselves both physically and psychologically, they may also find themselves trading sex for drugs, or may have unprotected sex while intoxicated, and this can increase the risk of certain infections such as HIV, hepatitis B and C, and others.

Again, it is important to invite women to discuss the aspects of the session topic that they recognize in their own lives or perhaps in the lives of female relatives (e.g., mothers, grandmothers, aunts) or other women they may have known. Group members may have specific medical or health questions regarding substances. The therapist ought to answer these to the best of her ability. She should try to avoid using "medical jargon" and answer questions in as straightforward a way as possible. If it turns out that she does not know the answer to a question about a particular effect of a substance on women's health, she should tell the group that she does not know the answer but will check on it and get back to them the next week.

The therapist can also remind the group that Participant Sheet PG.3 that was provided during the pre-group meeting lists reading and resources to learn more about specific health effects. The final main point of the session is that *substance problems can lead to self-neglect* and *recovery* (abstinence from all substances including alcohol) *enhances self-care.* The therapist can refer to the WRG's central recovery rule that "Recovery means taking care of yourself." This will also tie in with this week's skill practice (Participant Sheet 1.3).

Open Discussion

Topics may include ongoing discussion of today's specific topic, such that the discussion that began about self-care from the session topic may move naturally into the open discussion part of the group session. Again, other recovery-focused topics can be discussed during this time including discussion of issues brought up during the check-in. Remember that the therapist can summarize themes, and can relate the content of participants' discussion to the group theme of self-care or to other session topics of the WRG; this is a good way to jump-start discussion either at the beginning of open discussion or at any time when the discussion lags.

Wrap-Up and Reading of Take-Home Messages

Recap any themes of the open discussion and relate them to WRG themes (e.g., from this session one focus would be what participants can do to be as healthy as possible), distribute Participant Sheet 1.2, and transition to reading of the session topic's Take-Home Messages. Participants then take turns going around the group, with each reading one take-home message; alternatively, the therapist can read them if this is more clinically appropriate.

Distribution and Description of This Week's Skill Practice

Distribute this week's Skill Practice Sheet (Participant Sheet 1.3). Quickly read through the skill practice sheet and encourage participants to do it themselves before the next group and bring it with them to review at the next session.

Check-Out

Pass around the Check-Out Sheet and have each member answer orally the single question: "What will you do this week to take care of yourself?" When check-out is complete, thank the members for coming and tell them you look forward to seeing them next time.

How to Manage Triggers and High-Risk Situations

Learning to identify one's own triggers and high-risk situations, and how to manage them effectively without using drugs and alcohol, is a critical element of relapse prevention. The goal of this session of the WRG is to assist women in identifying their own triggers and high-risk situations and to generate possible alternative strategies to manage these without using substances. This session reviews gender-specific triggers, that is, triggers that are often salient for women, as well as strategies for managing these triggers. Other subsequent sessions will focus on specific triggers and high-risk situations that are especially relevant for women (such as Session 3, Overcoming Obstacles to Recovery; Session 4, Managing Mood, Anxiety, and Eating Problems without Using Substances; Session 5, Women and Their Partners; Session 6, Coping with Stress; and Session 7, Women as Caretakers). Subsequent sessions will also focus on developing specific skills to manage these triggers without using substances (such as Session 6, Coping with Stress; Session 8, Using Self-Help Groups to Help Yourself; Session 13, Can You Have Fun without Using Drugs or Alcohol; and Session 14, Achieving Balance in Your Life). Today's session topic provides a first introduction to the topic of triggers and alternative ways to manage these without using substances. As is the case with each session, detailed information is included in the next section, "Background Information." The therapist should read this section while preparing for this session.

Background Information

A "trigger" is anything, anyone, or any place that increases your urge to use drugs or alcohol. Triggers are sometimes also called "high-risk situations." A trigger can be *internal* (such as feelings and thoughts) or *external* (such as people, places, situations, and things). Internal triggers could include feeling sad, lonely, angry, depressed, or anxious, or thinking things like "I feel so bad I deserve to use" or "What difference does it make if I use?" External triggers could include people you once used with or bars where you used to drink before becoming abstinent, among many others.

It is important to know that there will always be triggers! The key is learning to identify *your own triggers* and *your own ways to positively manage them.*

More about High-Risk Situations

High-risk situations are those situations that can jeopardize your sense of control and increase your risk of relapse. Identifying high-risk situations and learning how to manage them are important parts of recovery.

High-risk situations that may cause one person to relapse may not affect another person in the same way. In general, however, there are certain high-risk situations that many people with SUDs commonly associate with a greater risk of relapse. Some examples of general high-risk situations that are associated with an increased risk of relapse are listed below:

1. *Internal*
   a. *Feelings*: loneliness, depression, anger, hopelessness, anxiety, exhaustion.
   b. *Thoughts*: "What difference does it make if I use just once?" or "No one cares about me."
   c. *Physical discomfort*: hunger, fatigue, acute or chronic physical pain.
2. *External*
   a. *People*: seeing your drug dealer, seeing other people use drugs or drink alcohol, being with people who you used to use with, seeing a friend/relative who always criticizes you.
   b. *Places*: passing by a bar or a liquor store, passing by a house or other place where you often bought or used drugs.
   c. *Things*: money, cigarettes, liquor bottles, drug paraphernalia such as mirrors, spoons, and needles.
3. *Interpersonal conflict*: arguments with family/partner/friends or difficulties with employer/coworkers/other students.
4. *Social pressure*: family/partner/friends putting pressure on you to drink or use drugs.

Do Women and Men Face Different Kinds of Triggers?

There is evidence that women may be more likely to relapse than men when faced with certain high-risk situations. Women sometimes show a tendency to relapse when they are in a negative mood state, such as depression, while men are more likely to relapse when they are in a positive mood state. For some women, negative mood states associated with the premenstrual phase of the menstrual cycle have also been associated with triggers to use. Additionally, women often say that being with a significant other who uses is their major trigger, and partner relationships can therefore play an important triggering role for women. Finally, women are often in caretaking roles and may be triggering when they feel overwhelmed by others' demands on them.

Drug and/or Alcohol Availability as a High-Risk Situation

Drug and/or alcohol availability is another high-risk situation that can have a powerful effect on your desire to use alcohol or drugs. Alcohol and drugs themselves, as well as the internal and external experiences associated with their use, are referred to as *conditioned cues*. Your reaction to a conditioned cue is referred to as the *conditioned response* (or the thoughts, feelings, and behaviors that result from exposure to the cue, based on your prior experiences with the cue). For example, a woman goes to visit her friend who is struggling to remain abstinent from marijuana. When she arrives, she sees her friend rolling a marijuana cigarette and smells the odor of marijuana in the air. She suddenly has a strong desire to smoke marijuana and decides to have a few puffs of marijuana because it will make her depression better.

What are the conditioned cues in this case? The *conditioned cues* would include her friend, the availability of marijuana, the smell of the drug in the air, and the act of rolling the marijuana cigarette. *The conditioned responses* would be both her strong desire for and her actual use of marijuana.

Managing High-Risk Situations and Triggers

Recovery and long-term sobriety would be simple if there were no high-risk situations in your life. Although it is not realistic to expect that you can arrange your life so you *never* face a high-risk situation, you certainly can *try to avoid* high-risk situations whenever possible. If a high-risk situation is unavoidable, your objective is to learn how to manage your response to the high-risk situation to prevent relapse to substance use. *How do you avoid high-risk situations?*

First, identify high-risk situations and work on plans to avoid them. For instance, if your route to and from home or to and from school includes passing a bar or a drug dealer's house, find another route even if it adds time to your daily commute. If your friends invite you to a party or a social gathering where you know substances will be used, turn down their offer and make plans with a sober friend instead. You should remember that while high risks can be extremely difficult to avoid, they are usually not impossible to avoid.

What if you identify a high-risk situation that you cannot avoid? A good rule of thumb for a high-risk situation you cannot avoid is, "If you can't avoid the high-risk situation, *don't face the situation alone*." For example, if you have had problems with prescription painkillers for migraine headaches in the past, going to your doctor's office can be a high-risk situation. Your best defense in this situation is to bring a sober friend to the doctor's office with you so you cannot ask for painkillers to treat your migraines or you can explain your risk and ask for alternatives. Similarly, if you are required to go to a work or college function where alcohol is served, bring a sober friend with you so you will be less likely to drink.

Sometimes, you may face an unavoidable high-risk situation without having anyone to face it with you. In these circumstances, *distracting yourself with self-nurturing activities* can take your mind off of the high-risk situation. For example, if you used substances at a certain time of day, make plans to attend a self-help group meeting, spend time with a sober family member/friend, or participate in an activity that you like to do (e.g., walking or listening to calming music) at that time of day. *Creating structure in your day by scheduling tasks and activities will help keep your focus away from high-risk situations.* Additionally, activities such as exercise or other pursuits you enjoy can help improve negative mood states like depression and anxiety by giving you a feeling of purpose and helping you overcome the sense of isolation these negative mood states can cause.

While having someone with you or having activities to distract you will not make it *impossible* for you to return to substance use, it will make it a little more *difficult* to relapse, which may be all that it takes to get you through a high-risk situation successfully. Identifying high-risk situations and learning how to avoid or manage them can be difficult at first because you feel awkward or because others in your life may feel angry or disappointed about your choices. You yourself may not feel you are making the right choices until sometime after the situation has passed. It might help to think about these feelings and triggers as wants or desires that come and go. Although there may be a strong one, it will pass. The short-term, difficult feelings you may experience and tolerate when you avoid or manage a high-risk situation will be worth it in the end when gradually these get less and less, and you experience the longer term positive feelings associated with ongoing recovery.

Examples of Some Triggers and Coping Strategies Identified by Women in Recovery

(Note to therapist: This outline of triggers and alternative coping strategies is also handed out to participants in Participant Sheet 2.1 and will be referred to as part of this week's skill practice in Participant Sheet 2.3. It is here for you to review in preparation for this session. The therapist can refer to these triggers and alternate ways to cope during the session and have participants read through them on Participant Sheet 2.1 during the topic review.)

Triggers

- Being in restaurants.
- Anxiety.
- Making dinner.
- Relationships or a particular relationship.
- Anger.
- Writing a letter that is difficult to write.
- Anniversary of a death.
- Watching a partner drink or use.
- Hurtful action by someone else (such as forgetting your birthday).
- Feeling sorry for yourself.
- Anger from relatives directed at you.
- Powerful, strong, difficult feelings (such as hatred).
- Guilt.
- Feeling imperfect.
- Drugs and alcohol being used by other people in the household.
- Separation.
- Doing paperwork (want to use to get through it).
- Family/children's/parents'/sibling's/partner's demands/needs.
- Dreaming about using.
- Nightmares.
- Depression.

Ways to Cope with Triggers

- Take care of others (but not at the expense of taking care of yourself).
- Exercise (unless this is not good for you due to another health condition).
- Make lists.
- Go to the gym (unless this is not good for you due to another health condition).
- Read.
- Take a bath.
- Get a massage if you can.
- Go to the movies.
- Be with people you like (who don't use).
- Get additional treatment if needed for substance use disorders or other psychiatric disorders (can include individual therapy, the WRG, self-help, etc.).
- Take care of responsibilities (will give you a feeling of accomplishment).
- Get rid of bottle of wine in the fridge or other alcoholic drinks at home.
- Get rid of other substances that are around you.
- Start a journal or, if you already use one, write in your journal.
- Do something positive to commemorate a loved one who is gone.
- Go to work or school.
- Write a goodbye note to someone you need to separate from.
- Talk with your significant other about what is going on or what you are feeling.
- Sleep a lot if you need to.
- Rent movies or watch a favorite TV program.
- Find/go to an Alcoholics Anonymous (AA) or other self-help meeting you really like.
- Altruism: do something for others to take your mind off yourself.
- Take time for yourself to do something you like.
- Garden.
- Go to church, synagogue, or other house of worship or service.
- Practice mindfulness.
- Do yoga.
- Practice meditation.
- Take a walk.
- Listen to music you enjoy.
- Use your sponsor if you have one.
- Limit your access to money that you would spend on alcohol or drugs.
- Get rid of any drug paraphernalia.

Therapist Overview

Goals of This Session

- To learn how to identify high-risk situations and triggers.
- To explore triggers and high-risk situations that women commonly experience.
- To learn how to manage high-risk situations and triggers by avoiding, distracting, or using other coping strategies.

Session 2 Outline

- **Introduction** (*If Needed*) (5 minutes).
- **Check-In** (15 minutes).
- **Review of Last Week's Skill Practice and Topic** (5 minutes).
- **Presentation of This Week's Topic and Distribution of Topic Overview** (25 minutes): Provide Participant Sheet 2.1.
  - Internal triggers.
    - Feelings, thoughts, physical discomfort.
  - External triggers.
    - High-risk situations, people, places, things.
  - Common triggers for women.
  - Identifying your own triggers.
  - Dealing with unavoidable triggers.
    - Distraction.
  - Creating positive alternatives.
  - Feelings and urges will pass.
- **Open Discussion** (30 minutes).
- **Wrap-Up and Reading of Take-Home Messages** (2 minutes): Provide Participant Sheet 2.2.
- **Distribution and Description of This Week's Skill Practice** (3 minutes): Provide Participant Sheet 2.3.
- **Check-Out** (5 minutes).

Session-Specific Materials Needed

- Bulletin Board Outline and Take-Home Messages for Session 2.
- Participant Sheet 2.1: Overview: How to Manage Triggers and High-Risk Situations.
- Participant Sheet 2.2: Take-Home Messages.
- Participant Sheet 2.3: Skill Practice: How to Manage Triggers and High-Risk Situations.

Introduction (If Needed)

As in the previous session, provide an introduction to the group if there are new members.

Check-In

Pass around the Check-In Sheet (see Appendix B) and ask each member to respond orally to the three check-in questions.

Review of Last Week's Skill Practice and Topic

From the check-in, the therapist should have a sense of who has done the skill practice and commented on whether or not it was helpful. The therapist can build on the check-in by asking if anyone would like to comment on the skill practice and what she learned. The therapist can also comment on the main highlights from last week's topic. The therapist can then transition to presentation of this week's topic.

Presentation of This Week's Topic
and Distribution of Topic Overview

The therapist should distribute Participant Sheet 2.1 and introduce the session topic: "Today's topic is about managing high-risk situations and triggers. The two terms are actually inter-changeable, and people generally use them to refer to the same things, that is, people, places, things, feelings, and internal states that lead to drug and alcohol craving and urges to use." At this point the therapist might tie the session topic in with the themes from the day's check-in by saying something like, "Many of you were talking about the triggers or high-risk situations that you experienced this past week. Today's topic is about how to manage such triggers or high-risk situations. . . ."

To begin this session, the therapist might start by saying that the bottom-line take-home messages for today are:

- Avoid high-risk situations or triggers whenever you can.
- In order to do that, you have to know what your own triggers are.
- Even knowing your own triggers, sometimes they can't be avoided.
- When you can't avoid them, you need to know how to manage them.

The therapist can stress here that it is important to know that *there will always be triggers*. That is why participants need to learn to *identify their own triggers* and how to manage them. This is very important to their recovery.

The therapist can then say that we sometimes describe triggers or high-risk situations as internal and external.

Internal Triggers

Internal triggers are most often *feelings, thoughts*, or *physical discomfort*.

- *Feelings*: Feelings such as anger, depression, hopelessness, and anxiety can all be triggers to use drugs or alcohol.
- *Thoughts*: Examples of thoughts that may be strong triggers to use are "What difference does it make if I use just once?" or "No one will know if I use now" or "I've been sober for 3 months now and I deserve a reward." In addition, some people have negative thoughts about themselves that may become triggers. These thoughts can accompany feelings of depression or anger and might be something like, "I am a bad person because . . ." or

"I always mess up, so why should this be different?" or "I've never been able to do this before, so why should this be different?"

- *Physical discomfort*: Physical discomfort can be a strong trigger to use drugs. Physical discomfort can be as routine as hunger and fatigue that can come from lack of self-care on a given day. These feelings can be triggers to use drugs or alcohol especially when someone has a past pattern of responding to these feelings by using. For some people, chronic pain (e.g., back pain, joint pain, recurrent headaches, dental pain) may be a strong trigger.

Discussion: After reviewing these *internal triggers*, the therapist should stop and ask the group if they relate to these types of internal triggers. It is helpful to encourage as many people as are willing to participate to identify and describe their own internal triggers of feelings, thoughts, or physical discomfort.

External Triggers

After this brief discussion of *internal triggers*, the therapist should tell the group that the other category of triggers or high-risk situations that people describe is *external triggers*. These can be people, places, or things. People who may be triggers can be drug dealers or other people participants used with. Places may be a bar participants drank at or a place where they used. Places might also include a party or an event where people are drinking or using drugs. One specific place that is common may be their own home. This may be specifically true for women's use of alcohol. Things may be money, cigarettes, a liquor bottle, or drug paraphernalia. Other high-risk or external triggers can be interpersonal conflict (e.g., fights, arguments, or stress with important people) or social pressure (e.g., family, partner, friends, or coworkers putting pressure on participants to use substances).

Discussion: After describing external triggers, the therapist should ask the group if any of these high-risk situations or triggers ring a bell for them and engage in brief discussion.

Common Triggers for Women

The therapist can then briefly describe several types of triggers that women describe more frequently than men. For example, while men more frequently describe relapse during a positive mood state, women tend to describe relapse during negative mood states, such as anger or depression. Negative mood states associated with the premenstrual phase of the menstrual cycle may also serve as a trigger for women. Additionally, women often describe a partner or a significant other who uses alcohol or drugs as a major trigger for their own use.

Identifying Your Own Triggers

The therapist can then say that the most important thing is for each woman to identify her own triggers or high-risk situations. These will not be the same for everyone, and it is important for each woman's needs to identify which triggers put *her* at the highest risk for using. Once a woman understands her own particular triggers and high-risk situations, she can begin to figure out a way to manage them without using. There are several key steps to this process. The first is to figure out which triggers are avoidable and which ones are not. Women should try to avoid high-risk situations whenever they can. Avoidable triggers might include a route home that passes a liquor store, drug dealer's house, or former place of use; a party where everyone is drinking and using; or a family event where there is likely to be friction that stirs up urges and cravings. In some instances, high-risk situations are not avoidable, and in these instances it is important that the woman doesn't face the situation alone. The woman should try to go to such events or places with someone who knows she is in recovery and can help support her. Also, she should develop an "early escape plan," planning to leave after a short period of time or if she feels that the situation is stirring up the urge to use. If she brings someone with her who is supportive of her recovery, that person can help her leave early or at the appropriate time. Other unavoidable triggers may be negative feelings or thoughts. Developing skills and alternative behaviors to manage these and not use alcohol or drugs is important and can include distraction and creating positive alternatives. The therapist can ask participants to refer to Participant Sheet 2.1 and ask if any of these external or internal triggers are ones that they have experienced.

Dealing with Unavoidable Triggers

Distraction

The therapist can tell group members that if they are in an unavoidable high-risk situation and are alone, they can try to distract themselves with self-nurturing activities to take their minds off the high-risk situation (e.g., take a walk, read a book, attend self-help, listen to music).

Creating Positive Alternatives

Creating structure in their days to help them during a difficult time of day or keep their focus away from high-risk situations can also be a key way to manage triggers. For example, attending a meeting or exercising at a gym during a specific time of day that the woman knows is difficult is one way to create a positive alternative. The therapist should tell group members that it is most important that they create positive alternatives that they can really do and not hypothetical ones that they know they will never do. If there are specific physical problems or mood states that may be triggers, they might seek the help of a doctor or other health care provider to try to find alternatives to relieve these states.

Feelings and Urges Pass

Finally, the therapist should remind group members that no feeling lasts forever. If they can tolerate a feeling without using, it will pass. The therapist can then ask group members to reflect on their own triggers and high-risk situations and then try to think of one alternative way to manage this trigger that they can actually do. Again, the therapist can refer to Participant Sheet 2.1 and ask participants if any of these alternate ways of coping are ones they use or might be helpful.

Open Discussion

Topics may include ongoing discussion of today's specific topic. The discussion that begins about triggers from the session topic may move naturally into the open discussion part of the group session. Again, other recovery-focused topics can be discussed during this time including discussion of issues brought up in the check-in.

Wrap-Up and Reading of Take-Home Messages

In wrapping up this session, the therapist can summarize the take-home messages by focusing on the importance of group members *identifying their own triggers and high-risk situations and developing their own realistic plans to manage these.* Distribute Participant Sheet 2.2. Then, as in previous sessions, the take-home messages can be reviewed by having members each read one of the messages in turn.

Distribution and Description of This Week's Skill Practice

Distribute the Skill Practice Sheet (Participant Sheet 2.3). This week's skill practice invites group members to list avoidable and unavoidable triggers and ways to manage them, as well as to list triggers that come up during the week and alternative ways to manage them. The session-specific overview (Participant Sheet 2.1) that was distributed earlier in the group has a list of triggers that previous WRG members identified, as well as some alternative ways they found to cope with and manage these triggers. The skill practice also has a wallet-size card that says "I take care of myself because. . . ." with lines for participants to fill in. The purpose of this card is for group members to write down the central reason(s) they want to be in recovery. When completed, participants can clip out the card and place it in their wallet or another location that is useful to them. Another alternative is to take a photo of the filled-in card with a smartphone if participants have one and put the photo on the phone's wallpaper or just in the photo file to be retrieved. The card (as hard copy or as a photo on a phone) can be referred to when participants are confronted with a trigger and need to remind themselves why they want to manage their triggers in ways other than using substances.

Check-Out

Pass around the Check-Out Sheet and ask each participant to answer orally the one-question check-out. Thank members and tell them you will see them next time.

Overcoming Obstacles to Recovery

This session presents internal and external obstacles that are especially relevant for women with SUDs that often prevent their seeking treatment and may also impede their ability to complete or stay in treatment. These obstacles include ascribing substance problems to family problems or to problems with mood or anxiety, societal stigma, lack of information about treatment that works, and familial or social barriers such as lack of family or partner support to seek treatment or lack of financial or child care resources. These barriers to accessing and completing treatment have specific relevance for women and are important to address because they can interfere with relapse prevention and sustained recovery. As is the case with each session, detailed information is included in the next section, "Background Information." The therapist should read this section while preparing for this session.

Background Information

What are the types of barriers women often find in both seeking treatment and being in recovery? Not all women will experience each and every one of these obstacles or barriers to treatment. However, women often report many of these experiences interfere with their ability to get themselves into substance abuse treatment or, once in treatment, to stay there and continue in recovery. Below are descriptions of some of the obstacles and barriers women commonly report.

Stigma

Women often perceive that there is a long-standing "double standard" in our culture such that women with substance problems are more negatively perceived by others than are men with substance-related problems. For example, there have been long-standing taboos against women's intoxication with substances; these may be related to certain attitudes that traditionally have placed a high value on women's "sexual virtue" or their roles as "nurturing caregivers." Substance problems are perceived to compromise these aspects of women's traditional role expectations directly, and such ideas may have contributed to increased societal stigmatization of women with substance problems. This can interfere with women feeling empowered enough to seek help and treatment for their substance use disorder. Sometimes women may worry that in seeking substance abuse treatment they will expose themselves to disapproval from others or to their own feelings of embarrassment. Some women also perceive that social attitudes are more rejecting of women who are intoxicated or high than of men with this same behavior, and they may not wish to obtain treatment because of fear of being "labeled" and/or judged "immoral" or "neglectful." Women are also more likely than men to experience a personal sense of shame or embarrassment related to entering and staying in treatment. Some women have experienced men's attitudes that women's use of substances and intoxication is a sign of sexual availability or is an acceptable excuse for men's expression of violence against women. Such experiences may also give rise to increased feelings of shame or embarrassment. Sometimes women who use substances will incorporate these socially stigmatizing attitudes into perceptions of themselves. This in turn can lead to lower self-esteem and become another barrier to seeking treatment for drug and alcohol problems.

Substance Use Disorders Are Not Only about Family Problems, Problems in Relationships, or Stressful Life Events

Women are often more likely to perceive that their substance problem is really not their main problem but rather is a *consequence* of other personal problems. They are less likely than men to define their personal problems as substance-related. Instead, women often feel that their substance problems have to do with their relationships, partner, spouse, or children. They may feel that a recent stressful event such as the loss of a job, marriage, parent, or friend is the root of the problem. In this way, women are more likely to seek mental health treatment to help them understand or cope with these other difficulties. They may feel that they use substances *because* of these problems and that if they can fix these problems, they will be able to stop using drugs and alcohol. Because of the way they have defined their problem, women may minimize both to themselves and to other people (including clinicians to whom they have gone for help) the extent and negative consequences of their substance use. They may not understand that these other types of difficulties are made worse by substance use and that it is necessary to try to address both of them at the same time.

Feeling That the Problem Is Not Really about Substances but about Mood or Anxiety

There is a greater prevalence of mood and anxiety problems among women with substance-related problems than among men. Some women may feel that their substance use is *a result* of their mood or anxiety symptoms. They feel that if they can get treated for mood and anxiety problems (with psychotherapy and/or medication), they will be able to stop using substances. They may therefore seek help from therapists, psychiatrists, or primary care doctors for these other problems. Because they feel that their substance use will get better as soon as the mood and anxiety symptoms are gone, they might not share their use of alcohol or drugs with their clinicians; even if they do discuss it, they may find themselves minimizing the use and its consequences. They may not understand that mood and anxiety disorders *can worsen substance disorders* but *substance disorders can also worsen mood and anxiety disorders*. Because of this fact, it is important that these problems be addressed at the same time.

Conflicts between Taking Care of Yourself by Getting Support for Your Recovery and Other Roles or Responsibilities as Workers, Caretakers, or Both

Women also find themselves trying to balance many different roles as workers, as well as caretakers of families, children, and/or elder relatives. Some women will find that trying to balance these obligations already strains their personal resources. Considering adding SUD treatment to this already delicate balance may seem overwhelming. Women may perceive that the economic or time costs may be too high for them to engage in treatment. In such cases, women may find themselves in a "vicious cycle." While their use of substances may be an attempt to "cope" with these other stressful life situations, in reality it actually worsens some of their personal circumstances and makes it difficult for them to deal as effectively as they could if they were not drinking or using drugs. Because of their substance use, they feel like they are losing ground, and this may lead to more feelings of being overwhelmed and "out of control," thereby making it even more difficult to imagine how to fit treatment into this picture.

Logistical Problems Such as Lack of Child Care or Elder Care

Women who are the primary caregivers for dependent children or elders may find it hard to work out additional support for these responsibilities while they seek treatment. They may be unaware of resources within their own communities that might be helpful in this regard.

Lack of Financial Resources

Women are often concerned that treatment will be too expensive and take too much time and that they will not have the financial resources to support it. Women with substance problems often do have fewer financial resources or less income than men with substance problems. Women who are employed outside the home are more likely than employed men to say that they are worried about losing a job and that this is a significant barrier to seeking treatment for substance disorders. Sometimes in this situation it is difficult to see that substance use impairs job performance, makes losing a job more likely, and may limit other possibilities of becoming more financially secure. In addition, some of these thoughts and feelings may come from a limited knowledge about the types of treatment that are available that may be less costly or require less time. Finally, the time invested in treatment up front often results in more time to invest in longer term life planning, as well as improved financial security (which some women report feeling after they enter a process of recovery).

Lack of Support from a Partner

Women who have substance-related problems are more likely to have a partner addicted to substances than are substance-dependent men. For example, heterosexual women with alcohol or drug problems are more likely to be living with drug-dependent men, compared with heterosexual drug-dependent men who are more likely to be living with non-drug-using women partners. Of course, this is not always the case, but women in SUD treatment are more likely to report that a substance-using partner at home is an obstacle to ongoing recovery than are men in SUD treatment. Women also often find themselves with a substance-using partner who supports their continued use of substances, and therefore becomes a significant barrier to women seeking help for their own substance problems. Women may feel torn between getting themselves help and their commitment to their relationships.

Lack of Information about the Fact That Treatment Works and about the Range of Existing Treatment Options

Women with substance problems often say that they had trouble seeking help because they weren't sure treatment would work, didn't know what treatments were available, and didn't know where to go for help. Often in this situation women are aware of only one type of treatment or think there are no available treatments. This lack of knowledge and information can be an obstacle to seeking help for substance problems.

What to Do about Obstacles to Seeking Treatment and Being in Recovery

Women may identify with all or some of these barriers to seeking treatment, or may have experienced an obstacle not discussed above. Clearly, because the participants are in your group, they have overcome whatever barriers they experienced in seeking treatment. Nonetheless, some of these same barriers (or perhaps others) may get in their way as they try to maintain abstinence from substances and continue on in recovery. The question that then comes up for each participant for potential discussion in this group session is "*What can you do to help overcome these obstacles?*"

Therapist Overview

Goals of This Session

- To learn about obstacles to recovery that are common for many women in recovery.
- To identify the obstacles to their own recovery and learn how to get the support they need to stay in recovery.
- To help group members think through the ways they can overcome these obstacles.

Session 3 Outline

- **Introduction (*If Needed*)** (5 minutes).
- **Check-In** (15 minutes).
- **Review of Last Week's Skill Practice and Topic** (5 minutes).
- **Presentation of This Week's Topic and Distribution of Topic Overview** (25 minutes). Provide Participant Sheet 3.1.
  - Common obstacles or barriers to treatment and recovery for women.
    - Stigma about getting help for alcohol and drug problems.
    - Thinking that substance problems are only about family problems, problems in relationships, or stressful life events.
    - Thinking that the substance problems are only about depression and anxiety.
    - Feeling that you have to take care of others before taking care of yourself.

- ■ Having an unsupportive partner.
- ■ Lacking financial or child care resources.
- ■ Lacking information that treatment works and range of treatment options.
  - ○ Overcoming obstacles to recovery.
    - ■ Make an inventory of negative consequences that substances have caused you.
    - ■ Identify the obstacles that have gotten in the way of your recovery.
    - ■ Brainstorm strategies to overcome these obstacles.
- **Open Discussion** (30 minutes).
- **Wrap-Up and Reading of Take-Home Messages** (3 minutes): Provide Participant Sheet 3.2.
- **Distribution and Description of This Week's Skill Practice** (3 minutes): Provide Participant Sheet 3.3.
- **Check-Out** (5 minutes).

Session-Specific Materials Needed

- Bulletin Board Outline and Take-Home Messages for Session 3.
- Participant Sheet 3.1: Overcoming Obstacles to Recovery.
- Participant Sheet 3.2: Take-Home Messages.
- Participant Sheet 3.3: Skill Practice: Overcoming Obstacles to Recovery.

Introduction (If Needed)

As in the previous session, provide an introduction to the group if there are new members.

Check-In

Pass around the Check-In Sheet and have each member respond orally to the three check-in questions.

Review of Last Week's Skill Practice and Topic

From the check-in, the therapist should have a sense of who has done the skill practice and commented on whether or not it was helpful. The therapist can build on the check-in by asking if anyone would like to comment on the skill practice and what she learned. The therapist can also comment on the main highlights from last week's topic. The therapist can then transition to presentation of this week's topic.

Presentation of This Week's Topic and Distribution of Topic Overview

Distribute Participant Sheet 3.1 at this time, which provides an overview of this topic. One way to introduce the session topic is to reference themes from the check-in that relate to the topic of obstacles to recovery. For example, the therapist might say, "Many of you have brought up a variety of obstacles to your own recovery and seeking the support and help you need. You have discussed issues such as . . . [list the issues that have come up]. Today we are going to be discussing obstacles to recovery that women say they often experience. Some of the take-home messages that I hope that you get from today's session are:

- Women often have powerful obstacles to their recovery and these can include:
  - Stigma about getting help for drug and alcohol problems.
  - Thinking the problem is only about depression and anxiety.
  - Feeling that you must take care of others before taking care of yourself.
  - Having an unsupportive partner.
  - Lack of financial or child care resources.
  - Lack of stable housing.
  - Lack of reliable transportation.
  - Lack of information about the fact that treatment works.
  - These obstacles can be overcome by asking for help, getting treatment, and working to create your own network of support for your recovery, as well as other strategies a woman may find for herself."

The therapist can then go on to say that she would like first to review each type of obstacle to see if any of these are ones that group members recognize in their own lives. Using the bulletin board take-home messages as a guide, she can then review each type of obstacle in turn.

Stigma

Women often report that *stigma* is a barrier to getting into treatment and to seeking the support they need for recovery. The therapist can discuss the "double standard" in our culture and how women often feel "labeled" or "judged" because of their substance problem, which in turn can increase women's feelings of shame and embarrassment and be an obstacle to their recovery. Women may themselves have absorbed societal stigma and attitudes about women and addiction or that women's intoxication is a sign of sexual availability and provides a rationale for violence against women. Such experiences can lead to increased feelings of shame or embarrassment, lower self-esteem, and become another barrier to seeking treatment for drug and alcohol problems.

Substance Problems Are Not Only about Family Problems, Problems in Relationships, or Stressful Life Events

Another obstacle is *feeling that the problem is not really about substances but about family problems, relationship problems, or stressful life events.* Women are less likely to define their personal problems as substance-related than are men. Instead, women often see their substance problem as a consequence of problems related to their relationships with a partner, spouse, or children. They may think that if they fix these problems, the drug or alcohol problem will go away. Because of the way women may define their problem, they minimize to themselves or others (including therapists, physicians, and others to whom they have gone for help) the extent and negative consequences of their substance use. This belief may interfere with their ability to get help for themselves for their substance problems and to get support for their recovery.

Feeling That the Problem Is Not Really about Substances but about Mood or Anxiety

Similarly, the therapist can point out that women sometimes feel that their *substance problem is a result of a mood or anxiety problem*. Compared with men, there is a greater prevalence of mood and anxiety problems among women with SUDs. However, women may believe their SUD is a result of their mood or anxiety problem. They therefore may not share their use of substances with clinicians or doctors because they think that once their depression or anxiety is treated, the substance problem will automatically go away. They may also not understand that mood and anxiety disorders can *worsen substance disorders but substance disorders also worsen mood and anxiety disorders*. Because of this reality, it is important that both/all of these disorders are treated at the same time. Women may minimize to themselves and others the seriousness of their substance problems and may not get the help they need for their SUD and their recovery.

Conflicts between Taking Care of Yourself by Getting Support for Your Recovery and Other Roles or Responsibilities as Workers, Caretakers, or Both

In trying to balance many different roles as caretakers of families, children, and/or elder relatives, some women find that this burden already strains their personal resources and that adding treatment for substance use disorders to this delicate balance is overwhelming. Women may perceive that the economic or time costs may be too high for them to engage in treatment. This can result in a "vicious cycle" where women find themselves using substances to try to "cope" with these other stressful life situations, but in reality this substance use worsens these personal circumstances and makes it difficult for them to deal as effectively as they could if they were not drinking or using drugs. This may contribute to feeling overwhelmed, "out of control," and as if they are losing ground and may make it more difficult to imagine how to fit treatment into this picture.

Logistical Problems Such as Lack of Child Care or Elder Care

Women who are the primary caregivers for dependent children or elders may find it hard to work out additional support for these responsibilities while they seek treatment. They may be unaware of resources within their own communities that might be helpful in this regard.

Lack of Financial Resources

Women are often concerned that treatment will be too expensive, take too much time, and they will not have the financial resources to support it. Women with substance problems often do have fewer financial resources or less income than men with substance problems. Women who are employed outside the home are more likely than employed men to say that they are worried about losing a job and that this in itself is a significant barrier to seeking treatment for substance problems. Sometimes in this situation it is difficult to see that substance problems impair job performance, make losing a job more likely, and may limit other possibilities of becoming more financially secure. However, the time invested in treatment up front often results in more time to invest in longer term life planning, as well as improved financial security (which many women report feeling after they enter a process of recovery). Women may also lack stable housing or reliable transportation, which are other potential obstacles.

Lack of Support from a Partner

Women who have substance-related problems are more likely to have a partner who abuses substances than are men with SUDs. For example, a heterosexual woman with alcohol or drug use disorders is likely to be living with a drug-using man, compared with a heterosexual man with SUD, who is more likely to be living with a non-drug-using woman partner. Of course this is not always the case, but women in SUD treatment are more likely to report that a substance using partner at home is an obstacle to ongoing recovery than are men in SUD treatment. Women also often find themselves with a substance using partner who prefers that they continue to use substances with them, and therefore become significant barriers to women seeking help for their own substance problems. Women may feel torn between getting themselves help and their commitment to their relationships.

Lack of Information about the Fact That Treatment Works and about the Range of Existing Treatment Options

Women with substance problems often say that they had trouble seeking help because they weren't sure treatment would work, didn't know what treatments were available, and didn't know where to go for help. Often in this situation, women are aware of only one type of treatment or think there are no available treatments. This lack of knowledge and information can be an obstacle to seeking help for substance problems.

The degree to which the therapist may describe each of the obstacles described above will depend, in part, upon the therapist's knowledge of the group members. For example, in a group of women who are single parents, the therapist may spend more time discussing lack of child care and conflicts between women's role as caretakers and women's recovery. If the group members are mostly women without children or women with grown children, this obstacle may be mentioned in a sentence and the therapist may then spend more time discussing other obstacles. After describing these obstacles, the therapist should ask the group members if they identify with any of these obstacles either in the past or in their current lives and if so, which ones. The therapist should pause to invite brief discussion after discussing a few potential obstacles; then describe several more, invite discussion, and so on. It is important to invite discussion after describing several obstacles in order to make the presentation interactive. Then the therapist should invite discussion of the various barriers that are now affecting group members.

Overcoming Obstacles

After the obstacles that seem most important to group members have been reviewed, the therapist should say something like, "Now let's move on to ways of overcoming these obstacles." The therapist can then point out that the group members have already started the first step in the group by doing a *personal inventory of the negative consequences that substances have caused them* and by *beginning to identify the obstacles to their own recovery.* It is helpful for each woman to make an inventory of the ideas, feelings, and circumstances that may be obstacles to her recovery. These obstacles can be overcome by asking for help, getting treatment, and working to create a network of support for recovery, among other strategies. At this point, the therapist should invite the group members to discuss some of the ways they might find to overcome the obstacles to their own recovery. It would be helpful for group members to talk about any ways that they feel they have already overcome obstacles, as well as to discuss new ways they might plan to overcome obstacles they have identified. The therapist can point out that attending the WRG is a way that many in the group already may be building support for their recovery and overcoming a number of obstacles.

Open Discussion

Topics may include ongoing discussion of today's specific topic and the discussion that began about overcoming obstacles from the session topic may move naturally into the open discussion part of the group session. Again, other recovery-focused topics can be discussed during this time including discussion of issues brought up in the check-in.

Wrap-Up and Reading of Take-Home Messages

When summarizing this session, it is important for the therapist to emphasize the major obstacles that women have brought up during the session. The therapist can then especially highlight this session's Take-Home Messages 2 through 6, which encompass ways that women can identify past obstacles to their recovery and also circumstances that continue to be obstacles to recovery now. As in previous sessions, distribute the Take-Home Messages (Participant Sheet 3.2) and review the take-home messages by having members each read one of the messages in turn.

Distribution and Description of This Week's Skill Practice

Distribute this week's Skill Practice Sheet (Participant Sheet 3.3). This week's skill practice will help group members think through current obstacles and ways they can help themselves overcome them.

Check-Out

Pass around the Check-Out Sheet. Participants each answer orally the one-question check-out. Thank members and tell them you will see them next time.

Managing Mood, Anxiety, and Eating Problems without Using Substances

Mood, anxiety, and eating problems are prevalent among women with SUDs. In some instances, these psychiatric disorders are diagnosed while the substance problem is not diagnosed or, if diagnosed, is not necessarily concurrently treated. Similarly, women may be diagnosed with an SUD and receive treatment for it but not be properly diagnosed or treated for a co-occurring mood, anxiety, or eating disorder. It is important for women with SUDs to know that mood, anxiety, and eating problems are highly prevalent among women with SUDs and that appropriate concurrent treatment for these other problems will help women in their recovery from substances. This session provides women with information regarding these other prevalent psychiatric disorders and helps them assess whether symptoms of these disorders have interfered with their recovery and how to get help. As is the case with each session, detailed information is included in the next section, "Background Information." The therapist should read this section while preparing for this session.

Background Information

Women and Mood, Anxiety, and Eating Problems

Women with drug and alcohol disorders often have other psychiatric symptoms and illnesses such as depression, anxiety, and eating disorders. While psychiatric symptoms and illnesses are more common among people (of either gender) with substance disorders than among people without substance disorders, women are more likely to have mood, anxiety, and eating disorders than are men both in the general population and among those with SUDs. In addition, depression, anxiety, and eating disorder symptoms can be triggers to using drugs and alcohol and can worsen the course of SUDs. Sometimes women feel that the main problem they have is depression or anxiety or other negative emotional states. They feel that if they can overcome these illnesses, then their substance problem will also get better. Sometimes these beliefs can lead women to minimize to themselves and others the extent to which their substance problem is affecting their lives, which can make it harder to get help. Individuals with SUDs who also have problems of depression, anxiety, eating disorders, or other psychiatric illness need treatment for their substance disorder *and* the other co-occurring illness(es). Without such treatment, it is hard to get well from either/all of these disorders. Because women are more likely than men to have mood, anxiety, or eating disorders, these disorders are more likely to complicate the course or outcome of substance problems in women. This section reviews symptoms of depression, anxiety, and eating problems. It discusses the ways that these other conditions can distort thinking or become triggers for women to use substances. It also discusses developing *positive coping strategies and getting treatment for these other co-occurring psychiatric conditions.*

What Are Common Symptoms of Depression?

Depression is an illness characterized by a number of symptoms that occur for 2 weeks or more such as:

- Depressed mood most of the time.
- Feelings of guilt, worthlessness, or helplessness.
- Irritability, restlessness.
- Loss of interest in activities or hobbies once pleasurable, including sex.
- Fatigue and decreased energy.
- Difficulty concentrating, remembering details, and making decisions.
- Insomnia, early morning wakefulness, or excessive sleeping.
- Overeating, or appetite loss.
- Thoughts of suicide, suicide attempts.
  (National Institute of Mental Health, n.d.-a)

In order to be diagnosed with depression, you need to have experienced a number of these types of symptoms most of the day nearly every day for at least 2 weeks. People can also have more "minor" depressions where some of these symptoms are present continuously for much longer periods of time.

Depression can change your thinking and make it harder to use effective coping strategies. For example, depressive thinking is *irrational* even though it feels *rational.* It is important to realize that you may need to challenge your thoughts when you are depressed and be aware that although they feel true, in reality they may not be true or at the very least be distorted. Depression also leads to *pessimistic* thinking, which can, at its worst, turn to hopelessness. This is the feeling that makes people ask "Why bother?," "What's the use?," and feel like "throwing in the towel," not following through on their program, or just giving in to drug cravings they may be having. This type of thinking also leads to self-critical feelings or hearing criticism in what others say, even when it may not be there. Sometimes pessimistic feelings can lead to "self-fulfilling" prophecies. For example, when you tell yourself you can't accomplish something, you may not even try, or you may feel so badly about yourself that you do not do as well as you normally could. People with depression often experience self-fulfilling prophecies with regard to recovery as well. Depression can make it much more likely that you will feel that it is not worth doing many things on your own behalf including *taking care of your recovery.* Depression may also affect people's ability to *set priorities* or make decisions. Those affected by depression may become avoidant of other people, situations at work, and certain tasks because they feel that these activities would be overwhelming. As a result, depression can make people more isolated, which can again impair their ability to *take care of themselves and their recovery.* Because depression is more common among women than men, many women with SUDs will need treatment for their depression as well as treatment for their SUD in order to recover from both.

What Is Anxiety?

There are many types of anxiety disorders. Some of the most common anxiety disorders among people with substance disorders are social anxiety disorder (social phobia) and generalized anxiety disorder (GAD). In both of these common anxiety disorders people experience an unrealistic amount of fear or dread and these feelings are present for 6 months or more.

Social anxiety disorder (or social phobia) is characterized by having an extreme amount of anxiety and fear of being judged by others and being embarrassed in a setting in which one is observed by other people. This fear can be so strong that it interferes with going to work or school or doing other everyday activities, as well as in social situations or settings such as performing or speaking. Common symptoms include:

- Being very self-conscious in front of other people and feeling embarrassed especially in social situations or situations where you will be observed by other people.
- Being afraid that other people will judge you and you will feel humiliated.
- Having excessive fear and worry before an event or social situation.
- Avoiding places or situations that will cause this anxiety.
- This fear can be so strong it interferes with going to work or school.
  (National Institute of Mental Health, n.d.-c)

Generalized anxiety disorder (GAD) is characterized by having an extreme amount of anxiety that is difficult to control, is more extreme than is warranted by the situation, is focused on routine activities, and lasts for more than 6 months. Common symptoms of GAD include:

- Difficulty relaxing.
- Difficulty concentrating.
- Startling easily.
- Trouble falling or staying asleep.
- Physical symptoms such as fatigue, headaches, muscle tension, muscle aches, difficulty swallowing, trembling, twitching, irritability, nausea, sweating, lightheadedness, needing to use the bathroom frequently, breathlessness, and hot flashes.
  (National Institute of Mental Health, n.d.-b)

Relationship of Anxiety Disorders and Substance Use Disorders

Anxiety disorders can be triggers for using substances. People with social anxiety disorder have an irrational fear that other people will negatively evaluate them. Many people use substances like alcohol to decrease the anxiety they feel in social settings. In fact, about 25% of people with social anxiety disorder have an alcohol use disorder, and about 15% of all people with alcohol dependence have social anxiety disorder. Among those with social anxiety disorder, women generally have more severe fears than do men.

Anxiety problems often begin early in life, such as in adolescence. Many women learn to "manage" their anxiety by using substances or to use substances (e.g., pills such as benzodiazepines, opiates, or alcohol) to help relieve symptoms of irritability, anxiety, or sleep disturbance. Over time, they develop tolerance and dependence on the substances themselves. Women may then feel that since the anxiety problem came first, the substance problem will go away if they can find treatment for the anxiety. In that instance, women may seek out therapy or medication treatments for anxiety and minimize their substance use as a problem. Anxiety often leads women to avoid situations that provoke it, which is a pattern that can also become socially isolating and decrease effective coping strategies, which in turn leads to more substance use. Social anxiety disorder may increase women's avoidance of treatment such as group therapy or self-help and this can also increase isolation and decrease access to effective treatment and support for recovery. Substance use can often trigger increased anxiety (due to the effect of intoxication or the effect of withdrawal), and increased anxiety then becomes a trigger to use more substances. In order to break this vicious cycle it is necessary to have treatment for both anxiety and substance use disorders and stop using substances.

What Is an Eating Disorder?

Many types of eating problems are common among women, and there are a variety of eating behaviors, such as overeating or undereating, that some women use as a negative coping strategy to manage stress or other difficult feelings or mood states. Although these behaviors are unhealthy, they are not necessarily eating disorders. Three types of specific eating disorders are anorexia nervosa, bulimia nervosa, and binge-eating disorder. These disorders are common among women in many age groups and are present among a significant number of women who have SUDs.

Anorexia nervosa can be characterized by the following symptoms:

- Restricting calories in order to pursue extreme thinness and a weight that is significantly below normal.
- Having an intense fear of gaining weight or becoming fat.
- Having a distorted body image.
- Having a sense of self-esteem that is heavily influenced by perceptions of body weight and shape, or a having a denial of the seriousness of low body weight.
  (National Institute of Mental Health, n.d.-d)

Other symptoms of anorexia nervosa that can develop over time in women and girls include absence of menstruation (amenorrhea), thinning of the bones (osteopenia or osteoporosis), developing brittle hair and nails, dry or yellowish skin, mild anemia, muscle wasting and weakness, severe constipation, low blood pressure, slowed breathing and pulse, damage to the structure and function of the heart, infertility, among other symptoms.

Bulimia nervosa is characterized by the following symptoms:

- Having recurrent and frequent episodes of eating unusually large amounts of food (i.e., binge-eating episodes).
- Feeling a lack of control over these episodes.
- Engaging in behaviors following these binge-eating episodes that compensate for the overeating such as forced vomiting (e.g., purging), excessive use of laxatives or diuretics, fasting, excessive exercise, or a combination of these behaviors.
- These behaviors interfere with weight gain from overeating and individuals may maintain a normal body weight.
- Having excessive fear of gaining weight, wanting to lose weight, and feeling unhappy with body size and shape.
- Anorexia nervosa is not present.
  (National Institute of Mental Health, n.d.-e)

Bulimic behaviors such as binging and purging often occur secretly because they are accompanied by feelings of disgust or shame. The binge-eating and purging cycle can occur once each week to many times a day for 3 or more months. There are many potential negative physical consequences of bulimia including chronically inflamed and sore throat, swollen salivary glands in the neck and jaw area, damaged tooth enamel, increasingly sensitive and decaying teeth as a result of exposure to stomach acid, acid reflux disorder and other gastrointestinal problems, intestinal distress and irritation from laxative abuse, severe dehydration from purging of fluids, and electrolyte imbalance (too low or too high levels of sodium, calcium, potassium and other minerals) that can lead to heart attack.

Binge-Eating Disorder

Individuals with binge-eating disorder lose control over their eating but these periods of binge eating are not followed by compensatory behaviors such as purging, excessive exercising, or laxative use. As a result, some people with binge-eating disorder may become overweight or obese and are at higher risk for other physical disorders such as hypertension or cardiovascular disease. Individuals with binge-eating disorder also experience guilt, shame, and distress about these behaviors, and that can lead to more binge eating (National Institute of Mental Health, n.d.-f).

Eating disorders and eating problems are common among women throughout their lifetimes, but like mood and anxiety disorders, they often occur at a higher rate among women with SUDs. In addition, depressive disorders and anxiety disorders are more common among individuals with eating disorders. Craving, loss of control, and a preoccupation with substances (whether they are drugs, alcohol, or food) are hallmarks of both SUDs and eating disorders. Women with SUDs may have concerns about overeating, food restriction, weight, and body shape. Importantly, women with *both eating and substance disorders* may alternate back and forth between symptoms of the two disorders. For example, they may get their substance use under control but find that their craving for, and loss of control over, food increases. Or they may find that they stop binging and purging, but their use of substances increases. Overall, they may find that they always feel out of control with either one disorder or the other. Treatment for both disorders together can help recovery from both.

In early recovery, many women who do not have eating disorders find themselves coping with *eating issues* or *other eating behaviors*. An essential aspect of recovery is a healthy relationship with food and nutrition, so it is important to pay attention to proper nutrition and eating patterns, especially in early recovery. At this stage of early recovery, it is not uncommon for people to report substituting certain foods for alcohol or drugs or to find an increase in craving for certain foods. Healthy nutrition is an important element of self-care. It can be helpful not only in early recovery but also in maintaining long-term good health and well-being.

Coping with Other Psychiatric Illnesses such as Depression, Anxiety, and Eating Disorders

Because depression, anxiety, and eating problems and disorders are common in women with SUDs, it is important for women in recovery to develop strategies to manage other psychiatric illness while managing their SUD recovery. Here are some steps to take:

1. *Understand* and *accept* that the substance disorder and the other disorder or disorders (e.g., mood, anxiety, eating disorders) are *both/all* important and require attention and treatment. One will not disappear because the other is treated.
2. *Get treatment for both/all disorders.* This is the best way for you to feel better from either/both/all of them.
3. *Learn more* about the mood, anxiety, or eating disorder. Gather information about treatments that help with these disorders. Try to recognize the symptoms early on so you can report them and get help for them before they worsen.
4. *Recognize and change depressed or anxious thinking.* Depressive or anxious thinking often makes the world look darker and more difficult than it is. Recognize a thought as a depressed thought or an anxious thought. Write it down. Write an answer to that thought. For example, one way to help yourself is to imagine others having the same situation. What would you say to them? How would you counter that thought for someone else? For yourself?
5. *Don't use substances* to manage the other disorders.
6. *Don't let the other disorders stop you from your recovery* from your substance problem.
7. *Develop positive coping strategies* for the other disorders as well as for your substance disorder.
8. *Establish healthy eating habits* to help manage unhealthy urges and cravings for food.
9. *Take care of yourself* by getting the help you need for your recovery from your SUD and your co-occurring depression, anxiety, and/or eating disorders.

Therapist Overview

During this session, it will be important to review symptoms of each of the problems/disorders presented. Common symptoms of each of these disorders are summarized in Participant Sheet 4.1. The therapist can become more familiar with specific criteria for diagnoses by referring to the *Diagnostic and Statistical Manual for Mental Disorders* (5th ed.) (American Psychiatric Association, 2013). In preparing for this session, the therapist should read the "Background Information" above, which includes detailed information on this topic. The therapist should review the symptoms in advance of this group and have the participant overview sheet available for herself during the session. The amount of time the therapist spends discussing each disorder and its potential effect on recovery from SUDs and relapse prevention will depend on the therapist's familiarity with the experiences of the women in the group and her sense of what will be relevant for them. Because the therapist may not know that some women in the group are experiencing symptoms of one or another of these disorders, though, it is important to review all of them.

Goals of This Session

- To understand that mood, anxiety, and eating disorders and problems are common in women with drug and alcohol problems.

- To learn about the symptoms of mood, anxiety, and eating disorders.

- To learn that there are specific treatments available for mood, anxiety, and eating disorders.

- To understand that it is necessary to treat *both* the SUD *and* the other psychiatric disorders (mood, anxiety, and eating disorders) in order to have the best chance for each/all disorder(s) to improve.

Session 4 Outline

- **Introduction (*If Needed*)** (5 minutes).
- **Check-In** (15 minutes).
- **Review of Last Week's Skill Practice and Topic** (5 minutes).
- **Presentation of This Week's Topic and Distribution of Topic Overview** (25 minutes): Provide Participant Sheet 4.1.
  - Overview of women, mood, anxiety and eating problems.
  - Depression.
    - What is depression? Symptoms of depression.
    - How depression can affect recovery from SUDs.
  - Anxiety.
    - What is an anxiety disorder? Symptoms of social anxiety disorder and generalized anxiety disorder.
    - How anxiety disorders can affect recovery from substance use disorders
  - Eating disorders.
    - What is an eating disorder?
    - Symptoms of anorexia nervosa, bulimia nervosa, and binge-eating disorder.
  - Other eating issues or behaviors.
    - How to cope with psychiatric illnesses such as depression, anxiety, and eating disorders without using substances.

- **Open Discussion** (30 minutes).
- **Wrap-Up and Reading of Take-Home Messages** (2 minutes): Provide Participant Sheet 4.2.
- **Distribution and Description of This Week's Skill Practice** (3 minutes): Provide Participant Sheet 4.3.
- **Check-Out** (5 minutes).

Session-Specific Materials Needed

- Bulletin Board Outline and Take-Home Messages for Session 4.
- Participant Sheet 4.1: Managing Mood, Anxiety, and Eating Problems without Using Substances.
- Participant Sheet 4.2: Take-Home Messages.
- Participant Sheet 4.3: Skill Practice: Managing Mood, Anxiety, and Eating Problems without Using Substances.

Introduction (If Needed)

As in the previous session, provide an introduction to the group if there are new members.

Check-In

Pass around the Check-In Sheet and have each member orally respond to the three check-in questions.

Review of Last Week's Skill Practice and Topic

From the check-in, the therapist should have a sense of who has done the skill practice and commented on whether or not it was helpful. The therapist can build on the check-in by asking if anyone would like to comment on the skill practice and what she learned. The therapist can also comment on the main highlights from last week's topic. The therapist can then transition to presentation of this week's topic.

Presentation of This Week's Topic and Distribution of Topic Overview

Distribute Participant Sheet 4.1. As always, the therapist should try to highlight specific themes from the check-in that are related to the day's topic of managing mood, anxiety, and eating disorders and problems without using substances. If no one has brought up these issues during the day's check-in, the therapist can refer to themes related to this topic that may have come up in previous groups by saying something like, "A number of you have discussed struggles with depression (or anxiety or eating problems), and today we are going to talk about managing these types of illnesses without using substances." The therapist might also want to begin by reviewing the take-home messages of the session:

- Mood, anxiety, and eating disorders and problems are common in women with drug and alcohol problems.
- These other illnesses can make it difficult to get well from your substance problem.
- The substance problem can also make it hard to get well from your mood, anxiety, or eating disorder.
- Get treatment for *both* the substance disorder and the other disorder(s).

Overview of Depression, Anxiety, Eating Disorders, and Co-Occurring SUDs

First, the therapist should point out to group members that women with SUDs often have other psychiatric symptoms and illnesses. Illnesses such as depression, anxiety, and eating disorders and problems are more common among both women *and* men who have SUDs than women and men without SUDs; however, it seems that among women with SUDs these other illnesses are the most prevalent. Most importantly for women in recovery, symptoms of depression, anxiety, or eating disorders can be triggers to use drugs and can worsen the course of SUDs. Women sometimes feel that if they get treated for these disorders, then their SUD will go away. Sometimes thoughts like these can lead women to minimize, to themselves and others, the extent to which their substance problem is affecting their lives. Generally, women with SUDs who have depression, anxiety, eating disorders, or other psychiatric illness need treatment for their SUD *and* the other co-occurring illness(es). At this point, the therapist can pause and ask, "Does anyone recognize any of these from her own life?"

Depression

After the group has responded and reflected on their own experiences of these disorders and their SUD, the therapist can say, "Let's stop for a moment and review common symptoms of these disorders so that we are all clear what we are talking about when we refer to depression, anxiety, and eating disorders." Using Participant Sheet 4.1 (just distributed to group members) and the bulletin board outline, the therapist should then review the symptoms of *depression* and state that typically a number of these symptoms must be present together for at least 2 weeks in order for a patient to receive a diagnosis of major depression. The therapist can then note that depression can lead to *pessimistic* thinking that can give rise to thoughts such as "Why bother?" and "I may as well throw in the towel." Such thoughts can make recovery from SUDs much more difficult because such feelings and thoughts undermine behaviors that support recovery and abstaining from drugs and alcohol. Depression can also make it *harder to make decisions and set priorities* which can, in turn, make it harder for a woman to take care of herself and her recovery. The therapist can pause to ask if these symptoms are recognizable to anyone in the group or has anyone had experience with depression? The group can discuss briefly before moving on to anxiety disorders.

Anxiety Disorders

Next the therapist can use Participant Sheet 4.1 and the bulletin board outline to review the symptoms of two common anxiety problems or disorders: *social anxiety disorder* and *generalized anxiety disorder*. The therapist can point out that social anxiety and alcohol dependence often coexist. It is also useful to point out that anxiety problems usually begin early in life (i.e., adolescence) and that sometimes women have learned to "manage" their anxiety by using substances (e.g., alcohol, sedatives, or opiates) to help relieve symptoms of irritability or sleep disturbance. Over time, they can then develop tolerance and dependence on the substances themselves. Women sometimes think that if they have their anxiety treated the substance use disorder will go away. However, *substances themselves can often trigger anxiety,* and then increased anxiety can become a trigger for the use of more substances. This vicious cycle usually needs to be broken by *treatment of both disorders* concurrently. Finally, because anxiety can lead women to avoid situations that provoke it, they may become more socially isolated, making it harder to use effective coping strategies and to seek help for their recovery. As is the case with depression and SUDs, when both anxiety and SUDs are present, *each disorder will worsen the other if left untreated.*

Before going on to eating disorders, the therapist might pause here and ask the group members something like, "Does any of this relate to experiences that any of you have had with depression or anxiety and the way they may have affected your life or your use of substances?"

Eating Disorders

After the group has discussed this topic for a few minutes, the therapist can then point out that many types of *eating problems* are also common among women and that both overeating and undereating are sometimes used by women as a negative coping strategy to manage stress. These unhealthy eating behaviors may be problematic but are not necessarily eating disorders. However, there are also eating disorders such as anorexia nervosa, bulimia nervosa, and binge-eating disorder that can be more common among women with SUDs. The therapist can then proceed to review common symptoms of *eating disorders*, referring to the common symptoms listed in Participant Sheet 4.1 and the bulletin board outline. The therapist can ask, "Are any of these behaviors or symptoms familiar to anyone?" It may also be helpful to point out that eating problems are often clinically significant in SUD recovery even if bulimia, anorexia nervosa, or binge-eating disorder are not diagnosed by a clinician. In fact, 60% of eating disorders are currently diagnosed as "eating disorder not otherwise specified" (EDNOS) and so other eating problems may also be significant for any individual woman in recovery from SUDs.

The therapist might then point out that craving, loss of control, and a preoccupation with substances, whether drugs, alcohol, or food, are hallmarks of both substance use and eating disorders. Women with substance use and eating disorders can often find themselves alternating back and forth between symptoms of the two disorders. For example, a woman might find that when she is sober, she experiences a return of binge eating, or alternatively, that when she abstains from binge eating, it becomes more difficult to stay sober. Again, getting treatment for *both* eating disorders and SUDs is important in recovering from both. *Each disorder will worsen the other.* The therapist can ask if eating problems are familiar to group members and if anyone in the group has experienced any of these?

How to Cope with Psychiatric Illnesses such as Depression, Anxiety, and Eating Disorders/Problems without Using Substances

There are a number of strategies that women with SUDs and these other illnesses can develop so that they can manage their recovery from both. The first is to understand and accept that the SUD and the other disorder are both important and require attention. One will not disappear because the other is treated. *Each disorder can worsen the other.* The best way to recover is to *get treatment for both* the SUD and the other illness(es). *Participants can help the mood, anxiety, and eating disorders or problems* by recognizing the symptoms early and reporting them before they worsen. *They can learn strategies to change their depressive, anxious, or eating-disordered thinking. Most importantly, participants should avoid using substances to manage the other disorders AND avoid letting the other disorders interfere with their SUD recovery.* It is essential to develop positive coping skills for both/all disorders.

Because depression, anxiety, and eating disorders and problems are common in women with substance disorders, it is important for women in recovery to develop strategies to manage other psychiatric illness while managing their recovery. Here are some steps to take:

1. *Understand and accept* that the SUD and the other disorder(s) (i.e., mood, anxiety, eating disorders and problems) are *all* important and require attention. One will not disappear because the other is treated.
2. *Get treatment for both/all disorders.* This is the best way for you to recover from either/all of them.
3. *Learn more* about mood, anxiety, and/or eating disorders and problems. Gather information about treatments that help with these disorders. Try to recognize the symptoms early on so you can report them and get help for them before they progress.
4. *Change your thinking.* Depressive thinking or anxious thinking often makes the world look darker and more difficult than it is. One way to help with this problem is to imagine others in the same situation. What would you say to them? Would you think their situations were hopeless?
5. *Don't use substances* to manage the other disorders.
6. *Don't let the other disorders stop you from your recovery from SUDs.*
7. *Develop positive coping strategies* for each/all disorders.
8. *Establish healthy eating habits* to help manage unhealthy urges and cravings for food.

Open Discussion

Topics may include ongoing discussion of today's specific topic and the discussion that began during the topic presentation about depression, anxiety disorders, and eating disorders may move naturally into the open discussion part of the group session. Again, other recovery-focused topics can be discussed during this time, including discussion of issues brought up in the check-in.

Wrap-Up and Reading of Take-Home Messages

The therapist can summarize the types of other disorders members of the group have endorsed experiencing. For example, she can say, "It sounds as if most people have experienced some depression during their lives, as well as struggles with eating, and at least a few of you have also had anxiety as well. It is important if you have symptoms of these illnesses to work with your doctor or therapist to get treatment and to learn to manage these without using substances. One major take-home message is that both substance use disorders and the other illness(es) need treatment." Distribute this week's Take-Home Messages (Participant Sheet 4.2). As in previous sessions, the take-home messages can then be reviewed by having members each read one of the messages in turn.

Distribution and Description of This Week's Skill Practice

Distribute this week's Skill Practice Sheet (Participant Sheet 4.3). This week's skill practice will help group members think through symptoms of depression, anxiety, and eating disorders or other psychiatric symptoms that they have experienced, as well as develop strategies to manage these symptoms without using substances.

Check-Out

Pass around the Check-Out Sheet and ask participants each to answer orally the one-question check-out. Thank members and tell them you will see them next time.

Women and Their Partners

The Effect on Recovery

Because not all women in the group will have partners, the group will examine the ways in which "having a partner" and *not* "having a partner" can be helpful or hurtful to the recovery process. Another important overall theme of the group is to think about group members' partners in the past, present, and future. For example, a woman without a partner now might have had a partner in the past who was an obstacle to her getting treatment; she might also think through some of these issues for her future life when she may seek or have a new partner. As is the case with each session, detailed information is included in the next section, "Background Information." The therapist should read this section while preparing for this session.

Background Information

One major aspect of women's recovery from SUDs is that women *recover in connection* and not in isolation. Women interact in significant ways with many people in their family and in their community (e.g., parents, siblings, friends, others). Each of these relationships can have a unique influence on a woman's recovery from substance problems. However, it appears that insofar as a woman has an intimate partner, this relationship can play a particularly critical role in her process of recovery. This session will focus on (1) *understanding the role that intimate partners can play in recovery*, (2) exploring *past and present intimate relationships in the context of addiction*, and (3) exploring strategies to help you *use your intimate relationships to support rather than obstruct your recovery*.

What Is a Partner?

A "partner" is defined as an individual(s) with whom a woman is intimately involved. For example, this person could be a spouse, boyfriend, girlfriend, and/or father/mother of the woman's child(ren). The content of this section is meant to refer to both heterosexual and lesbian relationships, although there may be some differences that are not covered here. Some of the information available is based solely on heterosexual intimate relationships. When that is the case, this section will refer to "male partners."

What Kind of Influences Can a Partner Have on Women's Recovery?

Relationships and social connectedness tend to be very important to women. Relational influences are strongly linked with women's addiction and recovery. Women often have a great desire to be in relationships, and their sense of self often develops through their affiliation, interaction, and engagement with close and significant others. In fact, *lack or loss of close relationships* can trigger negative feelings that may lead women to use drugs or alcohol. Disrupted relationships or being isolated and disconnected can be associated with low self-esteem and anxiety, which can sometimes contribute to a woman's perceived need for an intimate partner who helps perpetuate the woman's continued substance abuse. Low self-esteem may also get in the way of a woman's development of healthier or more positive relationships and friendships.

Most importantly, intimate partners can play a critical role by contributing *positively* or *negatively* to *sustaining a woman's substance use*, by *promoting* or *obstructing* her efforts to *get treatment*, or by *facilitating* or *hampering* her *ongoing recovery*. The following are some *negative* ways that partners can influence the process of women's substance disorders and/or their recovery:

Initiation of Use of Drugs

- Often a woman is introduced to drugs by a male partner.
- Less is known about partner influence on the initiation of substance use among lesbian couples but estimates of SUDs in this population range in prevalence from 28 to 35%.
- A heterosexual woman with an alcohol or drug use disorder is more likely to have a male partner who uses alcohol or drugs than a man with an SUD is to have a woman partner with an SUD.

Perpetuation of Drug Use

- A partner may be the supplier of a woman's drugs.
- A bond may have developed when both partners used drugs, and drug use may be the main focus of the relationship.
- A woman may fear that if she stops drinking or using drugs, she'll lose her partner.
- Sexual activity between the partners may have always been in the context of drug or alcohol use.
- Women may use alcohol and drugs as a way to maintain the relationship.
- A heterosexual woman may rely on a male partner to maintain her addiction either because he supplies the drug or because he supervises or coerces other illegal activities (e.g., prostitution, theft) that support the addiction.

Setting Up Obstacles to a Woman's Getting Treatment for Her Substance Problem

- A partner may have a negative attitude toward a woman getting treatment because he/she uses alcohol or drugs and fears losing the relationship if she gets into recovery.
- A partner may have a negative attitude toward a woman getting treatment because their sexual activity takes place in the context of substance use.
- A woman may be financially dependent on a partner who uses drugs and fears abandonment and loss of financial resources if she gets into treatment or stops using.
- A woman may be physically threatened by her partner and fear getting into treatment.

Role in Relapse

- Women more often relapse to drugs and alcohol in the context of using with a male partner.
- Women are prone to relapse after difficult emotional or interpersonal experiences, often with intimate partners.
- Women's desire to be in relationships may trigger them to use again to reconnect with a partner.
- If a woman's partner lives with her and he/she uses substances, the woman may relapse because the substance is freely available at home.

The following are some *positive* ways that partners can influence the process of women's treatment for SUDs and/or their recovery:

- Partners who do not use drugs can be instrumental in helping women enter treatment and remain in recovery.
- Partners who live with women can help by making sure that the home is drug- and alcohol-free and they can also not use themselves.
- Partners can engage in treatment themselves, as is individually appropriate. They may participate in family or education groups to learn about addiction and the process of recovery. Alternatively, they may engage in couple counseling to focus on any relationship difficulties that might contribute to a woman's past substance use or vulnerability to relapse, or that might have occurred as a result of the woman's substance use.
- Partners who themselves use drugs and/or alcohol can engage in their own SUD treatment.
- Treatment can also help partners to understand that as a woman becomes sober and is in recovery, certain roles and responsibilities that may have evolved as a result of her substance problem will likely change. This may help the couple adapt positively to changing roles and responsibilities.

What Kind of Influence Can the Absence of a Partner Relationship Have on Women's Recovery?

Women may find that *not* having an intimate partner when they enter recovery can be positive and/or negative. The following are some *negative* ways that absence of a partner can influence women's SUD and/or their recovery process:

- If a woman wants to have an intimate partner and she doesn't, loneliness or a sense of abandonment (if a relationship recently ended) can be a trigger for relapse.
- Absence of a partner may make a woman feel more isolated or leave her without social or other types of support, which can serve as a trigger to use.
- If a woman does not have a partner but wishes to seek one, sometimes common meeting places can involve alcohol and/or drugs (e.g., bars, parties, clubs), and these can pose a high risk for relapse.

The following are some *positive* ways by which *absence of a partner* can influence the process of women's recovery from an SUD.

- Women without partners may find themselves more flexible about getting to and making time for recovery activities.
- Women without partners may more easily be able to make their homes a drug- and alcohol-free zone.
- When women enter a new relationship in recovery, they can "start from the beginning" without drugs or alcohol; there is no past history or expectations for drinking or drug use.

What Can You Do?

Examine your past and present intimate partner relationships by asking yourself the following questions:

- Have you had intimate partners in the past who have introduced you to drugs or alcohol, facilitated your drug or alcohol use, or been an obstacle to your treatment and recovery?
- Have you had intimate partners in the past or present who have helped you get into treatment or facilitated your recovery?
- If you have an intimate partner now, is he or she a positive or negative force in your recovery?

Examine the positive and negative roles that your current partner plays in your recovery:

- Does your partner use alcohol or drugs?
- Does your partner support your treatment?
- Does your partner invite you or insist that you use drugs or alcohol with him or her?
- Does your partner supply the alcohol or drugs?
- Are there difficulties in the relationship that contribute to your own distress that may present high-risk situations for you and trigger you toward relapse?

What are some of the things that you could do that might be helpful?

- If your partner uses, is he or she willing to give up his or her own drug or alcohol use?
- Is your partner willing to make your home an alcohol- and drug-free zone?
- Is your partner willing to engage in some form of treatment either with you or on his or her own?

Therapist Overview

Goals of This Session

- To discuss the role of partners in the recovery process.
- To discuss the ways that *not* having a partner can be helpful to recovery or can be an obstacle to recovery.
- To discuss the ways that having a partner can be helpful to recovery or can be an obstacle to recovery.
- To explore past and present intimate relationships in the context of addiction.
- To explore strategies to help women use their intimate relationships to support rather than obstruct their recovery.

Session 5 Outline

- **Introduction (*If Needed*)** (5 minutes).
- **Check-In** (15 minutes).
- **Review of Last Week's Skill Practice and Topic** (5 minutes).
- **Presentation of This Week's Topic and Distribution of Topic Overview** (25 minutes): Provide Participant Sheet 5.1.
  - What is a partner?
  - What kind of influences can a partner have on women's recovery? These can be positive or negative.
    - Negative: Initiation and perpetuation of drug use; obstacles to getting treatment; role in relapse.
    - Positive: Support; helping make home drug- and alcohol-free; engaging in their own treatment if indicated.
  - What kind of influences can the absence of a partner have on women's recovery?
    - Negative: Sense of loneliness; isolation; common meeting places can present risks/triggers.
    - Positive: Flexibility for recovery and other activities; make home drug- and alcohol-free; new relationships can begin without drugs or alcohol being part of them.
  - Examining past and present intimate partner relationships.
- **Open Discussion** (30 minutes).
- **Wrap-Up and Reading of Take-Home Messages** (2 minutes): Provide Participant Sheet 5.2.
- **Distribution and Description of This Week's Skill Practice** (3 minutes): Provide Participant Sheet 5.3.
- **Check-Out** (5 minutes).

Session-Specific Materials Needed

- Bulletin Board Outline and Take-Home Messages for Session 5.
- Participant Sheet 5.1: Women and Their Partners: The Effect on Recovery.
- Participant Sheet 5.2: Take-Home Messages.
- Participant Sheet 5.3: Skill Practice: Women and Their Partners: The Effect on Recovery.

Introduction (If Needed)

As in the previous session, provide an introduction to the group if there are new members.

Check-In

Pass around the Check-In Sheet and ask each member to respond orally to the three check-in questions.

Review of Last Week's Skill Practice and Topic

From the check-in, the therapist should have a sense of who has done the skill practice and commented on whether or not it was helpful. The therapist can build on the check-in by asking if anyone would like to comment on the skill practice and what she learned. The therapist can also comment on the main highlights from last week's topic. The therapist can then transition to presentation of this week's topic.

Presentation of This Week's Topic and Distribution of Topic Overview

The therapist should first distribute Participant Sheet 5.1. If she has identified themes from the day's check-in that relate to the effect partners can have on the recovery process, these can be used as an introduction. If not from the check-in on this particular day, participants may have previously discussed issues relating to recovery and their partners (both positive and negative), and the therapist can refer to these issues when she introduces the topic. Again, it is important to emphasize that the session will discuss the ways partners can be both positive and negative forces in women's recoveries, and similarly that not having a partner can also be positive or negative. If in the course of this session women describe intimate partner violence, the therapist is referred to Session 10 on Violence and Abuse: Getting Help. If intimate partner violence is current, Session 10 provides guidance on assisting women in receiving immediate help to place themselves in a safe environment.

What Is a Partner?

The therapist can discuss the goals of the session and then move on to define what we mean by a "partner." The therapist should strive to be as inclusive as possible to encompass the breadth of women's experiences and should define the partner as an intimate partner such as a spouse, boyfriend, girlfriend, and/or father/mother of a woman's children. The therapist should also say that the content of the session is meant to refer to both heterosexual and lesbian relationships, although there may be some differences that are not covered here. Some of the information available is based solely on heterosexual intimate relationships, and when this is the case, the therapist will refer to "male partners."

What Kind of Influences Can a Partner Have on Women's Recovery?

The therapist can then go on to say that *relationships and social connectedness tend to be very important to women and that relationships are strongly linked to women's addiction and recovery.* Women often have a great desire to be in relationships, and their sense of self often develops through affiliation, interaction, and engagement with close significant others. The lack or loss of close relationships can trigger negative feelings that can lead women to use drugs or alcohol. Disrupted relationships can lead to feelings of isolation, which can be associated with anxiety or low self-esteem and can sometimes contribute to women's perceived need for an intimate partner who helps perpetuate continued substance use. Low self-esteem can get in the way of women's development of healthier, more positive relationships and friendships.

The therapist can go on to say that she will first present some ways that intimate partners can contribute positively and negatively to a woman's recovery.

On the Negative Side

Initiation of Drugs

- Women are often introduced to drugs by a male partner.
- Less is known about the role of partners in the initiation of substance use among lesbian couples but SUDs are estimated to range in prevalence from 28 to 35% among lesbians.
- A woman with an SUD is more likely to have a partner who uses alcohol or drugs than is a man with an SUD.

Perpetuation of Drug Use

- A partner may supply the woman with drugs.
- A bond may have developed when both partners used drugs and/or alcohol, and drug and/or alcohol use may be a main focus of the relationship.
- A woman may fear that if she stops using drugs, she'll lose her partner.
- Sexual activity between partners may always have taken place in the context of drug and/or alcohol use.
- A woman may use alcohol and drugs as a way to maintain the relationship.
- A heterosexual woman may rely on a male partner to maintain her addiction either because he supplies drugs or supervises or coerces other illegal activities that support the addiction (e.g., prostitution, theft).

Setting Up Obstacles to the Woman's Getting Treatment

- A partner may have a negative attitude toward a woman getting treatment or being in recovery because he fears loss of the relationship.
- A partner may have a negative attitude toward a woman getting treatment because their sexual activity takes place in the context of substance use.
- A woman may be financially dependent on a partner who uses and fears abandonment and financial loss if she stops using.
- A woman may be physically threatened by a partner if she tries to get into treatment.

Role in Relapse

- Women more often relapse in the context of using with a male partner.
- Women are prone to relapse after difficult emotional or interpersonal experiences, often with an intimate partner.
- Women's desire for relationship may trigger them to use again to reconnect with a partner.
- If the woman's partner lives with her and he/she uses substances, the woman may relapse because the substance is freely available at home.

At this point, the therapist should pause and ask the group if any of these situations with partners in the past or present are recognizable to them and if they can relate to any of these. The therapist should encourage discussion among the women and help facilitate and balance discussion between women with different life circumstances. After some discussion, the therapist can say that she would like to now look at some *positive* ways that partners can influence women's recovery and she would then like to discuss ways that *not* being in a partner relationship can also affect recovery, again both positively and negatively.

On the Positive Side

- Partners who don't use drugs can help women enter treatment and remain in recovery.
- Partners who live with women can help by making and keeping the home drug- and alcohol-free.
- Partners can engage in treatment themselves, as is appropriate, through family or education groups; couple work or other counseling for any ongoing relationship or family issues may also be helpful.
- Partners who use drugs or alcohol themselves can engage in their own SUD treatment.
- Treatment can also help partners understand how things can change in their relationship with a woman as she recovers and how certain roles and responsibilities might change now that she is no longer using substances.

What Kind of Influences Can the Absence of a Partner Have on Women's Recovery?

The therapist can then go on to say, "What about *not* having an intimate relationship when you are entering recovery? Women may find that the absence of having an intimate partner when they enter recovery can be both positive and negative."

On the Negative Side

- If a woman wants to have an intimate partner and she doesn't, loneliness or a sense of abandonment (if a relationship just ended) can be a trigger to relapse.
- The absence of an intimate partner may in some instances make a woman feel more isolated or leave her without social or other types of support, which can also serve as triggers to using.
- If a woman does not have a partner but wishes to seek one, sometimes common meeting places can involve alcohol and/or drugs (e.g., bars, parties, clubs), and these can pose a high risk for relapse.

On the Positive Side

- Women without partners sometimes find themselves more flexible about getting to and making time for recovery and other positive activities.
- Women without partners may be able more easily to make their own home an alcohol- and drug-free zone.
- When a woman enters a new relationship in recovery, she can "start from the beginning" and enter a relationship without drugs or alcohol; there is no past history or expectations of drinking or drug use.
- For women who have been in a negative relationship that has recently ended, the absence of the partner may enhance feelings of safety, security, or freedom to pursue treatment or other self-care activities.

Examining Past and Present Intimate Partner Relationships

At this point, the therapist can pause and ask again if there are experiences that women in the group recognize in terms of positive roles of partners, or how the absence of a partner may influence recovery both positively and negatively.

The therapist can then point out steps women can take in examining past and present intimate partner relationships including asking themselves the following questions:

- Do you currently have or have you in the past had partners who use, have introduced you to substances, or continue to get in the way of your recovery?
- Do you currently have or have you in the past had partners who helped you get into treatment or helped with your recovery?
- Do you have a partner in your life currently? If so, is he or she a positive or negative force in your recovery? Does he or she use alcohol or drugs?; support your treatment?; invite or insist that you use alcohol or drugs with him or her?; supply you with alcohol or drugs?

- Are there difficulties in your current relationship that might trigger you to relapse? If you're not currently in a relationship, have you ever been in one that triggered you to relapse?
- If your partner uses, is he or she willing to get treatment or give up his or her own use?
- Is your partner willing to make your living situation a drug- and alcohol-free zone?
- Is your partner willing to engage in treatment either with you or on his/her own?
- If you don't currently have a partner, have you ever had one with whom you've engaged in treatment?

Open Discussion

These questions about the positive and negative aspects of having or not having an intimate partner may very well transition easily into the open discussion part of this session. Again, during open discussion, other recovery-focused topics can be discussed, including discussion of issues brought up in the check-in.

Wrap-Up and Reading of Take-Home Messages

Based on this discussion, the therapist should now summarize some of the themes that the women have discussed regarding their partners or absence of partners as positive and negative forces in recovery. Distribute this week's Take-Home Messages (Participant Sheet 5.2). As in previous sessions, these take-home messages can then be reviewed by having members each read one of the messages in turn.

Distribution and Description of This Week's Skill Practice

Distribute this week's Skill Practice Sheet (Participant Sheet 5.3). This week's skill practice will help group members consider their experiences with and without intimate partners and the way these experiences have in the past affected as well as currently affect their recovery.

Check-Out

Pass around the Check-Out Sheet and ask participants each to answer orally the one-question check-out. Thank members and tell them you will see them next time.

Coping with Stress

The theme of this session is similar to the themes in "How to Manage Triggers and High-risk Situations" and in "Overcoming the Obstacles to Recovery," as well as themes in other sessions in this book. The basic purpose is to identify situations or feelings that may contribute to women's urges and cravings for substances and might increase the risk for relapse and to begin to think through each woman's particular circumstances to find alternative ways to manage stress rather than to use substances. In this session, the group will explore sources of stress and alternative coping skills to manage stress. As the therapist perceives themes from other sessions that have examined ways to manage triggers or ways to overcome obstacles, she can point these out to the group. Session 2, "How to Manage Triggers and High-Risk Situations," also discusses alternative ways to cope with triggers than using drugs, and Participant Sheet 2.1 has a list of possible alternate ways of coping with triggers. In addition, exposure to violence and/or abuse is an extreme stressor often associated with posttraumatic stress disorder (PTSD). The topic of getting help for violence and abuse is the focus of Session 10. Stress is a topic with which most people can identify. It is important in this group to continue to emphasize ways that group members can *identify their use of substances in response to stress and can think about alternate coping to respond to such stress.* As is the case with each session, detailed information is included in the next section, "Background Information." The therapist should read this section while preparing for this session.

Background Information

Life stress and stressful events are major contributors to the initiation and continuation of substance use, as well as to relapse. Therefore, identifying and coping with stress is an important part of recovery and long-term sobriety.

The Different Causes of Stress

External stressors can be broken down into two categories: (1) ordinary stressors that are common and part of everyone's life, and (2) extraordinary events that are less common and often more extreme in nature.

Examples of *ordinary stressors* include conflicts with family and friends, educational or occupational difficulties, financial problems, and illness in self or in family members. They may also include daily hassles, such as bad weather, traffic, and deadlines for work or school. Examples of *extraordinary stressors* include death of a family member, job loss, exposure to violence, and homelessness, among others.

Internal stressors are the negative feelings and attitudes that arise from an individual's experience of the outside world. These internal pressures include perfectionism, pessimism, negativism, fear of others' opinions, and need for control.

Stress from external or internal sources, from life events or from internal pressures, can be specific types of triggers to use drugs and alcohol or to relapse to drugs and alcohol. Understanding the sources of stress in one's own life and the role stress plays in one's own urges and cravings for substances is an important part of recovery.

Stressors Associated with Women's Roles

In addition to these common sources of stress, women often experience stress specifically associated with their gender roles. Some examples include being the primary caregiver for children, significant others, and/or elder relatives; managing the household; and providing the primary or secondary income for themselves and/or their families. The resulting stress women feel may be worsened by an inability to make changes in these situations. Financial constraints that limit access to child or elder care, single motherhood (where all household responsibilities can only be handled by one person), and minimal or no household support from a partner/family member who is unable or refuses to help with household responsibilities are all factors that can contribute to women's stress.

Additionally, women may be reluctant to acknowledge their own difficulties because they believe the problems of others are more important than their own. Since she gives other people's problems top priority, a woman may find herself in a cycle of helping others and ignoring herself. Women may feel a greater sense of shame regarding their substance problems than men because of pervasive stigma associated with women's addiction. Not surprisingly, the stress associated with women's roles has been associated with substance use, poor health, role dissatisfaction, and a sense of vulnerability to illness.

The emotional consequences of all types of stress include depression, low self-esteem, anxiety, shame, guilt, and anger. These negative emotional states can lead to the initiation of substance use, provide a rationale for continued substance use, or lead to relapse. Additionally, women are twice as likely as men to experience depression; therefore, women in recovery are more likely than men to experience depression. These symptoms can also be associated with shame and guilt that may, in turn, make women more vulnerable to relapse.

Coping with Stressful Situations

Stress is an inevitable part of life. While some stressful situations may be changed or relieved (e.g., asking for an extension for a school project, asking a sibling to help care for aging parents), changing other stressful situations may be more difficult (e.g., single parenthood, balancing full-time employment and family responsibilities) or impossible (e.g., chronic medical conditions, death of a family member).

Therefore, it is important to develop and have healthy *coping skills* to manage stressful situations. Coping can be divided into two categories: *unhealthy* and *healthy*. While unhealthy coping may provide a temporary escape from stressors, once this temporary relief has ended the stressful situation still exists and may even have worsened. Unhealthy coping does not provide women with a model for resolving or managing the stressor at hand or the stressors they will face in the future. *For women in recovery, it is important to understand that the use of drugs and alcohol may have been an unhealthy way of coping with life stress.*

There are other types of *unhealthy coping* that women (and men) can find themselves using, especially in early recovery when they are learning to be sober from drugs and alcohol. One very common one is *smoking* cigarettes and other tobacco use (either starting for the first time, relapsing to cigarettes after being abstinent, or increasing the number of cigarettes per day from a previous level of use). It is important to know that this is an unhealthy coping strategy that is also a type of SUD (i.e., nicotine dependence) and has serious health risks and consequences. *Getting clean from tobacco is an important (but often neglected) part of recovery.* There are many effective treatments for nicotine dependence, and they can be discussed with a primary care clinician, psychiatrist, or therapist. Having this conversation would be an excellent example of self-care. A helpful website for women who wish to be tobacco-free and to quit using tobacco is *http://women.smokefree.gov.*

Another common unhealthy coping strategy for some people in recovery is *increasing food consumption*, which is also very common, especially in the first year of recovery, and may lead to the unintended consequence of unwanted weight gain. It is important to be clear that in some cases women have substituted drugs for food and have lost weight and had unhealthy nutrition. In this instance, increasing food consumption through healthy eating and weight gain is an example of self-care and healthy coping. In addition, for women with a co-occurring eating disorder, focusing on healthy eating may require additional help, guidance, and treatment. For some women in recovery, though, compromised nutrition has not been an issue, and increasing unhealthy food consumption may result in undesired weight gain and contribute to other medical problems. The desire for carbohydrates is not uncommon in recovery. One strategy to try to manage this problem is to substitute lower calorie, healthier carbohydrate snacks for those that are higher in calories.

In contrast, healthy *coping skills* can not only help a woman resolve or manage the current stressor but also provide her with a model she can use to cope with future stressors. For example, a woman who is dependent on marijuana smokes a joint to decrease her anxiety after a fight with her partner, only to find that the anxiety is still there after the high is over and that she has no plan about how to work out the difficulties in her relationship. If, instead, a woman in the same situation uses a healthy coping skill (e.g., calls a supportive family member/friend and talks about the situation), she may experience decreased anxiety and may be able to come up with plans about how to address the problems in her relationship (e.g., go to counseling, talk with a therapist).

One particular coping skill for internal stress is to decrease unrealistic self-expectations. This can decrease feelings of internal pressure. One way to do this is to set realistic goals so that one does not find oneself failing to meet one's own goals or expectations. There are other types of self-care practices that can decrease feelings of stress such as yoga, exercise, meditation, and mindfulness, among others. Participant Sheet PG.3 lists resources including a book on stress-reducing activities. Some people use cell phone apps that assist with daily meditation or mindfulness to relieve feelings of stress. Other examples of unhealthy coping skills and alternative healthy coping skills are listed below:

Unhealthy Coping Skills

- Setting unrealistic goals for yourself.
- Complaining about a problem but doing nothing.
- Criticizing yourself/others for the situation.
- Punishing yourself (e.g., over/under eating, excessive exercise).
- Striving for perfection.
- Developing harmful relationships or isolating yourself from others.
- Passivity.
- Selfishness.
- Having high expectations of yourself in every situation.

Healthy Coping Skills

- Setting realistic goals.
- Making a plan to handle the problem.
- Seeing humor in the situation.
- Engaging in pleasurable, healthy activities (e.g., reading, hobbies).
- Accepting your limitations.
- Developing positive relationships.
- Assertiveness.
- Helping others.
- Changing expectations to be realistic in each situation.

What Can You Do to Help Cope with Stress?

- Make a list of the current and past stressful situations that have led you to use unhealthy coping, including using substances. As you make your list, consider stressors relating to relationships, family, general health, mental health, and work.
- Divide the list into those sources of stress you can change and those you can't change.
- Develop alternative coping skills for the different types of stressful situations.
- Consider different types of coping for changeable versus unchangeable stressors.
- Consider practices that lower stress responses such as exercise, yoga, meditation, mindfulness, and other self-care activities.
- Quit smoking cigarettes (resource: *http://women.smokefree.gov*).
- Use telephone app if available for mediation, mindfulness, or other stress-relieving activities.

Therapist Overview

Goals of This Session

- To help group members understand internal and external sources of stress.
- To examine stressors women say they experience in their daily lives.
- To understand how group members may have used substances as an unhealthy way to cope with stress.
- To learn healthy coping skills to manage stress rather than using unhealthy coping such as abusing substances.
- To learn that smoking can be a form of unhealthy coping and helpful quit sites for women such as *http://women.smokefree.gov*.

Session 6 Outline

- **Introduction** (*If Needed*) (5 minutes).
- **Check-In** (15 minutes).
- **Review of Last Week's Skill Practice and Topic** (5 minutes).
- **Presentation of This Week's Topic and Distribution of Topic Overview** (25 minutes): Provide Participant Sheet 6.1.
  - Different types of stressors: External and internal stressors.
  - Coping with stressful situations.
  - Unhealthy and healthy coping.
- **Open Discussion** (30 minutes).
- **Wrap-Up and Reading of Take-Home Messages** (2 minutes): Provide Participant Sheet 6.2.
- **Distribution and Description of This Week's Skill Practice** (3 minutes): Provide Participant Sheet 6.3.
- **Check-Out** (5 minutes).

Session-Specific Materials Needed

- Bulletin Board Outline and Take-Home Messages for Session 6.
- Participant Sheet 6.1: Coping with Stress.
- Participant Sheet 6.2: Take-Home Messages.
- Participant Sheet 6.3: Skill Practice: Coping with Stress.

Introduction (If Needed)

As in the previous session, provide an introduction to the group if there are new members.

Check-In

Pass around the Check-In Sheet and ask each member to respond orally to the three check-in questions.

Review of Last Week's Skill Practice and Topic

From the check-in, the therapist should have a sense of who has done the skill practice and commented on whether or not it was helpful. The therapist can build on the check-in by asking if anyone would like to comment on the skill practice and what she learned. The therapist can also comment on the main highlights from last week's topic. The therapist can then transition to presentation of this week's topic.

Presentation of This Week's Topic and Distribution of Topic Overview

The therapist should distribute Participant Sheet 6.1 and try to highlight specific themes from the check-in that relate to the topic of coping with stress without using substances. Then the therapist can say something like, "Life stress and stressful events can contribute to substance use and to relapse. So today we will be focusing on identifying and coping with stress without using substances. This is an important part of recovery and long-term sobriety." The therapist should use the take-home messages to highlight important points. The therapist can say, "Some of the important take-home messages we will discuss in today's sessions include":

- Stress can be caused by routine life circumstances, such as bad weather, deadlines, or traffic.
- Stress can be caused by more serious life events, such as loss of a job, death of a family member, or illness.
- Stress can also be caused by internal states such as feelings, thoughts, and attitudes (e.g., perfectionism, negative thoughts).
- There are many ways to cope with stress. Some of these, like using drugs and alcohol, are *unhealthy*.
- There are many alternative *healthy* ways of coping with stress.
- You can help your recovery by learning and practicing as many healthy ways to cope with stress as you can think of and that work for you.

Different Types of Stress

After summarizing these messages, the therapist can then say that we sometimes think of stress as being *external* or *internal*. Stress that is *external* can be either "extraordinary" or "ordinary." "Extraordinary" stress involves events or circumstances that are less common and more extreme in nature, such as the death of a family member, an accident, job loss, homelessness, or another change in life circumstances like retirement, divorce, or the birth of a child. An extreme form of stress is exposure to violence and abuse. The therapist can indicate that there will be an entire session on this specific topic. "Ordinary" stress involves the stress of daily life, such as routine illnesses, traffic, work problems, and minor conflicts with family or friends, among others. Both ordinary and extraordinary external sources of stress can make sobriety difficult and contribute to relapse. The therapist can pause here and ask the group members if they can think of *external stressors* that have made their recovery difficult or stressful circumstances that are current challenges.

After discussion of life stress that is a challenge for group members, the therapist can say something like, "We have been talking about ordinary and extraordinary external stress, but there are also *internal* sources of stress that can make recovery hard. This internal stress can be from negative feelings, such as perfectionism, pessimism, negativism, or fear of others' opinions. Examples of other possible internal sources of stress are the need to please others and the need for control, which can contribute to a feeling of pressure that can be a risk for relapse." The therapist can then ask, "Do any of these *internal sources of stress* sound familiar to any of you? Are these stressors ones that you may have experienced?"

After the group members have a chance to discuss this topic, the therapist can then say that women in recovery have reported certain types of stress associated with women's roles in our society. These *common sources of stress for women* may include being the primary caregiver for the family, managing the household, providing primary or secondary income for themselves and/or family, financial constraints, minimal or no support from partner or family members for household responsibilities, among others. These roles themselves, or feeling an inability to change them, may cause stress. In addition, women may place the needs of others they care for above their own, which may contribute to a cycle of ignoring and neglecting self-care. The emotional consequences of stress, which may include depression, low self-esteem, anxiety, shame, and guilt, can lead to relapse or continued substance use. Individuals can use these stressors and resulting feelings as a rationale for continued use or they can provoke initiation of use or relapse in someone who has already achieved sobriety. Again, the therapist can ask, "Does anyone recognize any of these sources of stress that are commonly reported for women as part of their own lives? Can anyone identify ways that she may have used substances to manage stress?"

Coping with Stressful Situations

After the group has an opportunity to discuss this topic, the therapist can say something like, "You have all been discussing stress that is both external and internal, and one of the things that is important in this group is learning ways to manage this stress other than by using substances."

Healthy and Unhealthy Coping

The therapist can then go on to say that *coping* can be divided into *unhealthy* and *healthy* coping. Substance use is one *unhealthy* way to cope. Although it may provide a temporary escape from stress, after intoxication the stressful situation still exists and sometimes is worse because of the substance use or because the situation wasn't directly dealt with in the first place.

There are other types of *unhealthy coping* that women (and men) can find themselves using, especially early in recovery when they are becoming sober. One very common one is *smoking* cigarettes and other tobacco use (either starting for the first time, relapsing to cigarettes after being abstinent, or increasing the number of cigarettes per day from a previous level of use). It is important here to say that this is an unhealthy coping strategy that is also a type of SUD (i.e., nicotine dependence) and has serious health risks and consequences. *Getting clean from tobacco is also an important (but often neglected) part of recovery.* There are many effective treatments for nicotine dependence, and these can be discussed with a primary care physician, psychiatrist, or therapist. Doing so would be an excellent example of self-care. A helpful website for women who wish to be tobacco-free is *http://women.smokefree.gov*. This site is also included in the resource list provided at the pre-group meeting.

Another common unhealthy coping strategy for some people in recovery is *increasing food consumption*, which is also very common, especially in the first year of recovery, and may lead to the unintended consequence of unwanted weight gain. It is important to be clear that in some cases women have substituted drugs for food and have lost weight and had unhealthy nutrition. In this instance, increasing food consumption through healthy nutrition and weight gain is an example of self-care and healthy coping. In addition, for women with a co-occurring eating disorder, focusing on healthy eating may require additional help, guidance, and treatment. For some women in recovery, though, compromised nutrition has not been an issue, and increasing unhealthy food consumption may result in undesired weight gain and contribute to other medical problems. The desire for carbohydrates is not uncommon in recovery. One strategy to try to manage this problem is to substitute lower calorie, healthier carbohydrate snacks for those that are higher in calories.

Healthy coping skills not only help a woman resolve or manage current stress but also provide a model to manage stress in the future without using substances. The therapist can list unhealthy coping strategies and alternative, healthy ways to cope. She should use the bulletin board materials and participant sheets to provide these examples. One particular coping skill that is important for managing internal stress is to decrease unrealistic self-expectations. In other words, it is important for women to *set realistic goals for themselves* so that they don't perceive themselves as failing to meet goals or expectations that were not realistic in the first place. There are other types of self-care activities that can lower feelings of stress such as yoga, exercise, meditation, mindfulness, or other similar activities. The therapist can remind group members that Participant Sheet PG.3 (that participants received during the pre-group meeting) lists resources including a book on stress-reducing activities. Some people use cell phone apps that assist with daily meditation or mindfulness to relieve feelings of stress. The therapist may ask women, "Are there healthy coping skills or strategies that anyone has used?" It is useful at this time to have a discussion of specific coping skills and strategies that the women might use in response to stress that they have described.

Open Discussion

After this discussion, the group can transition into open discussion of specific coping skills that the women might use in response to stress that they have described. Overall, the therapist should try to include as many members of the group in the discussion of different kinds of stress, the ways group members have used substances to manage this stress in the past, and other ways to cope that group members might find in their recovery. The greater the number of group members who participate in this discussion, the more fruitful it is likely to be. Again, during open discussion, other recovery-focused topics can be discussed, including discussion of issues brought up in the check-in.

Wrap-Up and Reading of Take-Home Messages

As always, the therapist should summarize the participants' discussion, which will in this case include some of the external and internal sources of stress that have been identified by the participants, as well as the unhealthy coping and healthy coping strategies group members have said they have used. As in previous sessions, distribute this week's Take-Home Messages (Participant Sheet 6.2), which can then be reviewed by having members each read one of the messages in turn.

Distribution and Description of This Week's Skill Practice

Distribute this week's Skill Practice Sheet (Participant Sheet 6.3). This week's skill practice will help group members consider their experiences with two stressful situations they have confronted and to write down coping strategies to change the situation as well as coping strategies to manage situations that they cannot change.

Check-Out

Pass around the Check-Out Sheet and ask participants each to answer orally the one-question check-out. Thank members and tell them you will see them next time.

Women as Caretakers

Can You Take Care of Yourself
While You Are Taking Care of Others?

Because not all women in the group will be "caretakers" or "caregivers" in the most traditional sense, this group emphasizes the caretaking role in whatever ways it may exist for each woman in the group. Taking care of other people in their immediate family, social circle, or wider community is a role often assumed by women. This role has been referred to at times as being a "caretaker" and more recently as being a "caregiver." In this session, these two terms are used interchangeably and the emphasis in this session is that it is necessary for women to care for themselves (i.e., self-care) in order to be able to take care of others. Caretaking can be both positive and negative in a woman's life and recovery, and this group session tries to encompass all of those experiences and their relationship to recovery. This session also gives consideration to the ways in which caretaking roles may shift over time. For example, a woman without caretaking responsibilities now might have had them in the past, and these may have been an obstacle for her to get treatment; she might also think through some of these issues for her future life. It is important for the therapist to keep in mind the different life phases and circumstances of participants within a specific group and to try to help balance the discussion so that each woman's experience can be shared and validated within the group. For example, if most women in the group have children and discuss mothering and one woman has no children but has a job where everyone depends on her, the therapist will need to balance the discussion so that the woman without children, who is depended on by others but not within the family context, has her experience validated and does not feel isolated during the discussion. Other types of caretaking (or caregiving) can be for elders, friends, or others in the community. As is the case with each session, detailed information is included in the next section, "Background Information." The therapist should read this section while preparing for this session.

Background Information

Women's Role as Caretakers

Women often serve an important role as caretakers in our society. Relationships are generally valued strongly by women, and their caretaking role can often be a source of self-esteem and fulfillment. On the home front, women may be caretakers of children, elders, partners, and families. On the work front, women often find themselves in caretaking roles as well, caring for coworkers, supervisees, or entire groups of people within a particular organization. In communities, women again may find themselves taking care of other community members (e.g., in neighborhoods, schools, religious groups). Young women may find themselves trying to take care of friends or siblings who need them or others who depend on them.

This social connectedness is often a source of strength and value for women, and disconnection from these roles and relationships can lead to feelings of isolation and lack of support. Even though these relationships and *the role of caretaker* can be *sources of value, self-esteem, and motivation* for women, they can *also interfere with women's ability to take care of themselves.* In the case of women with substance problems, the caretaking role can often interfere with women's ability to get into treatment or to do the things necessary to help themselves recover.

There are a number of ways that caretaking roles can interfere with women's ability to care for themselves and either get into treatment or maintain their recovery. According to the 2012 National Survey on Drug Use and Health, over 42% of the 41.5 million illicit drug users in the United States were women. Additionally, almost half of all reported alcohol users were women (85.5 million), and there were 7.5 million women over the age of 12 that had a SUD (Substance Abuse and Mental Health Services Administration, 2013). While not all women are mothers, being a mother is one of the most common caretaking roles. Some of the ways in which the role of mother may interfere with women's self-care, treatment, and recovery are the same as ways in which other caretaker roles can interfere. Thus, we will first start by using the role of "mother of children" as an example. For other caretaking roles, it is possible to substitute for the word *mother,* the word *caretaker,* and wherever it says "child," substitute the name of the person or type of person who is dependent on a woman's caregiving (e.g., parent, parent-in-law, sibling, friend, partner, employee, department, work team) and some of the same issues apply. These issues include the belief of having no time, feelings of shame and guilt, and the difficulty of taking care of oneself while taking care of others.

The Belief of Having No Time

Women sometimes have the belief that they do not have the time to seek treatment or to do the things they need to do to take care of themselves and keep their recovery going. This may be because they think:

- They need to put the needs of other people who depend on them first.
- They need to minimize the time spent at treatment/recovery.
- That drugs or alcohol enhance their ability to cope with the demands of parenting or other caregiving roles.

These perceptions can contribute to ambivalence regarding seeking help.

The Role of Guilt and Shame

Women may feel guilty and ashamed because of their actual or perceived neglect of their children or others who depend on them. Sometimes women with SUDs who are mothers have in fact neglected their children because they were using drugs or alcohol. Sometimes this is not so obviously the case, but women may feel that during the time they were using drugs or alcohol they were not as available physically, emotionally, or both. Women may have feelings of guilt and shame if their substance problems have interfered with other caretaking roles they have played for other people who have depended on them such as elders, parents, partners, friends, or colleagues. Women may find themselves avoiding these feelings, which thereby inhibits them from seeking treatment.

Fear of Losing Custody or Another Important Role

Some women fear that if they enter treatment they will lose legal custody of their children, and this can cause them to defer getting treatment. If delays in getting care are long enough, substance use problems can worsen to the point that there is a need for someone else to care for the children or for the intervention of child protection services.

Women who do not have children, but have other caretaking roles, may experience similar fears, such as the fear of losing a job or an important role in an organization, community, or family.

How Can You Be a Caretaker and Take Care of Yourself?

There are several things that are important to *learn*, *acknowledge*, *accept*, and then *apply* to your own life:

- You *cannot be the best caretaker* (or caregiver) that you can be *when you are using drugs or alcohol.*
- The desire to *be the best caretaker* and to get the most value and enjoyment from these relationships is *dependent on not using drugs or alcohol.*
- *Using drugs or alcohol is very time-consuming* and diverts your attention away from important relationships with those for whom you care.
- *Waiting until you have time does not work.* It only delays getting help and allows your substance use problem and all of its effects to worsen.
- *You do have the time to get help and to do the things that you need to do* (e.g., going to meetings, treatment, appointments) to continue your recovery. It takes more time to use and recover from the effects of using than to do your own recovery work.

Therapist Overview

Goals of This Session

- To help women think through the pros and cons of caretaking (or caregiving) roles.
- To help women identify that although being the caregiver for others can be rewarding, it can

sometimes be an obstacle to taking care of themselves and doing what is necessary for their recovery.

- To explore the belief of "having no time" and the role of guilt and shame.
- To help women identify that they do have time to take care of themselves.

Session 7 Outline

- **Introduction (*If Needed*)** (5 minutes).
- **Check-In** (15 minutes).
- **Review of Last Week's Skill Practice and Topic** (5 minutes).
- **Presentation of This Week's Topic and Distribution of Topic Overview** (25 minutes): Provide Participant Sheet 7.1.
  - Women's role as caretakers.
  - Caretaking can interfere with self-care and recovery.
    - Belief of having no time.
    - Role of guilt and shame.
    - Fear of losing custody or other important role.
  - How can you be a caretaker and take care of yourself?
- **Open Discussion** (30 minutes).
- **Wrap-Up and Reading of Take-Home Messages** (2 minutes): Provide Participant Sheet 7.2.
- **Distribution and Description of This Week's Skill Practice** (3 minutes): Provide Participant Sheet 7.3.
- **Check-Out** (5 minutes).

Session-Specific Materials Needed

- Bulletin Board Outline and Take-Home Messages for Session 7.
- Participant Sheet 7.1: Women as Caretakers: Can You Take Care of Yourself While You Are Taking Care of Others?
- Participant Sheet 7.2: Take-Home Messages.
- Participant Sheet 7.3: Skill Practice: Women as Caretakers: Can You Take Care of Yourself While You Are Taking Care of Others?

Introduction (If Needed)

As in the previous session, provide an introduction to the group if there are new members.

Check-In

Pass around the Check-In Sheet and have each member respond orally to the three check-in questions.

Review of Last Week's Skill Practice and Topic

From the check-in, the therapist should have a sense of who has done the skill practice and commented on whether or not it was helpful. The therapist can build on the check-in by asking if anyone would like to comment on the skill practice and what she learned. The therapist can also comment on the main highlights from last week's topic. The therapist can then transition to presentation of this week's topic.

Presentation of This Week's Topic and Distribution of Topic Overview

The therapist should first distribute the session overview (Participant Sheet 7.1). If she has identified themes from the day's check-in that relate to the topic of learning to take care of yourself while you take care of others, she can say something like, "Many of you have brought up a number of issues about taking care of other people in your life such as your children, partners, elder relatives, siblings, friends, community, and so on. Today we are going to be discussing how these roles can sometimes be rewarding but can also be difficult and feel like an obstacle to caring for yourself. Some of the take-home messages that I hope that you get from today's session are":

- You do have time to take care of yourself.
- Use the strength of your role as caretaker and your desire to be the best you can be as a motivation to seek the help you need for treatment and for ongoing recovery.
- Learn to ask for/find help if you need it in some of your caretaking responsibilities.

Women's Role as Caretakers (or Caregivers)

Women often serve an important role as caretakers in our society. Taking care of other people in their immediate family, social circle, or wider community is a role often assumed by women. This role has been referred to at times as being a "caretaker" and more recently as a "caregiver." In this session, these two terms are used interchangeably and the emphasis in this session is that it is necessary for women to care for themselves (i.e., self-care) in order to be able to take care of others. Relationships are generally valued strongly by women, and their caretaking role can often be a source of self-esteem and fulfillment. On the home front, women may be caretakers of children, elders, partners, siblings, and families. On the work front, women often find themselves in caretaking roles as well, caring for coworkers, supervisees, or entire groups of people within a particular organization. In communities, women again may find themselves taking care of other community members (e.g., in neighborhoods, schools, religious groups).

This social connectedness is often a source of strength and value for women, and disconnection from these roles and relationships can lead to feelings of isolation and lack of support. Sometimes having an SUD leads some women to social disconnection from some of these roles. However, even though these relationships and *the role of caretaker* can be *sources of value, self-esteem, and motivation* for women, they can *also interfere with women's ability to take care of themselves.* In the case of women with substance problems, the caretaking role can often interfere in women's ability to get into treatment or to do the things necessary to help themselves recover. The therapist can point out that this session topic directly relates to the WRG theme, "Recovery means taking care of yourself."

Caretaking Can Interfere with Self-Care and Recovery

One of the advantages of these caretaking roles is the social connectedness they bring, which is often a source of strength and value for women. As such, disconnection from these roles and relationships can often lead to feelings of isolation and lack of support. Nonetheless, even though these roles may be necessary in women's lives and/or give them a sense of value and strength, there are ways that they may interfere with women's ability to care for themselves. There are a number of ways that caretaking roles can interfere with women's ability to care for themselves and either get into treatment or maintain their recovery. According to the 2012 National Survey on Drug Use and Health, over 42% of the 41.5 million illicit drug users in the United States were women. Additionally, almost half of all reported alcohol users were women (85.5 million), and there were 7.5 million women over the age of 12 who had a substance abuse disorder (Substance Abuse and Mental Health Services Administration, 2013). While not all women are mothers, being a mother is one of the most common caretaking roles. Some of the ways in which the role of mother may interfere with women's self-care, treatment, and recovery are similar to ways in which other caretaker or caregiver roles can interfere. Women are also caretakers of others in their families and communities. You can substitute the name of the person or type of person who is dependent on you (e.g., parent, parent-in-law, partner, friend, sibling, employee, department, work team) for any other when considering the caretaking role. The therapist can pause here and ask people to reflect on their own caretaking or caregiving roles and the ways they may value these roles as well as whether they may interfere or create conflict with regard to self-care and recovery.

Belief of Having No Time

After a brief interactive discussion, the therapist can move on to say that with respect to their roles as any type of caretaker (or caregiver), women often have the belief of "having no time." They may:

- Think that they need to put the role of caretaker before their own needs.
- Minimize the time they spend in treatment or doing things to support their recovery.
- Think that using drugs or alcohol enhances their ability to cope with the demands of the caretaking role. This perception can contribute to ambivalence regarding seeking help.

The therapist can pause here and ask the group if they recognize any of these experiences or feelings and can relate them to their own lives.

Role of Guilt and Shame

After the women have time to discuss some of their own experiences, the therapist can then go on to point out that guilt and shame can also play a role in women's recoveries because they may feel guilty or ashamed at not fulfilling caretaking roles while using drugs. This may be because they were not available physically, emotionally, or both when they were using. Once they do decide to try to recover they may feel guilty or ashamed to take time away to get treatment. In order to avoid those feelings of guilt and shame, they may decide not to seek treatment or take care of themselves and their recovery. Again, the therapist can focus on the specific types of caretaking roles experienced by the women participants in the group. If all participants are mothers, much of the discussion will focus on the adverse effects of SUDs on the role of being a mother and the difficulty parenting responsibilities pose for engaging in treatment. If there are a variety of caregiving roles in the group, the discussion will more broadly address these.

Fear of Losing Custody or Other Important Role

For women who are parents, fear of losing custody of their children may make it harder to seek treatment or engage in recovery activities. For other women, there may be fear of losing a job or other important role. These fears and situations can often allow women to slip back into substance use, rather than allowing them to do the things they need to care for themselves and keep recovery going. Again, the therapist can pause here to encourage discussion and ask if any of the women recognize these feelings and experiences.

How Can You Be a Caretaker and Take Care of Yourself?

There are several things that are important to *learn*, *acknowledge*, *accept*, and then *apply* to your own life:

- You *cannot be the best caretaker* that you can be *when you are using drugs or alcohol.*
- The desire to *be the best caretaker* and to get the most value and enjoyment from these relationships is *dependent on not using drugs or alcohol.*
- *Using drugs or alcohol is very time-consuming* and diverts your attention away from important relationships with those for whom you care.
- *Waiting until you have time does not work*. It only delays getting help and allows your substance use problem and all of its effects to worsen.
- *You do have the time to get help and to do the things that you need to do* (e.g., going to meetings, treatment, appointments) to continue your recovery. It takes more time to use and recover from the effects of using than to do your own recovery work.

Open Discussion

The discussion that began with the presentation of caretaking (or caregiving) and the way in which taking care of others may interfere with self-care may very well continue into open discussion time. Women may reflect on their roles as parents, daughters, sisters, workers, partners, friends, community members, and so on and some of the responsibilities and role conflicts along with the ways in which these roles have made it difficult to obtain treatment and engage in recovery-oriented activities. Again, during open discussion, other recovery-focused topics can be discussed, including issues brought up in the check-in.

Wrap-Up and Reading of Take-Home Messages

The therapist should highlight themes from the group regarding common caretaking (or caregiving) roles and the ways the group has highlighted both the positive and negative aspects of these roles. Distribute this week's Take-Home Messages (Participant Sheet 7.2) and then review them by having members each read one of the messages in turn.

Distribution and Description of This Week's Skill Practice

Distribute this week's Skill Practice Sheet (Participant Sheet 7.3). This week's skill practice will ask group members to identify the ways they see themselves as caretakers (or caregivers) and to explore the ways they may value that role as well as ways that role may have been an obstacle in the past or currently to getting treatment or being in recovery, as well as ways to help themselves to take care of themselves. The therapist can point out that this is consistent with the group theme that recovery means taking care of yourself and it is important to do this even while caring for others.

Check-Out

Pass around the Check-Out Sheet and ask participants to each answer orally the one-question check-out. Thank members and tell them you will see them next time.

Using Self-Help Groups
to Help Yourself

Not all women will use self-help, and it is not an expectation or requirement of the WRG that women in the group attend self-help meetings. However, there is evidence that engaging in self-help groups can enhance long-term abstinence and recovery for those who do engage in self-help; this effect may have enhanced significance for women. This session therefore introduces women to different types of self-help groups and their potential utility as one means to enhance recovery support and engage in healthy coping with triggers and stressors. It is important for the therapist to acknowledge that not all women will engage in self-help groups, but for those who can and do there can be advantages for recovery. As is the case with each session, detailed information is included in the next section, "Background Information." The therapist should read this section while preparing for this session.

Background Information

Involvement in a self-help group can help you achieve and maintain long-term sobriety. Many people believe that Alcoholics Anonymous (AA) is the only self-help group available for substance-dependent individuals. While AA is the most widely recognized self-help group, it is not the only one. Some of the different self-help groups are outlined below.

Alcoholics Anonymous

Alcoholics Anonymous (AA) is an international fellowship of men and women who have had a drinking problem. AA is an abstinence-based organization. AA membership is open to anyone who wants to do something about problem drinking. Anonymity, or protecting the identity of AA members, is an important part of the organization's philosophy. AA meetings are held multiple times during the day in different areas of a town, city, state, or country. AA provides person-to-person service or "sponsorship" to its members and encourages establishing a support network among group members. The AA program, also known as the 12 steps, offers a way to develop a satisfying life without alcohol use.

AA meetings may be *open* or *closed*. Open meetings are open to individuals with or without drinking problems, while closed meetings are only open to individuals who have or may have a drinking problem. At *speaker meetings*, AA members speak about how alcohol has affected their lives and how their lives have changed because of their involvement in AA. *Discussion meetings* are led by one individual who speaks briefly about her or his experience with alcohol and then leads a discussion about AA, recovery, or any other drinking-related problem. *Step meetings* discuss one of the 12 steps and are usually closed. AA meetings are also held specifically for women, men, and teenagers/young adults, as well as for gays, lesbians, bisexuals, and transgender individuals.

Narcotics Anonymous, Cocaine Anonymous, Gamblers Anonymous

These groups were founded on the same principles as AA and are modeled on the 12-step program. All these organizations are fellowships of men and women who have problems with opioids, benzodiazepines, marijuana, or amphetamines (Narcotics Anonymous [NA]); cocaine (Cocaine Anonymous [CA]); or gambling (Gamblers Anonymous [GA]).

SMART Recovery

SMART (<u>S</u>elf-<u>M</u>anagement <u>a</u>nd <u>R</u>ecovery <u>T</u>raining) Recovery is an abstinence-based self-help program for people with problematic substance use. The purpose of SMART Recovery is to help individuals free themselves from addictive behavior by teaching them how to enhance and maintain their motivation for abstinence; cope with urges; manage thoughts, feelings, and behaviors; and balance short-term and long-term rewards. SMART Recovery bases much of its information and the skills they teach on a cognitive-behavioral model of addiction, viewing addictive behavior more as a complex maladaptive behavior than a disease.

Meetings are open to those who want, and those who think they want, to achieve abstinence. Group discussions may focus on achieving abstinence and how abstinence can help other areas of life. SMART Recovery believes that these abstinence-oriented discussions can help those individuals whose goal is moderating their use of substances if the individuals want to engage in a selected period of abstinence, or see their goal as abstaining from overinvolvement as opposed to all involvement.

SMART Recovery meetings are usually smaller than the 12-step groups, occur less frequently, and are not present in all geographical areas.

What Are the Pros and Cons of These Different Types of Self-Help Groups?

The Pros of 12-Step Groups (AA, NA, CA, GA)

1. *Education*: Sober individuals you meet at meetings can teach you the ways they became sober and how they maintain their abstinence.
2. *Hope*: You will see people at meetings who describe such difficult experiences with substances that it seems amazing that they are now doing well. If they can do it, so can you.

3. *Support*: People in self-help groups are part of a fellowship and support each other in different ways than friends, family, or professionals. Because 12-step groups encourage sponsorship and the establishment of a supportive relationship with group members, people in self-help groups *want* you to call and speak to them when you are feeling alone and desperate and want to use. They won't get mad and say, "There you go again." This understanding and acceptance can make the difference between using and staying clean and sober.

4. *Availability*: Twelve-step groups are generally available every day of the year, many times of the day, in nearly all locations throughout the country and throughout the world.

5. *Spirituality*: Twelve-step groups talk about God, spirituality, and a Higher Power; these concepts may fit with your personal beliefs.

6. *Effectiveness*: There are some studies supporting the effectiveness of 12-step programs in long-term recovery for women and men (Ullman, Najdowski, & Adams, 2012; Wells, Donovan, Doyle, & Hatch-Maillette, 2014).

The Cons of 12-Step Groups

1. *Isolation*: You may fear that people in the group already know each other and won't speak to you at meetings. You may see people hugging each other and feel uncomfortable because no one is saying hello to you.

2. *Unwarranted familiarity*: Conversely, people you barely know may come up and hug you, which also may make you feel uncomfortable. Women, in particular, may feel uncomfortable if they are approached by a man and can't be sure of his intentions.

3. *Spirituality*: Twelve-step groups talk about God, spirituality, and a Higher Power; these concepts may not fit with your personal beliefs.

4. *Language*: You may be offended by insensitive statements such as, "Take the cotton out of your ears and stick it in your mouth." Speakers may use curse words, slang, and language that is disrespectful to women, ethnic groups, religious groups, and/or individuals with different sexual orientations.

5. *"War stories"*: You may find other members' detailed stories of substance use, or "war stories," depressing or triggering rather than uplifting or inspiring.

The Pros of SMART Recovery

1. *Group size*: SMART Recovery meetings can be smaller than 12-step groups, increasing the likelihood that people will speak to you and you will have a chance to speak.

2. *Cognitive-behavioral approach*: SMART Recovery focuses on how you can change your own addictive thoughts and behavior, rather than relying on sponsors, the 12 steps, and/ or a Higher Power to help you in your recovery.

3. *Spirituality*: The concepts of God and spirituality are not part of the SMART Recovery philosophy.

The Cons of SMART Recovery

1. *Abstinence*: Although SMART Recovery is an abstinence-oriented program, there are sometimes discussions of moderating substance use as well. You may not find this approach helpful if you have tried moderating your use in the past and did not succeed and abstinence is the recommended goal for you.

2. *Support*: The cognitive-behavioral approach stressing reliance on changing your own thoughts and behaviors may lead you to believe you cannot call anyone in the group if you are in trouble.

3. *Effectiveness*: There are no studies examining the effectiveness of SMART Recovery for achieving and maintaining long-term sobriety.

4. *Availability*: SMART Recovery is not as widely available as 12-step groups and may not meet every day or multiple times each day. SMART Recovery may not be available in some cities and/or states and is not generally available worldwide.

5. *Spirituality*: The concepts of God and spirituality are not part of the SMART Recovery philosophy.

Are You More Likely to Have a Positive Experience in Women-Only Self-Help Groups?

Only you will be able to decide if a women-only self-help group is for you. The best way to determine if these single-gender meetings are a good fit is to attend different women-only and mixed-gender meetings. You should try to attend all types of women-only and mixed-gender meetings for 12-step groups. SMART Recovery has no gender-specific meetings, but that should not prevent you from trying it as well. Once you discover meetings you like, commit to attending a certain number of these meetings each week. When you are deciding the number of self-help groups you will attend each week, remember that it is better to make reasonable commitments to meetings than to make a commitment you cannot keep. For example, it is better to commit to two meetings a week and attend them rather than committing to six groups a week and attending very few or none. Keeping in mind that the ultimate goal is achieving and maintaining abstinence, work on finding the women-only and/or mixed-gender self-help group meetings that best suit your needs in recovery.

How Can You Use Self-Help Groups to Help Yourself?

- Review times and locations of women-only and mixed-gender self-help groups and identify ones you want to attend (refer to printed list of groups in your area or go to the AA, NA website, or SMART Recovery website).
- Ask your therapist or other group members to make recommendations about AA, NA, or SMART Recovery groups in your area that people have found helpful.
- After each meeting you attend, write down what you liked and disliked about each meeting.
- Keep track of when you attend meetings and how much you participate in them.
- Make a list of self-help meetings you find helpful and attend these.

Therapist Overview

Goals of This Session

- To learn about the different types of self-help groups.
- To learn about the availability of women-only self-help groups.
- To learn about the role of self-help groups in recovery.

Session 8 Outline

- **Introduction (*If Needed*)** (5 minutes).
- **Check-In** (5 minutes).
- **Review of Last Week's Skill Practice and Topic** (15 minutes).
- **Presentation of This Week's Topic and Distribution of Topic Overview** (25 minutes): Provide Participant Sheet 8.1.
  - Alcoholics Anonymous.
  - Narcotics Anonymous/Cocaine Anonymous.
  - SMART Recovery.
  - Pros and cons of 12-step groups (AA, NA, CA, GA).
  - Pros and cons of SMART Recovery.
  - Women-only self-help groups.
  - How do you use self-help groups to help yourself?
- **Open Discussion** (30 minutes).
- **Wrap-Up and Reading of Take-Home Messages** (2 minutes): Provide Participant Sheet 8.2.
- **Distribution and Description of This Week's Skill Practice** (3 minutes): Provide Participant Sheet 8.3.
- **Check-Out** (5 minutes).

Session-Specific Materials Needed

- Bulletin Board Outline and Take-Home Messages for Session 8.
- Participant Sheet 8.1: Using Self-Help Groups to Help Yourself.
- Participant Sheet 8.2: Take-Home Messages.
- Participant Sheet 8.3: Skill Practice: Using Self-Help Groups to Help Yourself.
- Self-help meetings lists (e.g., AA, NA, SMART Recovery), if available, to be distributed (therapist can print lists of local meetings from websites or distribute pamphlets and schedules if available).

Introduction (If Needed)

As in the previous session, provide an introduction to the group if there are new members.

Check-In

Pass around the Check-In Sheet and ask each member to respond orally to the three check-in questions.

Review of Last Week's Skill Practice and Topic

From the check-in, the therapist should have a sense of who has done the skill practice and commented on whether or not it was helpful. The therapist can build on the check-in by asking if anyone would like to comment on the skill practice and what she learned. The therapist can also comment on the main highlights from last week's topic. The therapist can then transition to presentation of this week's topic.

Presentation of This Week's Topic and Distribution of Topic Overview

In addition to distributing Participant Sheet 8.1, the therapist can provide lists or booklets of self-help groups or point out where these are available, depending on the clinical setting. The therapist may wish to print local lists from websites of self-help groups to distribute to group members. This can include AA/NA/Al-anon booklets or meeting lists, SMART Recovery meeting lists, or lists of other self-help meetings that may be available in the local area (e.g., Women for Sobriety). As always, the therapist should try to highlight specific themes from the check-in that relate to the day's topic of using self-help groups to help yourself. If self-help did not come up during the check-in but the therapist has heard group members mention self-help groups in previous sessions, the therapist can say something like, "A number of you have mentioned using AA, NA, or SMART Recovery groups, and today we are going to talk about using self-help groups to help yourself." It may also be useful to begin with the take-home messages or an abbreviated version of the take home messages. The therapist can say, "Some of the important take-home messages we will discuss in today's session are. . . ."

- Involvement in self-help groups can help you achieve and maintain long-term sobriety.
- There are different kinds of self-help groups, including some for women only.
- It is important to sample a number of different types of self-help groups before deciding if they are for you.
- Work on finding groups that best suit your recovery needs in terms of the type of meeting, location and timing of the meeting, and a membership with which you feel comfortable.

The therapist can then go on to point out that self-help groups can help women achieve and maintain long-term sobriety and that there are a number of different kinds and types of self-help groups for individuals with substance problems. The therapist may pause and ask if women have had experience attending self-help groups and engage a brief discussion about this topic.

Alcoholics Anonymous

Although AA is the most widely recognized and available of self-help groups, it is not the only self-help group available. AA was founded in 1935 by a stockbroker and a surgeon who both suffered from alcohol dependence. AA is open to anyone who wants to do something about problem drinking. Anonymity, or protecting the identity of the participants, is an important part of the organization. Person-to-person service, or sponsorship, encourages establishing a network of support among members. The AA program, also known as the 12-steps, offers a way to develop a satisfying life without alcohol use. The therapist can also point out that there have been research studies showing that involvement in AA is associated with long-term recovery from alcohol dependence.

The therapist can point out that meeting booklets/lists are available from the AA central office (and the therapist can distribute meeting booklets or lists or give the online website information or any other resources available within the treatment setting, clinic, or local area). In the meeting booklet/list, women can find a key about characteristics of specific meetings, such as whether a specific meeting is:

- *Open*: Open meetings are open to individuals with or without a drinking or drug problem.
- *Closed*: Closed meetings are open only to individuals with a substance use problem.
- *Speaker meeting*: Speaker meetings have members speak about how alcohol and/or drugs have affected their lives and how their lives have changed since stopping using?
- *Discussion meetings*: Discussion meetings are led by one individual who briefly speaks about her or his experience with alcohol and/or drugs followed by a discussion about AA, recovery, or any other drug- or drinking-related problems.
- *Step meeting*: A step meeting discusses one of the 12-steps of AA, NA, or CA.
- *Women only*: There are meetings for women only. There are also meetings that identify themselves as men only, teenagers/young adults, gays, lesbians, bisexuals, and transgender individuals, nonsmoking or smoking, or a combination of these characteristics.

Narcotics Anonymous, Cocaine Anonymous, Gamblers Anonymous

Narcotics Anonymous (NA), *Cocaine Anonymous* (CA), and *Gamblers Anonymous* (GA) were founded on the same principles as AA and are modeled on the 12-step program. All these organizations are fellowships of men and women who have problems with opioids, benzodiazepines, marijuana, or amphetamines (NA); cocaine (CA); or gambling (GA). NA, CA, and GA may also have women-only meetings available depending on the local area.

SMART Recovery

The therapist can now review the difference between the AA program and SMART Recovery. SMART stands for Self-Management and Recovery Training. SMART Recovery is an abstinence-based, self-help program for people with problematic substance use. SMART Recovery's purpose is to help individuals free themselves from addictive behavior by teaching them how to enhance and maintain their motivation for abstinence; cope with urges; manage thoughts, feelings, and behaviors; and balance short-term and long-term rewards. SMART Recovery bases much of its information and the skills they teach on a cognitive-behavioral model of addiction, viewing addictive behavior more as the result of complex, maladaptive thoughts and behaviors than a disease. Meetings are open to those who want, or think they want, to achieve abstinence. Group discussion may focus on achieving abstinence and how it helps in other areas of life. SMART Recovery believes that these abstinence-oriented discussions can help those whose goal is moderating their use of substances if the individual wants to engage in a selected period of abstinence, or see her or his goal as abstaining from overinvolvement as opposed to all involvement.

After describing AA, NA, and SMART Recovery, the therapist can ask the group something like, "Have people had experiences with any of these self-help groups, positive or negative?" The therapist should encourage a brief discussion of people's experiences with self-help.

Pros and Cons of 12-Step Programs

At this point, the therapist should say something like, "Let's review some people's perspectives on the pros and cons of 12-step groups and SMART Recovery. In our discussion I think many of you have said a number of things from your own experiences." Using the bulletin board outline, the therapist should then discuss the potential advantages or "pros" of 12-step groups (e.g., education, hope, support, spirituality, evidence for effectiveness, as well as availability every day, many times of the day, and in many different locations throughout the country and the world), and the potential disadvantages or "cons" (e.g., isolation, unwanted familiarity, spirituality, language, "war stories").

Pros and Cons of SMART Recovery

The therapist should also outline the potential advantages or "pros" of SMART recovery (e.g., group size, cognitive-behavioral approach, spirituality not part of program) and the potential disadvantages or "cons" (e.g., some discussion of moderation rather than abstinence, no studies of effectiveness, spirituality not part of the program, and more limited availability both in location and times).

One disadvantage some people note that is common to any self-help group is their worry that they will not be anonymous. An advantage that is common to all self-help groups (when people find ones with which they are comfortable) is that they provide ongoing support for recovery.

Women-Only Self-Help Groups

Finally, the therapist should discuss with the group the advantages that women often find in women-only self-help groups when they are available. Many women find that women-only self-help groups are smaller, have more consistent memberships, and tend toward more discussion. Some women find that mixed-gender groups may expose them to unwanted interactions from some participants or they may find it difficult to discuss specific details from their personal lives such as trauma or sexual assault. The therapist should encourage women to sample broadly among the different self-help groups, including women-only self-help, before making a decision about whether self-help is for them or not. Members can try different types of meetings and different locations. It is best for each woman to make a commitment that is realistic for her schedule and ability and try to stick to that commitment. Remind group members that *because the ultimate goal is achieving and maintaining abstinence, it is worthwhile to work on finding the women-only and/or mixed gender self-help group meetings that best suit their needs in recovery.*

How Can You Use Self-Help Groups to Help Yourself?

The therapist should acknowledge again that not all women will use self-help groups to help themselves. However, self-help groups can provide a source of both short- and long-term recovery support and are one means of healthy coping with triggers or stress. The therapist can then encourage women to experiment and find out whether self-help would be useful for them as a recovery tool by:

- Reviewing women-only and mixed gender self-help group lists and identify ones you want to attend (refer to printed list of groups in your area or go to the AA or NA/CA/GA websites or SMART Recovery website).
- Experiment with several different types of meetings (large vs. small, AA vs. SMART Recovery, open discussion, women-only vs. mixed-gender, etc.)
- After attending some of the meetings, write down what you liked and disliked about each meeting.
- Keep track of when you attend meetings and how much you participate in them.
- Make a list of self-help meetings you find helpful and attend these.

Open Discussion

It is likely that presentation of the topic led to discussion about group members' diverse experiences with different types of self-help groups including AA, NA, SMART Recovery, or other groups. Women may have experienced large open meetings or small step meetings or mixed-gender or women-only meetings. Some women may never have attended. Discussion of these experiences may continue through open discussion. As always, during open discussion, other recovery-focused topics can be discussed during this time, including discussion of issues brought up in the check-in.

Wrap-Up and Reading of Take-Home Messages

The therapist can summarize the types of self-help groups that women have used and the ways in which they have found them helpful. The therapist can also summarize the ways women have not found them helpful, as well as any feelings of ambivalence toward using self-help. The therapist can then emphasize the point that use of self-help groups can greatly enhance support and recovery. There are many types of self-help groups, and the therapist can encourage women to experiment and try as many of these as possible. Distribute this week's Take-Home Messages (Participant Sheet 8.2) and then review them by having members each read one of the messages in turn.

Distribution and Description of This Week's Skill Practice

Distribute this week's Skill Practice Sheet (Participant Sheet 8.3). This week's skill practice will ask participants to attend two self-help groups and to write down what they did and did not like about the meeting. It also asks participants to reflect on how they might make self-help part of their lives. If participants cannot attend self-help this week, the skill practice sheet will ask them to list for themselves the pros and cons of attending self-help groups. The therapist should also explain that if this week is a week they cannot attend a self-help group, they can do this a different week as well. The goal of the skill practice is to engage participants in trying self-help and considering how it might help them in recovery.

Check-Out

Pass around the Check-Out Sheet and ask participants to each answer orally the one-question check-out. Thank members and tell them you will see them next time.

Women's Use of Substances through the Life Cycle

Some WRG groups are characterized by great heterogeneity in the participants' ages and stages of life. It is possible that in any given WRG group several women will cluster in a particular life stage and then there will be several women in other stages (e.g., most women are middle-aged adults with a few women older and a few women younger); there may also be some WRG groups in which all of the women are at one life stage (e.g., all women in their early 20s, all women over age 60). It is therefore important for the therapist to stress that, as she talks about use of substances through each phase of the life cycle, depending on each woman's age, the material may differentially refer to her past, her present, or her future. The therapist should also make the point that it will be helpful for each woman to think not only about how the material relates to her current and past stages of life, but also to learn about how substances may affect future stages of her life as well. As with other sessions, while preparing for this session topic, the therapist should read the "Background Information" for this session, which follows here.

Background Information

Although substance use problems are usually a problem of early onset (i.e., in adolescence or young adulthood), like many other illnesses, the onset can occur or recur at any time during the lifespan. The pressures, triggers, and vulnerabilities to substance use may be different during different times in women's lives. Women may have had substance problems in adolescence or early adulthood and then stopped their substance use during their middle years, perhaps in response to marital, parenting, or work commitments. At a later stage of life, in the face of loss (e.g., loss of health, a partner, children as they leave home), they may find that the use of substances finds its way back into their lives.

In a different scenario, a woman may never have had any trouble with substances until later in life when she may find herself, for example, struggling to control her use of prescription drugs she once took as recommended by her doctor, and now finds that she uses to manage certain stresses of everyday life or feelings of depression or anxiety. Some women may have never had problems with substances until late life when, after suffering a major loss (e.g., the death of a spouse), they find themselves turning to drugs or alcohol as a way to cope with feelings of loneliness, grief, or isolation.

Each stage of life has its different potential rewards and challenges. It is important to understand the different risks and vulnerabilities through the life cycle and the ways these may affect substance problems and SUDs. A *risk factor* is a behavior or a part of a woman's history or her genetic makeup that may increase her chance of having a substance problem. There are some risk factors that are part of all life stages (e.g., genetics and family history), while others are specific to certain times in the life cycle.

Adolescence

Risks in adolescence include the following:

- *Social context*: Girls are influenced by peer alcohol and drug use or by the substance use of a partner. Group exposure contributes significantly to use of drugs and alcohol among adolescent girls.
- *Alienation or isolation*: Feelings of alienation or isolation especially among girls who are sexual minorities, girls who are bullied, or other girls who may experience marginalization or discrimination can increase the risk of using drugs and alcohol as a means of unhealthy coping or escape.
- *Depression*: Depression can have onset in adolescence and is a risk among teenage girls for substance problems.
- *Earlier age of first use* of cigarettes, marijuana, or alcohol increases the risk for substance problems.
- Smoking cigarettes is a *risk factor for other substance problems*, including problems with alcohol.
- *Sexual trauma* is a risk for onset of substance problems and SUDs.
- *Prescription drug use* is a risk for problems with prescription drugs, including developing opioid use disorders.

Adolescent girls who have substance problems may experience negative consequences, such as vulnerability to sexual assault, having higher rates of suicide attempts, having drunk driving arrests, having other consequences of binge drinking, and having other impulse-control problems.

Young Adulthood

Risks in the decades of the 20s and 30s include the following:

- The *presence of a partner with drug or alcohol problems* increases the risk for substance problems.
- *Depression*: The presence of a depressive disorder can increase the risk for SUDs.
- *Role-related issues*: Women in this part of the life cycle may experience life stressors

associated with work and family roles. One maladaptive coping style is the use of substances to manage role-related stress. Women may say they need to smoke marijuana, drink alcohol, or use drugs at the end of the day to "take the edge off," "relax me at night," "help me sleep," or "to give me more energy to manage everything."

- *Any substance use problem predisposes to problems with other substances*: Problems with prescription drugs, marijuana, other drugs, cigarette smoking, and alcohol problems can co-occur and each can increase the risk for the others.
- *Sexual trauma* is a risk for onset of substance problems and SUDs.
- *Prescription drug use* is a risk for problems with prescription drugs, including developing opioid use disorders.

Middle Years

Risks in the 40s and 50s include the following:

- The *presence of a partner who has drug or alcohol problems* increases risk for women's substance problems.
- *Depression*: The presence of a depressive disorder can increase the risk for SUDs.
- *Losses common to this stage of life*: Women can experience changes in their physical selves and experience these as loss; children grow up and leave home; loss of marriage through divorce or death; and other losses of relationships.
- *Feeling a lack of hope/pessimism about having new life roles* can also increase risk for substance use and problems.
- *Any substance use problem can predispose to other substance problems*: Problems with prescription drugs, marijuana, other drugs, alcohol, and cigarette smoking co-occur and can increase the risk for other substance problems.
- *Prescription drug use* is a risk for problems with prescription drugs, including developing opioid use disorders.

Older Age

Risks in the decades following age 60 include the following:

- *Presence of a partner who has drug or alcohol problems* is a risk factor.
- *Depression*: The presence of a depressive disorder is a risk factor for SUDs.
- *Prescription drug use*: Many women in this age group are prescribed a variety of medications. Some of these have addiction potential. Women can find themselves becoming dependent on these medications and using them in greater quantities or for purposes other than those for which they were originally prescribed.
- *Retirement*: Sometimes this is a welcome change. However, for some women retirement is associated with a loss of social networks, an important role from which they derived self-esteem, etc. For other women, the retirement of a partner may be disruptive to their lives or social networks that may have previously not included her partner.
- *Widowhood or other loss of a partner*: The loss of a long-term partner and the grief and sometimes loneliness associated with this grief can precipitate an increase in use of substances leading to onset of SUDs.

- *Other losses*: Women in older age may also experience other difficult losses, such as loss of health, friends, or social support. These losses may contribute to feelings of loneliness and isolation, which may put women at risk for substance problems and SUDs.
- *Changes in metabolism*: Older individuals have slower metabolism of drugs and alcohol. For example, some women may have been accustomed to drinking alcohol, for example, at a certain level each night (e.g., a glass or two of wine with dinner). In the older years, metabolism of alcohol declines, and a glass or two may actually be experienced as if it were twice as much. This may also precipitate the onset of an SUD.
- *Retirement communities*: Some women may move to retirement communities at this stage of life. In some instances, there is little access to alcohol or drugs within the community. In other communities, though, alcohol can be a major part of the community social life, and individuals may increase their drinking in response.

What Can You Do to Help Yourself?

Understand that use of substances changes throughout women's life cycle and that risks for substance problems can change through time.

- Be aware of specific risks that may be associated with your current stage of life.
- Understand these risks and construct ways to manage these situations that do not include using drugs or alcohol.

Therapist Overview

Goals of This Session

- To understand that the use of substances can change throughout a woman's life cycle and that risks for substance problems can change through time.
- To learn about specific risks that may be associated with each participant's current stage of life.
- To learn about ways to manage these situations that do not include using drugs or alcohol.

Session 9 Outline

- **Introduction (*If Needed*)** (5 minutes).
- **Check-In** (15 minutes).
- **Review of Last Week's Skill Practice and Topic** (5 minutes).
- **Presentation of This Week's Topic and Distribution of Topic Overview** (25 minutes): Provide Participant Sheet 9.1.
  ○ Overview of women's use of substances through the life cycle.
  ○ Adolescence.
  ○ Young adulthood.
  ○ Middle years.

      ○ Older age.

      ○ What can you do to help yourself at each stage of your life?

- **Open Discussion** (30 minutes).
- **Wrap-Up and Reading of Take-Home Messages** (2 minutes): Provide Participant Sheet 9.2.
- **Distribution and Description of This Week's Skill Practice** (3 minutes): Provide Participant Sheet 9.3.
- **Check-Out** (5 minutes).

Session-Specific Materials Needed

- Bulletin Board Outline and Take-Home Messages for Session 9.
- Participant Sheet 9.1: Women's Use of Substances through the Life Cycle.
- Participant Sheet 9.2: Take-Home Messages.
- Participant Sheet 9.3: Skill Practice: Women's Use of Substances through the Life Cycle.

Introduction (If Needed)

As in the previous session, provide an introduction to the group if there are new members.

Check-In

Pass around the Check-In Sheet and have each member respond orally to the three check-in questions.

Review of Last Week's Skill Practice and Topic

From the check-in, the therapist should have a sense of who has done the skill practice and commented on whether or not it was helpful. The therapist can build on the check-in by asking if anyone would like to comment on the skill practice and what she learned. The therapist can also comment on the main highlights from last week's topic. The therapist can then transition to presentation of this week's topic.

Presentation of This Week's Topic and Distribution of Topic Overview

Overview of Women's Use of Substances through the Life Cycle

The therapist should distribute Participant Sheet 9.1. As always, the therapist should try to highlight specific themes from the check-in that relate to the day's topic. It is possible that this topic will not have come up in the check-in on this particular day, but it is likely that themes of life-cycle-specific stressors have come up in previous sessions. For example, midlife issues (e.g., the loss that occurs when children leave home) or young adult issues (e.g., finding a partner when you are not drinking or using drugs) may have been brought up by the participants. It is helpful for the therapist to frame the session topic as one of "past, present, and future," meaning that the material will allow participants to reflect on use of substances in past phases of life, triggers associated with their current stage of life, as well as risks as participants strive for longer term recovery.

As always, it is helpful at this time to bring in any points brought up in the check-in that were related to the topic of women's use of substances through the life cycle. If there were no concerns related to the topic brought up on this particular day, the therapist may reference experiences that have been brought up by group members in previous sessions. For example, the therapist might say something like, "I know that some of you have talked about the challenges of having certain losses related to a particular phase of life. Some of you have mentioned that your substance use worsened when your last child left for college/for a job/etc., and we've also discussed how difficult retirement was for someone else. . . ." Alternatively, "Some of you have mentioned the stress you have felt when your adult child moved home" or " . . . that it was necessary for you to take on major child care roles for your grandchildren and that was unexpected. . . ." If the group is composed mostly of younger women, the therapist might say something like, "Some of you have talked about how hard it is to meet people and have a social life without drinking or without going to bars and clubs where there are a lot of drugs. . . ."

The therapist can then go on to say, "Today we are going to talk about women's use of substances through the life cycle. You will not all relate to everything that is mentioned with regard to each life stage. Likewise, because you are all at different stages of life, what for one woman is a past stage may, for another woman, be a future stage. So, it will be helpful for you to think of your past, your present, and your future as we review today's topic." As always it may be useful to begin by reviewing the take-home messages of the session and then to summarize that the group will be talking about *risks and triggers in women associated with adolescence, young adulthood, middle adult years, and older adulthood.*

The therapist can then proceed to discuss the fact that some women experience substance problems through their entire life cycle, from adolescence onward, while others find they develop a substance problem at a particular life stage. For example, some women may struggle with alcohol, cocaine, or marijuana problems from their teenage years onward, while other women may find they develop a problem with prescription medication or alcohol in their middle or later years even though they have never had substance problems in the past. Although some women may struggle with a single substance throughout their lifetime, other women may find that later in life they are having problems with a different substance than the one that was an issue at an earlier time in their life. For example, a woman in her 50s who had problems with marijuana in young adulthood may now be struggling with alcohol and prescription pain medications. A woman who has not had difficulties with any substances in her early life may find that in her midlife her alcohol use spiraled out of control. An older woman might report that following the death of a partner and a medical complication from surgery, her use of prescription opioid medication has become problematic. A young woman may describe having been introduced to marijuana in her early teens and finding that now in her 20s she is using both alcohol and prescription drugs.

After framing the discussion, the therapist can then proceed to discuss the major topics outlined in Participant Sheet 9.1. She can explain that the term "risk factor" refers to any behavior, part of a woman's history, or element of her genetic makeup (e.g., family history) that increases her chance of substance problems. The therapist can now go on to discuss risk factors for girls and women associated with life-cycle stages.

Adolescence

For adolescent girls, some risk factors for SUDs include peer alcohol or drug use and the opinion of members of the peer group including partners; the onset of depression, anxiety, or an eating disorder; earlier age of first use of cigarettes, marijuana, alcohol, or other drugs; and a history of sexual and/or physical abuse. For sexual minority girls, feelings of social isolation at home or at school may pose a risk for using substances. This is also true of girls who have been bullied. Substance problems in adolescent girls puts them at increased risk for a variety of negative consequences, including sexual assault, having higher rates of suicide attempts, drunk driving arrests, or other impulse-control problems. The onset of puberty itself and the beginning of the menarche (i.e., menstruation) is associated with hormonal changes that can create vulnerability for some girls and women to mood-related disorders as well as to substance use.

Young Adulthood

Women in young adulthood (20s or 30s) have a number of different risk factors for substance problems. One is having a partner or spouse who has a problem with drugs or alcohol. Another is the presence or onset of a depressive disorder, other psychiatric disorder, or history of sexual trauma or assault. Role-related issues may also become risk factors. For instance, during this phase of life some women may begin a maladaptive pattern of coping with stressors associated with work and family roles by using alcohol or drugs. Women may say that they need to use these substances to "take the edge off the day," "relax," or "help them sleep"; other thoughts and feelings may also contribute. Binge drinking is also a major risk for women between the ages of 18 and 34 (Centers for Disease Control and Prevention, 2013). In addition, problems with one substance can predispose to problems with other substances at this stage. Women with alcohol problems may find themselves at greater risk of having problems with prescription drugs, for example.

After reviewing risk factors for substance use among women in these two phases of life, the therapist should stop and ask the group if they recognize any of these things as applying to themselves now or in the past. Depending on the age range of the group, this discussion may be longer or shorter, as participants may or may not relate to these stages-of-life issues.

Middle Years

After some discussion the therapist should say, "Let's move on to discuss the middle years and older age." In the middle years, a partner with a drug or alcohol problem remains a common risk factor for use. As is discussed in other sessions, the presence of such a partner can pose a significant risk to a woman's recovery. As in younger adulthood, the onset or presence of depression remains a risk. Many women find themselves using substances on which they eventually become dependent in response to untreated or undertreated mood disorders. There are also losses associated with the middle years. For example, women with children may have a sense of loss when children grow up and leave home, or marital or partnered status may change through separation, divorce, or death. There may be losses of other long-standing relationships, as well. Women face shifts in their physical selves, and some may experience such changes as a loss. There are also endocrine changes associated with the perimenopause and menopause to which some women may respond by using substances in maladaptive ways. Maladaptive coping at this stage of life may lead to substance use and substance problems in response to some of these stressors, mental and physical symptoms, and risk factors.

Older Age

In older age, women face some of the same risks as in the middle years, but there are additional risks that are specific to older age. Among those similar to the younger and middle years are a partner with substance problems and the onset or presence of mood disorders. In addition, many women in this age group receive a variety of prescription medications. Some medications have addiction potential, and women are at risk for becoming dependent on these medications. Furthermore, retirement from employment or community responsibilities may be a welcome or unwelcome change. For some women it represents the loss of social networks, work they enjoy, or occupational prestige. For other women, the retirement of a spouse or partner may be disruptive to her daily life or social network that may not have previously included her partner or spouse. Other losses that may pose risks include loss of health and loss of social relationships and support through death of partners, spouses, family members, or friends. These losses may contribute to loneliness and isolation, and women in this age group may find themselves turning to substances to "numb" out these feelings, provide an "aid" for insomnia, or other maladaptive use patterns. Changes in metabolism may also be a specific risk for this age group. Metabolism of alcohol and certain prescription medications slows with increasing age and may predispose women to becoming dependent even on doses or amounts they previously tolerated well. One drink per night in a woman's forties may seem like two or three times that amount when she is in her sixties. Finally, social life in retirement communities may include drinking. For women in recovery or for those trying not to drink or use other substances, this can pose a risk.

The therapist should again open up the session for discussion and ask, "Does anyone recognize any of these risks and triggers that I have described for the middle and older years?" She should wait for responses and encourage participation and discussion. If there are not a lot of responses, the therapist can bring up material from past sessions that relate to this topic (e.g., partners, mood disorders, stress). She could also ask whether any younger women in the group are concerned about any of these risks or triggers in their future or recognize them from their own families or others in their social networks.

How Can Women Help Themselves through the Life Cycle?

After some discussion, the therapist should then pose the question, "What can individuals do to help themselves with the risk factors of each life stage?" She might then ask the group to think through and share ideas for coping strategies that are alternatives to using substances in the face of these risk factors. After some discussion, she can highlight the healthy coping strategies that the participants have described. The therapist can also stress these particular messages: women should understand that use of substances occurs through the life cycle and that risks for substance problems change with time; be aware of specific risks that may be associated with women's current stage of life as well as those in the future; and develop alternate coping strategies to manage these risks, care for themselves, and not use substances.

Open Discussion

This topic may have begun a variety of discussions about different ages and stages of life and risks for substances. This discussion may continue into the open discussion period. Again, as in previous sessions, during open discussion other recovery-focused topics can be discussed during this time, including discussion of issues brought up in the check-in.

Wrap-Up and Reading of Take-Home Messages

The therapist should summarize the experiences of different life stages discussed by the group members, as well as any themes of vulnerabilities or rewards that influence addiction and recovery during each phase of life. As in previous sessions, distribute this week's Take-Home Messages (Participant Sheet 9.2), and review them by having members each read one of the messages in turn.

Distribution and Description of This Week's Skill Practice

Distribute this week's Skill Practice Sheet (Participant Sheet 9.3). This week's skill practice will ask participants to identify their current stage of life, the main risks and triggers for their substance use, whether they think these are related to their stage of life, and then list three things they can do to help themselves manage these triggers.

Check-Out

Pass around the Check-Out Sheet and ask participants each to answer orally the one-question check-out. Thank members and tell them you will see them next time.

Violence and Abuse

Getting Help

Many women in the U.S. population and worldwide have experienced childhood and/or adult-hood sexual or physical assault, and many others have experienced emotional abuse. In addition, domestic violence is a very important public health problem that affects women's mental and physical health. Women with histories of childhood sexual and/or physical assault are at an increased risk of onset of SUDs, other psychiatric disorders (e.g., PTSD, depression, anxiety disorders, eating disorders), and at higher risk of again experiencing abuse or sexual assault. The proportion of women in SUD treatment with histories of sexual and physical abuse is greater than the prevalence of these histories in the general population. Therefore, it is important to address the way in which histories of violence, sexual abuse, and assault affect women's addiction and recovery. As always, while preparing for this session, the therapist should read the "Background Information" that follows.

Background Information

Women and Histories of Violence and Abuse

Many women in SUD treatment programs have experienced abuse or violence either as children or as adults. Between 30 and 75% of women in SUD treatment programs say that they experienced sexual abuse as children. Some investigators report that adult women with histories of childhood sexual abuse are up to five times as likely as those without this history to have problems with drugs and twice as likely to have problems with alcohol. It may be that some women use drugs and/or alcohol to numb or mask the pain or shame associated with past histories of sexual abuse. Addressing the feelings associated with past histories of abuse may help women who are recovering from alcohol and drug problems.

Some women with earlier histories of sexual or physical abuse may also be more at risk for violence in adulthood, which may take the form of physical assault, emotional abuse, domestic violence, sexual abuse, or rape. Again, these experiences in adulthood (whether childhood maltreatment existed or not) may contribute to feelings of shame, worthlessness, and social isolation that can predispose women to substance problems and increase risk of relapse to substances for women who have entered recovery.

Certain feelings and illnesses are particularly common among women with histories of violence and abuse, regardless of whether an SUD is present or not. When women experience these problems along with SUDs, we say that the disorders "co-occur." One such disorder is *posttraumatic stress disorder* (PTSD). Women who have PTSD may experience intrusive thoughts, nightmares, or other reexperiencing of their past abuse. Such experiences can lead to avoidance of situations or places that may be associated with the traumatic experience.

There are other co-occurring disorders that women with substance problems and histories of violence can experience. Depression and anxiety are more prevalent among women with SUDs, and histories of trauma and abuse may also contribute to an increased vulnerability to these disorders. These disorders can be triggers for relapse to substances, and attention to these is also important in recovery.

Other Feelings Associated with Histories of Violence and Abuse

In addition to certain disorders such as depression, anxiety, and PTSD there are a number of other feelings that can be associated with histories of violence and abuse that can create obstacles for women in recovery. Women with histories of violence often experience feelings of shame and guilt and may develop avoidant coping strategies that can make them more vulnerable to relapse to drugs and alcohol. In addition, experiences of violence can inhibit feelings of trust and affect women's relationships with family and others. Emotional, physical, or sexual abuse may also contribute to low self-esteem or feelings of stigmatization among women. Such feelings may have a number of consequences for women. These feelings may:

- Predispose women to using substances to mask or numb the negative feelings.
- Reinforce choices of partners or other relationships that may be unhealthy or destructive.
- Inhibit choosing healthier friendships and social connections.
- Lead to women's feeling more socially disconnected and isolated.

All of these consequences can serve as triggers to relapse and obstacles for recovery.

Emotional, Psychological, and Verbal Abuse

These forms of abuse can coexist with other forms of either physical or sexual abuse, or they may occur on their own. Emotional, psychological, and verbal abuse can take a number of forms. When a partner controls a woman's choices or there is a clear difference in the power within the relationship, this may be one form of emotional or psychological abuse, and it may or may not be associated with verbal abuse. All of these forms of abuse can lead to women's feelings of shame, humiliation, and lower self-esteem. They can also lead to depression and anxiety and to alcohol and drug problems. One study found that 46.7% of women reported being subjected to emotional abuse by an intimate partner, and 2.9% experienced physical abuse at least one time by their partner (Murty et al., 2003). In another group of women being treated for alcohol or drug problems (ages 18–73), more than 60% reported being subjected to emotional abuse in their home growing up and rated it "very distressing" (Berry & Sellman, 2001). Other studies of women with alcohol and drug problems have also found a large majority of women reporting physical and sexual abuse. In one such study, 20% of women reported physical abuse only, 4% experienced sexual abuse only, and 57% suffered from both physical and sexual abuse (Liebschutz et al., 2002). Thus, childhood abuse (including emotional abuse) may make women more vulnerable to alcohol and drug problems later in life. Emotional or psychological abuse in adulthood may also predispose women to using alcohol or drugs and can also be an obstacle to getting treatment and being in recovery.

Domestic or Intimate Partner Violence

Domestic violence, or intimate partner violence (IPV), is more common in our society than is generally thought. There are clearly other factors beyond substance problems that contribute to domestic violence. One possibility is cultural norms that may sanction violence and especially violence toward women. Another factor that may contribute to violence between intimate partners is perceived inequality between the partners. For example, differences in employment, income, finances, or family roles may sometimes contribute to a perceived inequality within a couple such that the couple perceives one member to be more dominant or in control. The other member of the couple may feel powerless and may in fact have fewer resources to help her express her autonomy within the relationship or to leave the situation.

While these factors listed above make their own contribution to the incidence of domestic violence or IPV, the risk of such violence is even greater in the setting of substance use and substance problems. Domestic violence episodes are more severe when one or both partners have been drinking than if both individuals were sober (Graham, Bernards, Wilsnack, & Gmel, 2011). Domestic violence and IPV are not restricted to male–female pairs but also occur in gay and lesbian couples and is similarly higher among those using alcohol or other drugs. There are a number of ways to understand this link between substance problems and domestic violence.

Women who experience domestic violence or IPV may use substances to cope with their feelings. The substance use may in turn make them less able to defend themselves and also contribute to feelings of guilt and shame. These patterns can perpetuate a *vicious cycle* where violence and abuse gives rise to more substance use and substance use gives rise to more violence. Any and all of these patterns can *inhibit* women's ability to *seek out treatment for their substance problems* and to get help to *get themselves to a place of safety* and *stop the violence*.

Relationship of Abuse and Violence to Problems with Substances
- Women who experience abuse and/or violence may use substances to cope with the trauma of the abuse and/or violence.
- Women who use substances may be more vulnerable to violence because partners may stigmatize them as being "reasonable" targets of abuse and violence.
- Women who are intoxicated may be less able to defend themselves against abuse and violence because of impaired judgment, vigilance, ability to react, etc.

- Women who use substances may feel guilt and shame about their substance use, as well as about the abuse and violence itself, and this may make them feel less deserving and less able to get help to stop the abuse and/or violence.
- Women (whether they abuse substances or not) who are with substance-dependent partners are at greater risk for domestic violence and IPV and abuse because substances can decrease the partner's ability to control aggressive and violent impulses.

What Can You Do to Help Yourself?

The first and most important part of helping yourself is to *assess for yourself* and *communicate with your clinicians (your doctors, therapists, and other clinicians working with you on your recovery) your own experience of violence and abuse* before you were in treatment and recovery, while you are now in treatment and recovery, and after treatment when you are in recovery and maintaining abstinence. Self-assessment at each of these stages is listed below:

Before Recovery

Have you experienced sexual, physical, or emotional abuse or violence before your drug or alcohol problem and/or before seeking treatment for your drug or alcohol problem? If so, in what way do you think this may have contributed to your starting to use drugs, continuing to use drugs, and any difficulties in seeking treatment or entering recovery?

During Treatment and Recovery

Now that you are in treatment and have entered recovery, are sexual, physical, or emotional abuse or violence a current part of your experience? If so, in what way(s) do you think these experiences are currently inhibiting your recovery? Some questions you may begin to ask yourself about this are:

- How often does your partner show disapproval toward you?
- When was the last time you felt threatened or controlled by or afraid of your partner?
- How often does someone hurt you?
- How often does your partner use words that put you down and make you feel bad about yourself?

Considering the answers to these questions, if you are *not* physically *safe*, it is important to *seek a safe place*. If you are *not* physically *threatened or in physical danger*, it may be time to *consider* whether *counseling* for you with or without your partner would be useful.

After Treatment and While Maintaining Abstinence

Are there ongoing abusive relationships in your life? If so, what would be the best way to take care of yourself? Do you need to find a place to be physically safe? Otherwise, do you need to find alternatives with or without your partner? Were there relationships that were violent or abusive, that you experienced in the past either before using drugs or while using drugs and before seeking treatment, or during your treatment and beginning of recovery? If so, what do you think the effects of these experiences are for you now? To what extent do you feel that grief and loss play a role in your current abstinence and recovery?

These self-assessments and communication with clinicians are very important and can lead to any or all of the following important steps:

- Taking care of yourself physically and emotionally.
- Getting yourself physically safe if physical safety is not part of your life now.
- Addressing the consequences of emotional or verbal abuse that took place in the past or may be occurring now.
- Grieving losses that may have come from abuse and violence.

Therapist Overview

Goals of This Session

- To understand that histories of violence and childhood and adult abuse are common for many women in recovery from SUDs.
- To identify the illnesses (e.g., PTSD, mood disorders, and anxiety disorders) and feelings (e.g., shame, difficulty with trust, and low self-esteem) that are common experiences for those with histories of violence and abuse.
- To understand that these feelings can all lead to women's feeling more socially isolated and disconnected.
- To encourage women to do a self-assessment regarding history of abuse before recovery, or during treatment and recovery, and to communicate whether this is a past and/or current problem.
- To encourage women to get help to get physically safe if physical safety is not a current part of their lives.
- To convey the importance of learning over time to address the emotional consequences of any abuse.
- To begin to learn strategies for managing feelings and consequences of experiences of violence and abuse without using substances.

Session 10 Outline

- **Introduction (*If Needed*)** (5 minutes).
- **Check-In** (15 minutes).
- **Review of Last Week's Skill Practice and Topic** (5 minutes).
- **Presentation of This Week's Topic and Distribution of Topic Overview** (25 minutes): Provide Participant Sheet 10.1.
  - ○ Women and histories of violence and abuse.
  - ○ Feelings associated with histories of violence and abuse.
  - ○ Emotional, psychological, and verbal abuse.

- ○ Domestic and intimate partner violence.
- ○ Relationship of abuse and violence to problems with substances.
- ○ How can you get help to help yourself?
- **Open Discussion** (30 minutes).
- **Wrap-Up and Reading of Take-Home Messages** (2 minutes): Provide Participant Sheet 10.2.
- **Distribution and Description of This Week's Skill Practice** (3 minutes): Provide Participant Sheet10.3.
- **Check-Out** (5 minutes).

Session-Specific Materials Needed

- Bulletin Board Outline and Take-Home Messages for Session 10.
- Participant Sheet 10.1: Violence and Abuse: Getting Help.
- Participant Sheet 10.2: Take-Home Messages.
- Participant Sheet 10.3: Skill Practice: Violence and Abuse: Getting Help.

Introduction (If Needed)

As in the previous session, provide an introduction to the group if there are new members.

Check-In

Pass around the Check-In Sheet and have each member respond orally to the three check-in questions.

Review of Last Week's Skill Practice and Topic

From the check-in, the therapist should have a sense of who has done the skill practice and commented on whether or not it was helpful. The therapist can build on the check-in by asking if anyone would like to comment on the skill practice and what she learned. The therapist can also comment on the main highlights from last week's topic. The therapist can then transition to presentation of this week's topic.

Presentation of This Week's Topic and Distribution of Topic Overview

Distribute the Topic Overview (Participant Sheet 10.1). The therapist can introduce the topic by saying that this session is important in order to help women understand that violence and abuse are experiences that are common among women in the general population but are especially prevalent among women with SUDs. The purpose of the session is not to ask participants to discuss their specific experiences of violence and abuse but rather to present common feelings and illnesses, types of abuse, the need to secure physical safety, and the need to help oneself develop strategies to maintain sobriety in spite of these feelings related to histories of abuse and/or symptoms of other related illnesses.

Women and Histories of Violence and Abuse

Certain feelings and illnesses are particularly common among women with histories of violence and abuse, regardless of whether substance problems are present or not. When women experience these problems along with substance problems, we say the disorders "co-occur." One such disorder is PTSD. Women who have PTSD may experience intrusive thoughts, nightmares, or other reexperiencing of their past abuse. Such experiences can lead to avoidance of situations or places that may be associated with abuse.

There are other co-occurring disorders that women with SUDs and histories of violence can experience. Depression and anxiety are more prevalent among women with SUDs, and histories of abuse may also contribute to an increased vulnerability to depression and anxiety. These disorders can be triggers for relapse to substances, and treatment for these co-occurring disorders (e.g., PTSD, depression, anxiety) is also important for recovery.

Other Feelings Associated with Histories of Violence and Abuse

In addition to certain disorders such as depression, anxiety, and PTSD a number of other feelings associated with histories of violence can create obstacles for women in recovery. Women with histories of violence often experience feelings of shame and guilt and may develop avoidant coping strategies that can make them more vulnerable to relapse to drugs and alcohol. In addition, experiences of violence can inhibit feelings of trust and affect women's relationships with family and others. Emotional, physical, or sexual abuse may also contribute to low self-esteem or feelings of stigmatization among women. Such feelings may have a number of consequences for women. These feelings may:

- Predispose women to use substances to mask or numb them.
- Reinforce choices of partners or other relationships that may be unhealthy or destructive.
- Inhibit choosing healthier friendships and social connections.
- Lead to women's feeling more socially disconnected and isolated.

All of these consequences can serve as triggers to relapse to substances and present obstacles for recovery.

The therapist can present some of the basic information about the prevalence of violence and abuse, which often lead to certain types of consequences. First, the therapist can explain that women with histories of abuse may experience other illnesses in addition to SUD, including PTSD, mood disorders, or anxiety disorders. In addition, women who have had experiences of violence and abuse may also have certain feelings, such as guilt and shame, lack of trust, and low self-worth. These feelings can lead to women feeling more socially disconnected and isolated, which can be an obstacle to recovery or can serve as triggers to relapse.

Emotional, Psychological, and Verbal Abuse

The therapist can then briefly describe the types of abuse and violence that women may have experienced. Emotional, psychological, and verbal abuse can coexist with other forms of physical or sexual abuse or violence and can take a number of different forms. One important and common circumstance occurs when a partner controls a woman's choices or there is a clear power difference in a relationship, which can provide a situation where emotional, psychological, or verbal abuse can take place.

Domestic or Intimate Partner Violence

Another common form of violence and abuse that women experience is domestic violence or intimate partner violence (IPV). There are a number of factors that can contribute to domestic violence, and the presence of substance problems is certainly one of them. The therapist can explain that 75% of all domestic violence incidents involve alcohol use by the partner, the woman, or both. Women who experience domestic violence or other abuse may use substances to cope with the feelings produced by these experiences. Using substances to mask or numb feelings can lead women to feel more guilt and shame and can also make them more vulnerable to further episodes of violence or abuse, thereby creating a vicious cycle. These patterns can also make it more difficult for women to get help for their substance problems and for symptoms of other disorders. Domestic violence and IPV is not restricted to male–female pairs but also occurs in gay and lesbian couples and is similarly higher among those using alcohol or other drugs. There are a number of ways to understand this link between substance problems and domestic violence.

Women who experience domestic violence may use substances to cope with their feelings. The substance use may make them less able to defend themselves and also contribute to feelings of guilt and shame. These patterns can perpetuate a *vicious cycle* where violence and abuse gives rise to more substance abuse and substance abuse gives rise to more violence. Any and all of these patterns can *inhibit* women's ability to *seek out treatment for their substance problems* and to get help to *get themselves to a place of safety* and *stop the violence*.

Relationship of Abuse and Violence to Problems with Substances

The therapist can review the following points that are also contained in Participant Sheet 10.1.

- Women who experience abuse and/or violence may use substances to cope with the trauma of the abuse and/or violence.
- Women who use substances may be more vulnerable to violence because partners may stigmatize them as being "reasonable" targets of abuse and violence.
- Women who are intoxicated may be less able to defend themselves against abuse and violence because of impaired judgment, vigilance, ability to react, etc.
- Women who use substances may feel guilt and shame about their substance use, as well as about the abuse and violence itself, and this may make them feel less deserving and less able to get help to stop the abuse and/or violence.
- Women (whether they use substances or not) who are with substance-dependent partners are more at risk for domestic violence or IPV and abuse because substances can decrease the partner's ability to control aggressive and violent impulses.

What Can You Do to Help Yourself?

The therapist should explain that the first most important part of helping yourself is to *asses* and *communicate with your clinicians (your doctors, therapists, and other clinicians working with you on your recovery) your own experience of violence and abuse* before you were in treatment and recovery, and now that you are in treatment and recovery, and maintaining abstinence. Self-assessment at each of these stages is listed below:

Before Recovery

Have you experienced sexual, physical, or emotional abuse or violence before your drug use and/or before seeking treatment for your drug use? If so, in what way do you think this may have contributed to your starting to use drugs, continuing to use drugs, and any difficulties in seeking treatment or entering recovery?

During Treatment and Recovery

Now that you are in treatment and have entered recovery, is sexual, physical, or emotional abuse or violence a current part of your experience? If so, it is important to seek help to get yourself to safety. In what ways do you think these experiences are currently inhibiting your recovery? Some questions you may ask yourself about this issue are:

- How often does your partner show disapproval toward you?
- When was the last time you felt threatened by, controlled by, or afraid of your partner?
- How often does someone hurt you?
- How often does your partner use words that put you down and make you feel very bad about yourself?

Considering the answers to these questions, if you are *not* currently physically *safe*, it is important to *seek a safe place* to be and to ask for help to get physically safe. If you are *not* physically *threatened or in physical danger*, it may be time to *consider* whether *counseling* for you with or without your partner would be useful.

After Treatment and While Maintaining Abstinence

Are there ongoing abusive relationships in your life? If so, what would be the best way to take care of yourself? How can you get help to find a place to be physically safe if you are in any physical danger? Do you need to find treatment for these issues with or without your partner? If there are no ongoing relationships that are violent or abusive, are there relationships that you experienced in the past that were violent or abusive either before using drugs, while using drugs, before seeking treatment, or during your treatment and beginning of recovery? If so, what do you think the effects of these experiences are for you now? To what extent do feelings of grief and loss play a role in your current feelings about substance use, treatment, and recovery?

These self-assessments and communication with clinicians are very important and can lead to any or all of the following important steps:

- Taking care of yourself physically and emotionally.
- Getting yourself physically safe if physical safety is not part of your life now.
- Addressing the consequences of physical, sexual, emotional, or verbal abuse that took place in the past or may be occurring now.
- Getting treatment for PTSD or other illnesses or feelings from abuse.
- Grieving losses that may have come from abuse and violence.

It is important for the therapist to emphasize the point that if women are not physically threatened, but are having ongoing problems with their partners, they should seek counseling. In addition, for women who have had a past history of abuse and/or violence, addressing the emotional consequences and grieving the losses can be helpful in recovery.

The therapist should emphasize that the first step in addressing violence and abuse is to *make sure that participants are physically safe now.* Women who are currently living in a setting where they are likely to experience abuse or violence should make sure they have a safe place to be. Women should be encouraged to assess their situation, enlisting the help of their clinicians in making this assessment, and determining ways to make their situations safer. It is important for the therapist to have a *list of resources in her local area* (e.g., shelters, clinics, crisis centers) that help women who are experiencing IPV or domestic abuse. The therapist should have these lists available to distribute if clinically appropriate.

The therapist should also stress the importance of finding healthy ways to manage feelings that are related to experiences of violence without using substances and to get treatment for co-occurring disorders such as PTSD. Maintaining abstinence from substances is key to recovery and to working through past experiences of violence and abuse.

Open Discussion

The length of interactive discussion during the presentation of today's topic will depend on the group members and their experiences with past or present trauma. It is possible in a group where many women have experienced trauma and abuse that the entire session topic presentation and open discussion will focus on this topic. In other settings, group members may not identify this as part of their experience even though they acknowledge that this is a common experience for many women. As always, the open discussion time may also focus on other recovery issues, including any issues that were raised during the check-in.

Wrap-Up and Reading of Take-Home Messages

As always, the therapist should sum up any themes that have come up within the group during the discussion. In addition, the therapist can again stress the need for physical safety in order to care for oneself and recover from addiction and to ask for help in getting physically safe. Reaching out to clinicians for help with symptoms is important. It is also important to emphasize that remaining abstinent from substances and learning ways of managing feelings related to histories of abuse and violence without using substances is critical to recovery. As in previous sessions, distribute this week's Take-Home Messages (Participant Sheet 10.2), and review them by having members each read one of the messages in turn.

Distribution and Description of This Week's Skill Practice

Distribute this week's Skill Practice Sheet (Participant Sheet 10.3). This week's skill practice will ask participants to write down whether they have experienced past violence or abuse and the possible effects it is has had on them and their recovery. It also asks participants to write down whether their life currently has any abuse or violence in it and options for safety as well as three ways they can support their recovery this week.

Check-Out

Pass around the Check-Out Sheet and ask participants each to answer orally the one-question check-out. Thank members and tell them you will see them next time.

The Issue of Disclosure

To Tell or Not to Tell?

This session covers the issues women face when deciding how, when, and to whom to disclose (or to tell other people) about their substance problem. Within the context of the WRG, women are encouraged to share within their comfort zone. However, outside of treatment, as women seek support for their recovery, they are often confronted with the issue about with whom they feel comfortable sharing knowledge of their substance problem and recovery. This session is meant to help women discuss the pros and cons of disclosing their substance problem as well as their perceptions of stigma and feelings of shame related to their disclosure. As always, in preparing for this session, the therapist should read the "Background Information" that follows.

Background Information

The issue of whether to disclose one's problem with substances is often quite complex and always personal. *Disclosure* means "revealing thoughts and feelings while stating crucial facts about oneself." Sometimes disclosure may be a *choice* or a *necessity*; it may happen *intentionally* or *unintentionally*. People with substance problems often find themselves facing the dilemma of *"to tell or not to tell."* One aspect of this dilemma is that a substance problem is the type of condition that can be "concealed," as opposed to another type of condition that is "immediately revealed" by appearance. That is to say, if your illness is under control and you can go about life and perform its tasks without disclosure, the decision about disclosing can be particularly difficult.

In some instances, disclosure can be prompted by situations that are outside the individual's control. For example, a new illness episode requiring treatment or a job change may push an individual to disclose her substance problem because of the need to gain accommodation in the work environment. Another disclosure that may be out of the individual's control is if someone else discloses her substance problem without her consent. An accidental meeting of an acquaintance at a self-help meeting might also prompt a disclosure that was unintended.

In many cases, individuals with substance problems who are in recovery find themselves confronted with the *dilemma of disclosure*. This dilemma can be described as *"secrecy and control versus getting it out in the open."* The feelings of secrecy and control can be described as wanting to control what others know about you and perhaps wishing to "put away" those darker moments when life felt out of control. The desire to "get it out in the open" often stems from a desire for increased support, as well as the sense that there might be relief in not having to be burdened with the secret of addiction and that it might be helpful if someone close knew about your history and your problems with substances.

The issue of disclosure is one that is personal, requires careful thought, and can be made best with prudence, restraint, and safety. In the end, the question "to tell or not to tell?" can only be answered by the person contemplating disclosure.

What Are Some of the Barriers to and Possible Disadvantages of Disclosure?

- *Fear of discrimination*: The term "discrimination" refers to actions that take place based on prejudice. Discrimination against a person who reveals her substance problem may take place in the workplace (in spite of federal regulations that prohibit this through the Americans with Disabilities Act) or elsewhere. Discrimination may be overt (not getting a promotion because of one's history) or more subtle (being left out of something because of one's illness or impairment).
- *Fear of stigma*: *Stigma* is defined as "a brand or mark of infamy" because of "an attribute that is deeply discredited." People who disclose their substance problems can feel that the disclosure makes the difference between being "regarded as a competent, productive, and accepted person" and "feeling a disbelief in one's ability to do the task." The effects of societal stigma may also be felt in the fear that family or friends will *no longer see you as a complete person* or will see you as somehow *defective*.
- *Feelings of shame*: Shame runs deep in the illness of addiction. Disclosing one's addiction to another person may provoke feelings of anxiety and shame.
- *Giving up of a feeling of privacy*: People often feel that their addiction and recovery are private issues. Giving up this privacy often feels filled with discomfort or peril.
- *Fear of rejection*: People can feel that disclosing one's addiction and recovery will prompt rejection by friends and family. In addition, women with addicted or substance-using partners may worry that revealing addiction and recovery to this partner will prompt a rejection because the partner may wish to continue to use and not understand the woman's desire and need for sobriety.

What Are Potential Benefits of Disclosure?

- *Recognition and acceptance can enhance recovery*: Sometimes women can discover that people in their lives are accepting of their illness and their recovery. This can enhance their sense of support in their environment and can help in recovery.
- *Gaining new supports and building new relationships*: Disclosing may reveal other people who are supportive of women's recovery and help to build a recovery-focused network.
- *Decreasing isolation*: Having disclosed can enhance feelings of connectedness and can

also provide women with supportive others who are available for social interaction and support.

- *Beginning and/or continuing the healing and recovery process*: When the individual herself has a feeling of readiness and a compelling sense that it is the right thing to do, disclosure may enhance self-acceptance and recovery.
- *Sharing new perspectives/helping others*: Sometimes a disclosure is helpful to others who may be struggling (or who know someone else who is struggling). This can lead to mutual support or a sense of making a contribution to others.
- *Obtaining reasonable accommodation in the workplace or at home*: Whether it is leaving work to get to a group or individual therapy appointment, or obtaining a leave of absence to attend a more intensive program, sometimes disclosure in the workplace can lead to enhanced accommodation to treatment needs. This, in turn, can lead to enhanced recovery and enhanced performance on the job. Similarly, at home it can be helpful for all members of the family to know about your recovery so that the home can become an alcohol- and drug-free zone and family members can accommodate your need for time to go to treatment or self-help meetings.

Some Issues That Come Up

In considering "to tell or not to tell," you might think about:

- How much do you want to disclose?
- To whom will you disclose? (Pick someone you trust.)
- To whom is it important that you *not* disclose?
- In what form will disclosure be made?
- When will you disclose?
- Why are you disclosing? What do you hope to gain?
- Where will you disclose? (Choose a safe environment.)

Some Dos and Don'ts of Disclosure

Think about and assess your own readiness and comfort with disclosure. Look for a compelling feeling that this is the right thing to do for yourself, with this person, and at this time.

- Choose carefully to whom you wish to disclose. Emphasize feelings of safety and comfort.
- Make sure the environment is right. Choose colleagues, partners, supervisors, and friends whom you think will be open, willing to listen, accepting, and supportive.
- Think carefully and discuss with someone else the pros and cons. Think about "what if" situations. "What if I disclose and this happens; how will I feel?"
- Disclose carefully, selectively, and wisely, not impulsively and generally.
- Remember that once you have disclosed personal information, you cannot take it back.

Therapist Overview

Goals of This Session

- To discuss the pros and cons of disclosing that you are in recovery.
- To learn that, if you choose to disclose, it is important to disclose wisely and carefully.
- To choose the time, people, and place to disclose so that your disclosure will help support your recovery.

Session 11 Outline

- **Introduction** (*If Needed*) (5 minutes).
- **Check-in** (15 minutes).
- **Review of Last Week's Skill Practice and Topic** (5 minutes).
- **Presentation of This Week's Topic and Distribution of Topic Overview** (25 minutes): Provide Participant Sheet 11.1.
  - The issue of disclosure: What is it? "To tell or not to tell?"
  - Barriers to disclosure.
  - Potential benefits of disclosure.
  - Some issues that come up with disclosure.
  - Some dos and don'ts of disclosure.
- **Open Discussion** (30 minutes).
- **Wrap-Up and Reading of Take-Home Messages** (2 minutes): Provide Participant Sheet 11.2.
- **Distribution and Description of This Week's Skill Practice** (3 minutes): Provide Participant Sheet 11.3.
- **Check-Out** (5 minutes).

Session-Specific Materials Needed

- Bulletin Board Outline and Take-Home Messages for Session 11.
- Participant Sheet 11.1: The Issue of Disclosure: To Tell or Not to Tell?
- Participant Sheet 11.2: Take-Home Messages.
- Participant Sheet 11.3: Skill Practice: The Issue of Disclosure: To Tell or Not to Tell?

Introduction (If Needed)

As in the previous session, provide an introduction to the group if there are new members.

Check-In

Otherwise, pass around the Check-In Sheet and have each member orally respond to the three check-in questions.

Review of Last Week's Skill Practice and Topic

From the check-in, the therapist should have a sense of who has done the skill practice and commented on whether or not it was helpful. The therapist can build on the check-in by asking if anyone would like to comment on the skill practice and what she learned. The therapist can also comment on the main highlights from last week's topic. The therapist can then transition to presentation of this week's topic.

Presentation of This Week's Topic and Distribution of Topic Overview

The Issue of Disclosure: What Is It? "To Tell or Not to Tell?"

As always, the therapist should try to highlight specific themes from the check-in that related to the day's topic of disclosure. It is possible that this topic did not come up specifically in today's check-in, but it is likely that themes about disclosure have come up before in other group sessions. For example, participants may have discussed whether to tell their partners they are in recovery or have had a substance use problem, how to manage in the workplace, whether to reveal a substance use problem to adult children, or what to do when someone "finds out" unintentionally. The therapist can make the transition to the session topic by saying something like, "Today we are going to talk about the issue of disclosure. Disclosure means telling something important about oneself. In recovery, when we refer to disclosure we're talking about whether to tell or not to tell someone about your substance problem and that you are in recovery. This issue comes up in many different ways for people in recovery." As always, the therapist can use additional details from Participant Sheet 11.1 and from the Background Information above to highlight important points.

The therapist should point out that the issue of disclosure is *personal*, requires *careful thought*, and can be made best in a setting that is emotionally and physically *safe*. Disclosure can be a *choice* or a *necessity*; it can happen *intentionally* or *unintentionally*. For some women in recovery there can be a *dilemma* of *choosing secrecy and control versus getting it out in the open and seeking support*. There is no right answer to disclosure; it is a matter of personal choice. The therapist can invite people to discuss whether they have now or have had in the past a dilemma about "telling or not telling" about their substance problem or about their recovery. After some discussion, the therapist can then go on to discuss the potential barriers to disclosure, the potential benefits, and some of the issues that come up for women thinking about disclosure. The bulletin board materials can be helpful in outlining these points for discussion.

For some people, disclosure is unintentional. For example, a woman's partner may tell their relatives, neighbors, friends, and work colleagues. This may happen for a variety of reasons, including the partner's seeking support for him- or herself or because he or she is angry, or for many other reasons. The woman herself may not have been ready to have others know about her recovery. Unintentional disclosure also could happen in the workplace if a woman shows up to work high or drunk, and is given the opportunity to keep her job as long as she receives treatment. When she returns to work, others in the workplace may know about her illness and recovery even if she did not intend for that to be the case.

Barriers to and Potential Disadvantages of Disclosure

For some, there is a need to decide whether to tell partners, parents, children, friends, acquaintances, or others. The potential barriers to disclosure include fear of discrimination, fear of stigma, fear of loss of custody or other legal proceedings, feelings of shame, giving up a feeling of privacy, and fear of rejection. It is important for the therapist to note that these are possible barriers that can sometimes occur when people disclose.

Potential Benefits of Disclosure

The potential benefits of disclosure include the recognition and acceptance of existing supports, gaining new supports and building new relationships, decreasing isolation, beginning and/or continuing the healing and recovery process, sharing new perspectives/helping others, and obtaining reasonable accommodations in the workplace and sometimes at home as well. For example, some women find it helpful to have a boyfriend/girlfriend, spouse, parents, or close friends know because they can lend support, not ask them if they want to use or to drink, not bring alcohol or drugs to their home, not expect them to drink at a social or family occasion, and so on. In other situations, women find that family or friends are critical of them and make them feel ashamed or self-conscious; these women will find it is best not to tell but instead sometimes to limit contact, have shorter visits, not attend or leave family gatherings or other social events more quickly.

Some Issues That Come Up with Disclosure

Some of the issues that come up about disclosure include how much to disclose; to whom to disclose; to whom is it important *not* to disclose; in what form disclosure is made; and when, why, and where to disclose. After reviewing these issues, it would be helpful then for the therapist to invite discussion by asking something like, "Has anyone experienced any of these issues either on the positive or negative side of disclosure? Do you recognize any of these issues?"

Dos and Don'ts of Disclosure

After some discussion, the therapist might then present the final part of the session topic by reviewing the "dos and don'ts of disclosure." These include:

- Think about your own readiness for and comfort with disclosure.
- Choose carefully to whom you wish to disclose. Emphasize feelings of safety and comfort.
- Make sure the environment is right.

- Think carefully and discuss the pros and cons with someone else you trust. Consider "what if" situations.
- Disclose carefully and wisely, and not impulsively.
- Remember that once you have disclosed personal information, you cannot take it back; if possible, consider and decide in advance, to whom, when, and how you wish to share this information.

Open Discussion

If time permits, as part of the topic presentation or as part of open discussion, the therapist can encourage role playing. She can ask someone to volunteer to be a woman in recovery and someone else to be a boss, family member, partner, etc. The role play could be hypothetical or can take the format of a disclosure issue that was raised by members of the group during the open discussion. If this does not seem appropriate to the group, or if there are other aspects of disclosure that the group is pursuing, open discussion can focus on these. As always, the open discussion time may also focus on other recovery issues, including any issues that were raised during the check-in.

Wrap-Up and Reading of Take-Home Messages

The therapist should summarize themes of disclosure that have come up during the group discussion both in terms of not disclosing because of shame or stigma and in terms of disclosing to gain support. If individuals have brought up disclosures they or others have made that were not helpful (or were hurtful), the therapist can summarize these here as well. The therapist can emphasize that considering how and when to disclose should be done thoughtfully so that the participant can best help her own recovery. As in previous sessions, distribute this week's Take-Home Messages (Participant Sheet 11.2), and review them by having members each read one of the messages in turn.

Distribution and Description of This Week's Skill Practice

Distribute this week's Skill Practice Sheet (Participant Sheet 11.3). This week's skill practice will ask participants to answer specific questions about experiences with disclosure if they have already disclosed their substance problems, treatment, and recovery to family, friends, or employers/coworkers (Questions 1–3). It will also ask participants if they have not yet disclosed but are considering disclosing to explore their thoughts and feelings about this (Questions 4–7).

Check-Out

Pass around the Check-Out Sheet and ask participants each to answer orally the one-question check-out. Thank members and tell them you will see them next time.

Substance Use
and Women's Reproductive Health

This session reviews the interaction of substances and women's health including women's reproductive health and the interaction of substances and hormonal changes during the menstrual cycle, pregnancy, and menopause. In addition, this session addresses the issue of safe sex and using protection to keep women healthy and to avoid transmission of sexually transmitted diseases (STDs) including HIV and hepatitis B and C, among others. As always, in preparing for this session, the therapist should review the detailed "Background Information" on the topic. In addition, the therapist should familiarize herself with the manual "Safer Sex Skills Building for Women," available from the NIDA (details below). During the session, the therapist can then use the Therapist Overview as a guide for presenting this topic.

Background Information

While substance use and substance problems can occur at any time in the life cycle, they are most common during the reproductive years, when women experience menstrual cycles, pregnancies, and the transition to menopause. Between the onset of menstrual cycles (average age 11 years) and menopause (average age 51 years), women experience monthly fluctuations in their hormone levels as part of the menstrual cycle. During the reproductive years, women who choose to have children also experience the hormonal changes of pregnancy and the postpartum period. During the menopause transition, women's hormones change markedly as menstrual cycles become unpredictable and then stop. For some women, mood problems and significant stress accompany these reproductive life events. Patterns of substance use and substance problems may change during these life events, and the hormonal changes that occur may influence the effects that substances have on women.

Before I discuss the relationship between substances problems and women's reproductive life cycle, I review the hormonal changes that occur during the major reproductive life stages in women's lives.

Menstrual Cycles

The average menstrual cycle is 28–32 days in length, with 3–7 days of menstrual bleeding. By convention, the first day of bleeding is considered Day 1. Ovulation occurs 14 days prior to the start of a menstrual bleed (e.g., in a 30-day cycle, ovulation occurs on Day 16). The *follicular phase* is the term given to the phase of the menstrual cycle between the start of menstrual bleeding and ovulation, and the *luteal phase* refers to the phase of the menstrual cycle between ovulation and the start of the next menstrual bleed. When estradiol (the strongest estrogen), progesterone, luteinizing hormone (LH), and follicle-stimulating hormone (FSH) rise and fall across the cycle, these hormonal changes effect the entire body, including the brain.

The "premenstrual" phase is usually considered to be the 7 days before onset of bleeding. It is during this premenstrual week that many women experience mild mood changes or physical discomfort (premenstrual mood syndrome [PMS]). In addition, a smaller number of women (approximately 3–8% of the population) experience severe mood problems, including depression and irritability (premenstrual dysphoric disorder [PMDD]). During the menstrual period, some women experience severe menstrual cramps (or dysmenorrhea). Problematic menstrual cramps are particularly severe in teenage girls, but painful periods can persist into adulthood.

There are a number of different reasons why menstrual cycles can become unpredictable and irregular in some women. Common reasons include pregnancy, breastfeeding, transition to menopause ("perimenopause"), and hormonal disorders, such as increased levels of the hormone prolactin. Excessive exercise, extreme weight loss that may occur in illnesses such as anorexia nervosa or other medical illnesses, and severe stress can also cause irregular cycles. Prescribed medications and addictive substances are other causes of irregular periods. When menstrual cycles are irregular, ovulation usually does not occur on a regular basis. This can make it difficult to get pregnant.

Birth Control Medications

Most birth control medications, or oral contraceptives, include a combination of estrogen and progesterone that is taken for 3 weeks and followed by a placebo, which is taken during the fourth week. Menstrual bleeding occurs during the fourth (placebo) week. Estradiol and progesterone levels are extremely high during the 3 weeks of active medication and then drop significantly during the placebo week. These hormonal changes affect the entire body, including the brain.

Pregnancy and the Postpartum Period

Estradiol and progesterone levels rise as pregnancy progresses and peak immediately before delivery. Estradiol and progesterone levels both drop substantially within the first few days after delivery. During pregnancy, another hormone, prolactin, also increases, but it remains elevated during the first few postpartum months. Prolactin is one of the hormones that is necessary for breastfeeding. Menstrual cycles can be skipped during the first few postpartum months, especially with breastfeeding, because of increased prolactin levels. This, however, does not mean that women cannot become pregnant following the postpartum period when ovulation and periods are irregular, so birth control is warranted to avoid unintended pregnancy during this time.

The fetus develops throughout pregnancy, starting immediately after conception. Many women do not know that they are pregnant until 2 or 3 weeks or more after conception, so significant exposure of the fetus to substances (including alcohol and nicotine) may occur even before women know they are pregnant. Most substances taken by pregnant women cross the placenta so that the fetus is exposed to them. During the first trimester, the major organs and body parts (e.g., heart, spinal cord, kidneys, limbs) of the fetus are formed. The brain continues to develop throughout the entire pregnancy and during the first 25 years of life. Substances taken during the first trimester have the potential to cause problems with organ development. Substances taken after the first trimester can have adverse effects on brain development, which can lead to learning and behavioral problems in children. Substances taken while breastfeeding can influence childhood development because many substances will be passed on to the baby through breast milk.

Menopause Transition

Menopause is reached when a woman has no periods for 12 months and the hormonal changes of menopause occur. The hormonal changes of menopause include a gradual increase in FSH levels and a decrease in estradiol levels. However, highly erratic levels of estradiol and FSH usually accompany the perimenopause, which precedes menopause. The hormonal changes of the perimenopause and menopause are experienced by the entire body, including the brain. During the years prior to menopause, most women experience several years of irregular periods, in which menstrual cycles become more frequent (e.g., shortening from 28 to 25 days) and then are skipped and occur only every few months. During this time, vasomotor symptoms or hot flashes are very common. The most common initial symptoms of menopause are hot flashes and are experienced by approximately two-thirds of women in the United States. Hot flashes are caused by lowered levels of estrogen and subsequent irregular bursts of gonadotropin-releasing hormone that affects the center in the brain that controls body temperature. Women experience a sensation of heat and perspiration that can last several minutes, may be accompanied by soaking sweats, and followed by chills. Hot flashes at night can interrupt sleep repeatedly. Many women find that the sleep disruption associated with hot flashes is bothersome, leading to daytime fatigue and irritability.

After menopause, menstrual periods stop, but hot flashes and sleep problems can persist. These menopausal symptoms usually subside within the first 2 years after the final menstrual period. Postmenopausal women have extremely low levels of estradiol and high FSH levels. In postmenopausal women, hormone levels no longer change, and the brain therefore stops experiencing changing levels. In the past, women were often prescribed hormone replacement therapy (HRT), which is usually a combination of estrogen and progesterone, during and after the menopause transition. HRT typically stabilizes the amount of estrogen and progesterone in the body and the brain. However, in two studies published in 2003, as well as in subsequent studies, the benefits of long-term HRT were called into question by new research findings, and many women were withdrawn from the treatment (Aderson, Judd, Kaunitz, Barad, Beresford, et al., 2003) . The current status of HRT for perimenopausal transition continues to be investigated.

Influence of Menstrual Cycle on the Amount of Substances Used

Some women report that they drink more alcohol during the week prior to the menstrual period (premenstrual). Alcohol use may increase premenstrually because of increased stress and mood problems, including severe PMS symptoms or PMDD. Many women attribute the premenstrual increase in alcohol use to a greater need for relaxation. An alternative explanation is that alcohol is processed differently premenstrually, which alters its effects and leads women to drink more during this time. If we look at blood levels of alcohol only, we would expect women to drink less alcohol premenstrually because alcohol blood levels are highest premenstrually. However, the variation in blood alcohol levels across the menstrual cycle may make it difficult for some women to predict how intoxicated they will be at different phases of their cycle.

We have less information about the effects of the menstrual cycle on other substances. The amount of marijuana smoked does not seem to vary across the menstrual cycle. Likewise, blood levels of benzodiazepines (e.g., minor tranquilizers) do not vary across the menstrual cycle. However, higher cocaine levels occur in the follicular than in the luteal phase (Terner & De Wit, 2006). In addition, some studies indicate that women may have greater success with quitting nicotine use in the follicular than in the luteal phase (Franklin et al., 2008).

Menstrual Irregularities and Altered Hormone Levels Caused by Substances

Some women with severe alcohol use disorders have irregular menstrual cycles or amenorrhea (no menstrual periods). Alcohol can cause menstrual problems by interfering with ovulation and disrupting hormones required for regular menstrual cycles. In premenopausal women, alcohol increases estradiol and prolactin levels and decreases progesterone levels. The higher prolactin levels in women drinking alcohol may be the cause of menstrual problems. It is not known how frequently alcohol use disorders lead to menstrual cycle irregularities.

Cocaine, marijuana, opioids, and possibly benzodiazepines can also cause menstrual cycle irregularities because they can interfere with ovulation and hormones, such as prolactin. It is not known how often dependence on these substances leads to menstrual cycle irregularities.

Safer Sex and Protection for Prevention of STDs, Including HIV

Regardless of a woman's hormonal status or intentions regarding pregnancy, it is important for her to learn about safer sex and protection and to use protection (e.g., condoms) for intimate sexual behavior. The use of condoms during heterosexual intercourse is a very important protection for women for prevention of HIV, hepatitis C, and other sexually transmitted diseases. Women can ask about and discuss the proper use of condoms and how to introduce them into their relationships with their internists, health care providers, therapists, and other health care clinicians. This is an important part of self-care. A manual-based treatment called "Safer Sex Skills Building (SSSB) for Women" has had good results in clinical trials (Tross et al., 2008) and is free and available for download on the NIDA website (*http://ctndisseminationlibrary.org/display/398.htm*). The SSSB for women has been designated a promising-evidence intervention by the Centers for Disease Control and Prevention (*http://www.cdc.gov/hiv/prevention/research/compendium/rr/complete.html*). The goal of the SSSB for Women intervention is to help women change behaviors that put them at risk of becoming infected with HIV (and other STDs) and to help women live healthy lifestyles. The intervention focuses on the importance of changing high-risk behaviors and teaches social and technical skills necessary to keep women from engaging in these high-risk behaviors.

Risks of Harmful Effects of Alcohol and Drug Use on the Pregnant Woman and Growing Fetus

The effects of drugs and alcohol on hormones and ovulation can make it difficult for women to get pregnant. Specifically, cocaine and marijuana are known to reduce fertility. Pregnant women who continue to use marijuana, cocaine, or alcohol are more likely to have a miscarriage than pregnant women who do not use these substances in pregnancy.

Many substances are known to cross the placenta and have potential to cause significant problems for the developing fetus. Here are some of the most notable effects on the fetus and longer term effects on development:

- Alcohol can cause fetal alcohol syndrome (FAS), which includes mental retardation, facial abnormalities, low birth weight, and other organ problems.
- Marijuana may be associated with low birth weight.
- Cocaine can cause premature delivery, miscarriage, rupture of blood vessels in the placenta (requiring emergent delivery and can lead to death of the fetus), and death of the pregnant woman. Cocaine can also lead to strokes (bleeding into the brain) in the fetus, problems with formation of several different organ systems, severe behavioral problems, and sudden infant death syndrome.
- Nicotine exposure during pregnancy has been associated with low birth weight.
- Heroin and other opioid use during pregnancy is associated with pregnancy complications such as preterm delivery and has also been associated with birth defects. Children exposed to heroin and other opioids can also have low birth weight as well as opioid withdrawal (e.g., neonatal abstinence syndrome) shortly after delivery, requiring treatment at birth.
- Benzodiazepines taken near to delivery can lead to sleepy babies; respiratory depression, which can put them at risk for breathing problems; and withdrawal symptoms in the first few days of life. There is evidence that certain benzodiazepines taken during pregnancy may be associated with cleft lip or cleft palate.

This is not an exhaustive or complete review of all of the evidence for the risks that drugs and alcohol have on the developing fetus or in development, in part because information on the short-term and longer term outcomes changes rapidly. Because of this, it is advisable to discuss the potential effects of any substance on fetal development with a physician. However, it is clear that there are potentially harmful effects on the pregnancy and fetal development either directly (e.g., direct effects on the fetus or the placenta) or indirectly (e.g., decreased likelihood of prenatal care) that can be caused by alcohol and drugs.

Because of the substantial risk of harm to the fetus, many women with substance problems will stop using alcohol and drugs during their pregnancy. However, some women are unable to stop and put themselves and their pregnancy at risk for health problems. Even women who do stop using drugs and alcohol when they learn they are pregnant may have inadvertently put the fetus at risk because they used substances before they knew they were pregnant. Discussion with your health care professional (e.g., your doctor, nurse, therapist) about avoiding pregnancy if you are using substances, getting treatment to stop using substances if you are intending to get pregnant, getting treatment for substance problems if you learn you are pregnant, and seeking help for yourself for substance problems and prenatal care if pregnant are very important types of self-care.

Effects of Alcohol and Drugs on Breastfeeding Infants

Many drugs and alcohol can be passed on to the infant through breast milk and can therefore affect the development of the baby. Little is known about potential long-term effects of exposure to certain substances through breastfeeding, but there is some information about immediate effects on breastfed infants. Alcohol can lead to sluggishness and problems with muscle development and muscle tone. Cocaine can cause irritability, vomiting, diarrhea, tremor, and seizure. High doses of benzodiazepines can lead to sleepiness in the infant. Any substance that causes sleepiness and sluggishness in babies can lead to breathing problems.

The Postpartum Period

It is also important to note that there are many changes in hormonal levels in women in the postpartum period. Most women have minor mood changes, the so-called baby blues, but a minority of women will have a major depression or postpartum depression. For some women these mood changes, whether minor or major, may be triggers to use substances or to relapse if a woman was already in recovery. It is important for women to seek treatment for postpartum depression and to report these mood changes to their doctor. In addition, for some women, the pregnancy provided a motivation to get clean and sober because they did not want to harm the pregnancy or developing fetus. They may feel that the pregnancy itself made them feel like not drinking or using drugs. However, once the baby is born, some women may find it harder to stay in recovery. All of these things may create a risk for relapse.

Contraceptive Medications Alter How Some Substances Are Metabolized

Women who take birth control or oral contraceptive pills (OCPs) metabolize alcohol and benzodiazepines more slowly than women who do not take OCPs. We therefore expect that women on an OCP are likely to have higher blood levels of alcohol and benzodiazepines than those not using an OCP. The effects of benzodiazepines on memory can be greater when women are taking an OCP medication.

Effect of Drugs and Alcohol on Menopause

Alcohol use disorders may lead to earlier menopause. Little is known about whether menopausal women drink more alcohol or increase their use of other substances during the menopause transition. However, although the research literature on this topic is sparse, clinically it is observed that some women find themselves having mood changes during menopause, which are likely associated with the hormonal fluctuations of menopause. In response to these mood changes, women who are already in recovery may find themselves feeling more triggered to use substances. Women in this age group who have not had histories of substance problems may increase their use of alcohol or other substances, sometimes in response to life events. It is unclear whether changes in patterns of use are related to menopause.

Alcohol Use Increases the Risk of Breast Cancer

High estradiol levels are a risk factor for breast cancer, and alcohol increases estradiol. Therefore, alcohol use may increase a woman's risk for developing breast cancer. Women who are heavy drinkers are at greater risk for developing breast cancer than women who do not drink alcohol. There is recent evidence that even low to moderate alcohol intake can increase a woman's risk for breast cancer.

What Can You Do about the Effects Drugs and Alcohol Have on Your Health and the Effects of Reproductive Life Events on Your Use of Substances?

Women may identify with all or some of these issues or they may not have experienced any of these reproductive health issues. By being in the WRG, women have expressed an interest in learning about how SUDs affect their well-being and how they can make the best and healthiest choices for themselves. Understanding the relationship between reproductive health and substance problems can help women to identify major concerns as they strive to maintain abstinence from substances and continue in recovery.

What Can Women Do about Their Reproductive Health to Support Their Recovery?

- *Know your body.* Keep track of your menstrual cycle patterns and premenstrual symptoms. Simple daily charting of your cycles and associated mood and physical symptoms can give you tremendous insight into the way your body works. Some women may not realize that their menstrual cycles have changed since they started having problems with alcohol and drugs. In addition, many women are not aware of the extent to which menstrual or premenstrual symptoms (e.g., cramps, pain, PMS, mood swings) influence their use of substances.
- *Seek professional help.* Gynecologists, primary care doctors, and endocrinologists can help you to regulate your menstrual periods and understand why your periods may be abnormal. Similarly, treatment is available for perimenopausal and menopausal symptoms. If you are pregnant, it is important to seek treatment for your SUD and to seek

regular prenatal care during the pregnancy to help have the healthiest pregnancy and delivery.

- *Practice safer sex.* Use protection when having intimate sexual relations to protect yourself from HIV, hepatitis C, and other STDs. Use the Safer Sex Skills Building (SSSB) for Women to help build skills for negotiating safer sex with your partner.
- *Use contraception.* Avoiding unplanned pregnancies is critical for women trying to maintain sobriety and establishing a stable environment for continued recovery.
- *Learn.* Seek information about your reproductive health and how it can be affected by alcohol and drugs.

Therapist Overview

Goals of This Session

- To learn that substances can affect women's hormones and health.
- To learn about changes in hormones over the life cycle that can also affect women's substance use.
- If you are of childbearing age, to learn that avoiding unplanned pregnancies can be important to maintaining sobriety and having a stable situation for continued recovery, as well as planning for a healthy pregnancy.
- To learn that practicing safer sex can help keep women healthy and avoid STDs, including HIV and hepatitis B and C, among others.
- To discover that knowing your body, learning more about hormones and health, practicing safer sex, and seeking professional help can be useful in keeping yourself healthy and managing hormonal changes at all stages of life.

Session 12 Outline

- **Introduction (*If Needed*)** (5 minutes).
- **Check-In** (15 minutes).
- **Review of Last Week's Skill Practice and Topic** (5 minutes).
- **Presentation of This Week's Topic and Distribution of Topic Overview** (25 minutes): Provide Participant Sheet 12.1.
  - Major Reproductive Life Events in Women.
    - Menstrual cycles.
    - Pregnancy and the postpartum period.
    - Menopause transition.
  - Menstrual cycles, reproductive hormones, and substance-related issues.
  - Risks of substance use in pregnancy, breastfeeding, and the postpartum period.
  - Safer sex and protection from STDs including HIV and hepatitis B and C.
  - What you can do about your reproductive health and your recovery.

- **Open Discussion** (30 minutes).
- **Wrap-Up and Reading of Take-Home Messages** (2 minutes): Provide Participant Sheet 12.2.
- **Distribution and Description of This Week's Skill Practice** (3 minutes): Provide Participant Sheet 12.3.
- **Check-Out** (5 minutes).

Session-Specific Materials Needed

- Bulletin Board Outline and Take-Home Messages for Session 12.
- Participant Sheet 12.1: Substance Use and Women's Reproductive Health.
- Participant Sheet 12.2: Take-Home Messages.
- Participant Sheet 12.3: Skill Practice: Substance Use and Women's Reproductive Health.

Introduction (If Needed)

As in the previous session, provide an introduction to the group if there are new members.

Check-In

Pass around the Check-In Sheet and have each member respond orally to the three check-in questions.

Review of Last Week's Skill Practice and Topic

From the check-in, the therapist should have a sense of who has done the skill practice and commented on whether or not it was helpful. The therapist can build on the check-in by asking if anyone would like to comment on the skill practice and what she learned. The therapist can also comment on the main highlights from last week's topic. The therapist can then transition to presentation of this week's topic.

Presentation of This Week's Session Topic and Distribution of Topic Overview

The therapist should first distribute the topic overview (Participant Sheet 12.1). She should then summarize any themes that have come up during the check-in or in previous sessions regarding hormonal changes and the way these might relate to substance use. For example, participants may have discussed premenstrual dysphoria as a trigger for substance use or changes in peri-menopause or menopause and its relationship to substance use. The therapist can say something like, "There is a complicated relationship between hormonal changes through the life cycle and women's substance use. Today's session will attempt to summarize and discuss some of these and to talk about women's reproductive health through the lifespan."

Major Reproductive Life Events in Women

The therapist should explain relatively briefly that SUDs can occur at any time in the life cycle, but are most common during the reproductive years when women experience menstrual cycles, pregnancies, and the transition to menopause. Between the onset of menstrual cycles (average age 11 years) and menopause (average age 51 years), women experience monthly fluctuations in their hormone levels as part of the menstrual cycle. During the reproductive years, women who have children also experience the hormonal changes of pregnancy and the postpartum period. During the menopause transition, women's hormones change markedly as menstrual cycles become unpredictable and then stop. For some women, mood problems and significant stress accompany these reproductive life events. Patterns of substance use may change during these life events, and the hormonal changes that occur may influence the effects that substances have on women.

The therapist can briefly review the hormonal changes that occur during the major reproductive life events in women including (1) menstrual cycles, (2) oral contraceptive medications, (3) pregnancy and the postpartum period, and (4) menopause transition. The therapist can provide basic information regarding hormonal changes that affect women throughout the life cycle. She should first review the menstrual cycle and the *follicular phase* (approximately first 14 days of the cycle from the first day of menses up to the day of ovulation) and the *luteal phase* (from the day of ovulation to the first day of the menses) as well as the premenstruum (the 7 days before the onset of bleeding). During the menstrual cycle there are fluctuations in reproductive hormones including estradiol, progesterone, luteinizing hormone (LH), and follicle-stimulating hormone (FSH). The rise and fall of these hormonal levels affect the entire body including the brain.

Next she should review hormonal changes during pregnancy and the postpartum period and use of oral contraceptives. The therapist can discuss that during the pregnancy and postpartum phase there are also profound changes in the levels of these hormones. Oral contraceptive medications usually include a combination of estrogen and progesterone. Women may be prescribed oral contraception to prevent pregnancies, to help regulate periods, or for other reasons. It is important to work with your health care provider to find the right oral contraceptive for you. It is also important to realize that oral contraception does not prevent the transmission of STDs such as HIV, hepatitis B and C, among others. Using protection (e.g., condoms) is important for safer sex. Finally, the therapist should describe hormonal changes during the perimenopause and menopause, which include a decrease in estrogen levels and an increase in FSH. When a woman has not had periods for 12 months she is considered to have entered menopause. As with pregnancy and the postpartum period, the changes in reproductive hormones during perimenopause and menopause are experienced by the entire body including the brain. The menopause transition can be short (under a year) or long (several years) and women's experiences vary. The menopause transition, or perimenopause, may be accompanied by a variety of symptoms including hot flashes (e.g., vasomotor symptoms) that can cause considerable physical discomfort for some women including sleep disruption. There are a variety of treatments that can be useful and women can seek treatment from their primary care physician, clinician, gynecologist, or other health care professional. The therapist can then pause and ask if anyone has any questions about these hormonal changes or other questions about women's reproductive health or these reproductive stages of women's lives.

Menstrual Cycles, Reproductive Hormones, and Substance-Related Issues

The therapist can then go on to present information on the relationship of substance use to women's hormonal status and reproductive life-cycle events. She can note that some women experience cravings and increased use of substances during the premenstruum or premenstrual phase (e.g., approximately 7 days before menses). This is particularly the case for alcohol, though there is some information available regarding how the premenstruum may affect cravings for other substances. The therapist can pause and ask if anyone has experienced changes in cravings or use during the premenstrual phase or during other reproductive life stages (e.g., perimenopause or menopausal transition).

The therapist can then go on to discuss how substance use can cause menstrual cycle irregularities. Women with severe alcohol use disorders can have irregular menstrual cycles or no menstrual periods at all (amenorrhea). In addition, cocaine, marijuana, opioids, and possibly benzodiazepines can also cause menstrual-cycle irregularities. These irregularities can influence women's ability to become pregnant. Furthermore, women who do become pregnant while using substances may be more likely to have a miscarriage. Also of concern is the fact that many substances cross the placenta and can cause problems for the developing fetus. In particular, alcohol and tobacco are associated with adverse fetal effects. Cocaine can also lead to adverse events in pregnancy, and certain benzodiazepines are associated with congenital abnormalities in the fetus. In addition, opioids and other drugs may lead to neonatal abstinence syndrome (NAS) (e.g., withdrawal from substances in the newborn).

Risks of Substance Use in Pregnancy, Breastfeeding, and the Postpartum Period

Pregnancy can be used as a motivation for women to become abstinent and be in recovery. Prenatal care is very important for both the mother and the developing fetus. After the birth of a newborn, significant support and ongoing treatment can help the mother maintain abstinence and remain in recovery. The postpartum period also brings significant hormonal changes that can lead to changes in mood, so it can be a period of vulnerability for women with regard to both mood disorders and relapse to substances. Support for this life transition, as well as treatment for mood symptoms and relapse prevention, can be helpful to women trying to make this transition and remain in, or begin, recovery. Asking for help if you are pregnant and need support to enter treatment to stop using drugs or support to remain abstinent, as well as to seek prenatal care, is very important for women's health and well-being. In addition, asking your doctor or therapist for help if you are having mood difficulties or cravings or urges to use drugs in the postpartum period (e.g., after the baby is born) is important for a woman's mental and physical health as well as the health of her baby. The therapist can pause and ask if anyone has experiences like these she wishes to share or if these experiences are familiar.

Safer Sex and Protection for Prevention of STDs, Including HIV

Regardless of hormonal status or intentions regarding pregnancy it is important for women to learn about safer sex and protection and to use protection (e.g., condoms) for intimate sexual behavior. The use of condoms during heterosexual intercourse (vaginal and anal) is very important for protection for prevention of HIV, hepatitis C, and other STDs. It is important to ask about and discuss with their therapists, internists, or other clinicians the proper use of condoms and how to introduce them into their intimate relationships. It is important for women who are sexually active to learn how to discuss condom use with male partners and to feel empowered to learn how to use condoms, why to use condoms, and how to discuss condom use with male partners so that condoms are used properly and women are protective of their health and well-being. One excellent resource that is in the Participant Sheet is the manual "Safer Sex Skills Building for Women." It can be downloaded without cost from the National Institute on Drug Abuse (see website in additional materials and participant overview). This helps women change behaviors that put them at risk for becoming infected with HIV (and other STDs) by focusing on changing high-risk behaviors and teaching social and technical skills to help prevent these high-risk behaviors. The therapist should familiarize herself with this manual and may discuss any of the skills with the group in the manual that are clinically appropriate for this specific group. For some groups, more time in this session may be spent focusing on safer sex skills building.

What Can You Do about Your Reproductive Health and Your Recovery?

After inviting discussion of the points made above, the therapist can then discuss what women can do about the impact that substances can have on health and reproductive life-cycle events. One aspect of self-care is for women to learn about their own bodies' patterns, including menstrual cycle patterns and premenstrual symptoms or perimenopause or menopausal symptoms. Women can track changes in their patterns, especially those that might occur in the presence of substance use. Another aspect of self-care is to seek professional help from primary care doctors, gynecologists, and other health professionals to understand any changes in their menstrual cycle and any other health concerns. Women can take care of themselves by using contraception to avoid unplanned pregnancies. In addition, practicing safer sex can help women avoid STDs, including HIV and others. Finally, good self-care includes women learning as much as they can about their bodies, their physical health and reproductive health, how substances can affect their health, and how recovery can help them stay well and be as healthy as possible.

Open Discussion

During open discussion, women may continue to pursue any aspect of today's topic. Women may have questions about their reproductive health and may explore experiences in the past as well as current experiences or concerns for their health now or in the future. As always, the open discussion time may also focus on other recovery issues, including any issues that were raised during the check-in.

Wrap-Up and Reading of Take-Home Messages

As always, the therapist should summarize any themes she has heard during the discussion related to this topic. She can then remind participants that taking care of their health is a major part of self-care and recovery. In particular, using protection and safer sex to prevent STDs including HIV is important. Seeking health care from primary care physicians and other health care professionals to evaluate any concerns regarding menstrual irregularities, menopausal symptoms, or other concerns is also important. Distribute Participant Sheet 12.2, and the take-home messages can then be reviewed by having members each read one of the messages in turn.

Distribution and Description of This Week's Skill Practice

Distribute this week's Skill Practice Sheet (Participant Sheet 12.3). This week's skill practice will ask participants to write down two reproductive health issues they have had that they think affected their patterns of using substances. It also asks participants to write down one thing they plan to do differently in their recovery with regard to their reproductive health.

Check-Out

Pass around the check-out sheet and ask participants each to answer orally the one-question check-out. Thank members and tell them you will see them next time.

Can You Have Fun
without Using Drugs or Alcohol?

The purpose of this session is to help women consider this aspect of "repair work." The central recovery rule of the WRG is that Recovery = Relapse Prevention and Repair Work. In other sessions, the group has focused on relapse prevention by identifying triggers and high-risk situations, obstacles to recovery, and stressors, and considered ways for developing skills and alternative coping strategies to manage these problems without using substances. As women engage in treatment and pursue recovery, they are confronted with considering ways to "repair" their lives. This often means finding ways to enjoy themselves without using alcohol or drugs. Especially early in recovery, women may find this goal a difficult task. In preparing for this session, the therapist should read the "Background Information" that follows, which contains additional detail relating to this topic.

Background Information

Recovery is hard work. Although each woman's recovery path is different, many women experience recovery (especially early-on) as effortful and requiring great time, energy, emotional commitment, and focus. In addition, often women in recovery are simultaneously experiencing losses. For example, once in recovery, women may begin to acknowledge and fully experience losses related to their prior substance problems (e.g., loss of partners, spouses, jobs, friends, children, possessions, and health). Additionally, in order to become clean and sober, each woman has to deal with the loss of the substance itself. Women may also find that they need to avoid people, places, and things that trigger their craving or place them at high risk to use. As a result, they may find that they have had to give up a partner who continued to use, close friends or a social network of people who used, places they liked to go where they used alcohol or drugs, going to parties or social events, entertaining, and so on.

At some point, women in recovery may wonder if it is all hard work and whether they ever will be able to enjoy themselves again. This session explores balancing the work of recovery (i.e., avoiding triggers, using coping strategies, attending treatment) with finding satisfaction and even fun in one's life.

The Work of Recovery

Recovery work includes both relapse prevention and repair work. Relapse prevention consists of all of the work that you do to identify triggers and high-risk situations in advance, plan to avoid them, and develop alternative ways to cope with them rather than using substances. Relapse prevention work also includes trying to make your environment as trigger-free as possible. This may mean making sure your home is an alcohol- and drug-free zone or changing work or social patterns so that you are not in high-risk environments. Relapse prevention also includes getting treatment for other disorders you may have (e.g., depression, anxiety) and attending treatment sessions and self-help groups to support your recovery.

Repair work focuses on repairing damage to self and relationships that may have occurred because of substances. This may mean working with a therapist to understand feelings of low self-worth, including the past life experiences that may have contributed to them. It may also mean repairing damage to close relationships with partners, children, family, or friends that may have occurred as a consequence of substance problems. This work may take place in a number of ways including in the context of individual, family, or couple therapy.

Focusing on all of these tasks simultaneously can often lead women to feel that it is hard to resume previous activities that were satisfying or fun. A second part of repair work is learning to enjoy your life substance-free.

Enjoying Your Life in Recovery

There are a number of areas of concern for women in recovery. Here are some questions about events or activities that can raise concerns for women who want to participate but are worried about their ability to do so and remain alcohol- and drug-free:

"Can I ever entertain people in my own home?"
"Can I attend a ball game or other sporting event?"
"Can I attend a music festival?"
"What should I do at the winter holidays, New Year's Eve, etc.?"
"How can I have the Memorial Day or July 4th barbecue at my house as I usually do without alcohol or drugs? Can I attend the Memorial Day or July 4th event I usually attend?"
"How can I see my friends/colleagues/coworkers when they always get together in a bar or always use when they are together?"
"Can I go to my book group (or other social gathering) if everyone drinks at our meetings?"
"What if I have to attend a lot of work meetings, receptions, etc., where alcohol is served?"
"I liked to go to jazz clubs or other music venues or clubs to relax, but there was always a lot of alcohol, cocaine, etc., around. Now what?"
"We always watch the Super Bowl at my house and serve beer. Now what?"
"All my friends use. They say they don't mind if I don't, but what if I'm not confident I can be with them and not use?"

"Everyone in my school drinks or uses drugs. How can I have a social life? How can I have friends and not use alcohol or drugs?"

"My nephew's wedding is coming up. There is always a lot of alcohol around. What do I do? What about toasts?"

"There is a lot of drug use where I live (my neighbors, people on my street). How can I avoid that and *not* be completely isolated in my house/apartment/room?"

These questions are not meant to be exhaustive but rather to be representative of the types of concerns that are often raised by people in recovery. There are a number of strategies that can be useful. *First*, identify the situations that place you at such high risk that you feel it would be impossible for you to participate, and realize that these situations most likely need to be avoided. It is important to note that avoidance of these situations may only be temporary (e.g., in early recovery when craving is high) or may persist over time. If there is something you must participate in and you know that it places you at high risk, several strategies are available. One is to bring someone with you who knows that you are not using and will support you and be with you. The other is to limit the amount of time you spend at the activity or to limit the event to the minimum essential activity (e.g., attend the wedding ceremony and skip the reception), and develop an exit strategy to leave when you need to go. Remember that sometimes these situations represent high risk early in recovery but that can change over time.

Second, there may be events and activities that could be high risk, but you can learn how to manage them and to *enjoy the actual event or activity* without substances. There are a number of strategies that may be useful. Again, these are not meant to be exhaustive but representative. These may not apply to everyone, and they may not apply to anyone all the time.

- At a dinner party or in a restaurant, turn your wine glass over. The server will usually take it away and not ask if you want alcohol.
- When you go to a reception or party or bar, as soon as you arrive get a nonalcoholic beverage to put in your hand. People will usually stop trying to give you alcoholic drinks.
- Attend sporting events, jazz clubs, musical events, other social events, etc., with at least one other person who knows about and is supportive of your recovery. Some music festivals now have "sober tents" where people in recovery can enjoy the music free from alcohol or drugs.
- Practice "substance refusal lines," such as "No, I can't smoke that because I am just getting over a lung infection" or "I am taking a medicine I can't use with alcohol" or "I'm not drinking anymore because of my health," or "I am trying to get healthy so I am not using that anymore," etc. Find some lines that flow off your tongue easily, and practice saying them.
- Make your own home a "substance-free zone." Begin "training" people who are frequent visitors to know that there isn't any alcohol, marijuana, or other substances in your home. If they want to see you, they'll come anyway. For most people without a substance problem, this is not an issue. If alcohol has been the issue, serve a variety of other cold and sparkling nonalcoholic drinks.
- Many colleges have dormitories that are alcohol- and drug-free and students living in them make a commitment not to use.

Third, there may be some activities that you find you really can't do or some people with whom you find you can't associate, and they may need to be given up. If this is the case, it is important to think of other activities, people, and events that you enjoy and begin to spend some of your leisure and free time engaging in these activities. For many women in recovery, there is a gain in possible recreational or family time because hours spent using or recovering from use are now freed up. You may find that you develop or rediscover interests that could not be pursued or had been given up because of using. Finally, women sometimes discover that there were people or activities or events that were only enjoyable while intoxicated. These are often most easily given up, but sometimes finding other activities that feel satisfying is more challenging.

The most important thing to remember is that slowly but surely it is possible to find yourself having fun and feeling satisfied with life in recovery. It may take some time and sorting out, but it *can happen*.

Therapist Overview

Goals of This Session

- To discuss having fun in your life while in recovery.
- To learn some strategies that will help women enjoy their lives, relationships, and social events drug- and alcohol-free.
- To practice and role play drug and alcohol refusal lines.

Session 13 Outline

- **Introduction** (*If Needed*) (5 minutes).
- **Check-In** (15 minutes).
- **Review of Last Week's Skill Practice and Topic** (5 minutes).
- **Presentation of This Week's Topic and Distribution of Topic Overview** (25 minutes): Provide Participant Sheet 13.1.
  - The work of recovery.
  - Enjoying your life in recovery.
  - Strategies for social settings.
- **Open Discussion** (30 minutes).
- **Wrap-Up and Reading of Take-Home Messages** (2 minutes): Provide Participant Sheet 13.2.
- **Distribution and Description of This Week's Skill Practice** (3 minutes): Provide Participant Sheet 13.3.
- **Check-Out** (5 minutes).

Session-Specific Materials Needed

- Bulletin Board Outline and Take-Home Messages for Session 13.
- Participant Sheet 13.1: Can You Have Fun without Using Drugs or Alcohol?

- Participant Sheet 13.2: Take-Home Messages.
- Participant Sheet 13.3: Skill Practice: Can you have fun without using drugs or alcohol?

Introduction (If Needed)

As in the previous session, provide an introduction to the group if there are new members.

Check-In

Pass around the Check-In Sheet and have each member respond orally to the three check-in questions.

Review of Last Week's Skill Practice and Topic

From the check-in, the therapist should have a sense of who has done the skill practice and commented on whether or not it was helpful. The therapist can build on the check-in by asking if anyone would like to comment on the skill practice and what she learned. The therapist can also comment on the main highlights from last week's topic. The therapist can then transition to presentation of this week's topic.

Presentation of This Week's Topic and Distribution of Topic Overview

The therapist should first distribute the topic overview (Participant Sheet 13.1). As always, the therapist should try to highlight specific themes from the check-in that relate to the day's topic of how to have fun and be in recovery. Insofar as participants have discussed issues in their own lives about how to attend social events or family parties, see friends, or go to work events and remain drug- and alcohol-free, the therapist can summarize these issues and say that these fit in well with today's topic. The therapist should use the bulletin board to highlight important points.

The Work of Recovery

The therapist can introduce this topic by saying that many women experience the work of recovery as *effortful*, requiring a good deal of time and energy. Coupled with this issue, women in recovery may experience a *feeling of loss* for the substances themselves, as well as for things related to the substances (e.g., relationships, partners, jobs, friends, health). Sometimes women ask if they can "ever have fun again" and wonder about *balancing recovery work with having fun in one's life. The therapist can point out that the WRG central recovery rule is that recovery work* includes both *relapse prevention* and *repair work. Relapse prevention* includes identifying triggers and high-risk situations, planning to avoid such situations, and developing coping skills to manage situations that can't be avoided. It also involves making one's environment as "trigger-free" as possible and getting treatment. *Repair work* includes a woman repairing the damage to herself and her relationships due to substances and learning how to enjoy her life substance-free.

In learning to enjoy their lives substance-free, there are a number of areas of concern many women have, which can include such things as: Can I ever entertain people in my own home? What should I do at the holidays? Can I attend a ballgame or sporting event? What about the July 4th barbecue? New Year's Eve? A music festival I used to enjoy? How can I see my friends when we always used together? How can I go out with my friends and not drink? The therapist should pause here and ask something like, "Does anyone recognize any of these questions or issues in her life?," and encourage the group to discuss some of their thoughts and struggles on this topic (as well as any strategies they have used for these types of events or situations). If this group session falls near a holiday, this approaching holiday can also be a focus for discussion.

Enjoying Your Life in Recovery

After some discussion, the therapist can call the group's attention to the fact that there are useful strategies they can think about and possibly try to use in their own lives. The therapist can mention that some of these strategies are the same as more general ones that group members have been learning throughout the WRG sessions (e.g., identifying high-risk situations and avoiding those they can, preparing in advance for situations that can't be avoided). So, each person will need to identify situations that she feels she may need to avoid at least for a time (e.g., in early recovery when craving is high). But in addition to these basics of relapse prevention in recovery, women can begin to think about other ways to spend leisure time by discovering or rediscovering interests that may have been given up or not developed because of substance use. There may also be some situations that women may have found enjoyable only while intoxicated, and they will need to find new activities to substitute for these. The therapist may pause here and ask participants if they have had activities they gave up because of substance use or activities they would like to have a chance to do because they have more "found time" now that they are not using drugs and alcohol.

Strategies for Social Settings

After some time for this discussion, the therapist can point out that there are some specific strategies that a woman might use to help in social settings. These can include turning her wine glass over at a restaurant or dinner party so she is not offered alcohol; immediately getting a nonalcoholic drink at a reception or social event so that she has a drink to carry and is not offered an alcoholic beverage; attending events with a person supportive of her recovery; making her own home a substance-free zone; and practicing substance (e.g., alcohol and drug) refusal lines that are comfortable for her.

The therapist should now ask people to offer any of their own substance refusal lines. It is important here to let group members first offer any specific substance refusal lines they may have used. The therapist can also ask group members to try out a refusal line and should encourage everyone in the group to participate if they would like to try. For those who might be reluctant to speak, the therapist might say something like, "It would be great if everyone could give at least one try with a substance refusal line. . . . Does anyone else have one?" The therapist can encourage the group members to write down these lines in order to remember them and perhaps practice them during the group or at another time and see if they might be helpful. The therapist can write down the lines on a blackboard or on a sheet of paper, which she can later photocopy and hand back out to the group members at the next group. This way the group can compile its own list of "substance refusal lines." Substance refusal lines include things like "No, thank you, I don't drink," or "No, I don't use that stuff anymore," or "That stuff is bad for me," or "I'm allergic to that," or "I'm on some medicine and can't use that anymore," and so on.

After everyone who is willing to participate has had an opportunity to say her line, the therapist could do some role play if that is appropriate to the group. For instance, the therapist could ask someone in the group to offer alcohol/cocaine/pills/a joint to another woman and have that woman practice her refusal line.

After doing the role play (if that is useful for the group), the therapist should move on to other strategies to have fun and enjoyment in life. The therapist can ask the group members about leisure or recreational activities they enjoy that they can do substance-free (e.g., going to the movies, playing sports, exercising, reading, listening to music, walking, visiting with friends and family) and if they have other thoughts or if they have ever used different strategies to enjoy themselves while remaining substance-free.

Open Discussion

During open discussion, women may continue to pursue any aspect of today's topic. The group can do additional role play of drug and alcohol refusal lines. As always, the open discussion time may also focus on other recovery, issues including any issues that were raised during the check-in.

Wrap-Up and Reading of Take-Home Messages

The therapist should summarize the themes of relapse prevention and repair work, as well as examples of fun and enjoyment that group members have had without using drugs and alcohol. In addition, the therapist can review some of the effective ways that the group members have practiced refusal of substances. The therapist can emphasize the importance of each participant practicing refusal lines, as well as finding ways to enjoy herself. Distribute Participant Sheet 13.2 and the take-home messages can then be reviewed by having members each read one of the messages in turn.

Distribution and Description of This Week's Skill Practice

Distribute this week's Skill Practice Sheet (Participant Sheet 13.3). This week's skill practice will ask participants to write a list of fun or satisfying events and activities that they enjoyed before recovery. Then the skill practice asks women to list events or activities that are too high risk to be included in their recovery life. Next participants will list fun or satisfying events and activities they can enjoy in their recovery life, as well as special strategies to use so that these events can be enjoyed and recovery also protected. It will also ask women to write down activities (new or old) that can be enjoyed without substances. The skill practice then asks women to write down in their own words one to three substance refusal lines that they would be comfortable using and to practice them.

Check-Out

Pass around the Check-Out Sheet and ask participants each to answer orally the one-question check-out. Thank members and tell them you will see them next time.

Achieving a Balance in Your Life

Women in recovery often find that, in addition to needing to balance a number of roles in their lives (e.g., as workers, partners, parents, caretakers, siblings, children, students, friends), they are also confronted by needing to balance these usual life tasks with recovery activities in order to create a lifestyle that promotes their recovery. This task can be quite difficult for some women. They can find that their recovery activities begin to feel like they crowd out other life priorities, or alternatively, that their other responsibilities make participating in recovery-oriented activities (e.g., appointments, therapy, self-help, exercise, meditation, medical appointments, good nutrition) very difficult. Either way, they feel life is out of balance. This problem can sometimes lead to stress, or avoidance of recovery activities, and increase the risk of relapse. Achieving a balance in your life focuses on "repair work" that is essential to recovery. The therapist can again emphasize the WRG central recovery rule that Recovery = Relapse Prevention and Repair Work. In preparing for this session, therapists should read the "Background Information" that follows for additional details.

Background Information

Early recovery can be a time when life can feel "out of balance." Sometimes women can feel that their life is filled with treatment or recovery-related activities and that this crowds out other activities that are also important to them. In order to gain perspective on this dilemma, I review the *course of recovery* and how things change from early recovery to longer term, more stable recovery. I talk about *dealing with ambivalence, setting priorities,* and *achieving a balance in your life*.

The Course of Recovery

The tasks of early recovery include learning about yourself, including your internal and external triggers to use substances, and learning positive coping strategies to manage those triggers and not use substances. Early in recovery, it is essential for women to have enough treatment support to help them learn ways to recognize triggers and manage urges and cravings. Treatment supports can include self-help groups, group treatment, individual treatment, and other meetings that support recovery. Sometimes making use of so many supports can lead to life feeling "out of balance."

Nevertheless, throughout recovery it is important to deal with any ambivalence there may be about sobriety, to set priorities, and to learn to achieve a balance. Sometimes ambivalent feelings about sobriety are specifically prompted by this feeling of "lack of balance." When this is the case, one way women sometimes act on their ambivalence is to drop out of treatment or activities that are supportive of their recovery. Unfortunately, this can be the road back to using substances. It is important (though sometimes hard) to remember that active substance problems take more time away from family, friends, work, or other important activities. That is to say, substance problems themselves make life be "out of balance."

One of the most important parts of *early recovery* is learning to recognize triggers, resist urges and cravings, and use other coping strategies. This process takes time and practice and may, in fact, mean prioritizing recovery activities and treatment. It may even require cutting back on some other activities for a while. Over time, though, certain things in your life that were difficult at first likely will become easier. When this happens, it is possible to put other activities back into your life without jeopardizing your recovery.

Dealing with Ambivalence

What Are Examples of Ambivalent Thinking and Behavior?

One example is wondering whether you really have a substance problem or if it is as serious as other people's substance problems. These questions can lead to thoughts such as "It really isn't that bad" and "I can do it on my own" or "I don't really need this group or that AA meeting or therapy." An example of an ambivalent behavior is missing your treatment or group sessions or individual therapy or self-help groups.

What Do You Do When You Have Ambivalent Thinking or Behavior?

Almost everyone has ambivalence sometime during her recovery. One important action to take is to *share the thoughts* with someone else or to let someone else know that you skipped a meeting or treatment. The second important action is to make sure you *stay in treatment* and *don't use substances* even if that is not what you feel like doing. Anytime you are considering changing your treatment by reducing it or dropping out, don't do it on your own. Make sure you have discussed the pros and cons with a treater, clinician, or sponsor and that you have *reached an agreement* about making these changes. Having this sort of conversation is a way to check yourself and make sure the change you want to make is in your best interest and is not acting on ambivalence. It is important to take care of yourself and make sure that changes you make help you with self-care and your recovery.

Setting Priorities

Another important part of recovery is learning to set priorities for yourself. Early in recovery, recovery activities need to be high on the priority list and may occupy more of your time than later in your recovery. The reason for this is that in early recovery, women encounter many situations and feelings that they need to *learn to manage without substances*. For many women, it is the first time in their adult life that they are managing certain situations while substance-free. That takes a lot of support and a lot of practice. For example, women may be learning how to get through an evening at home, cooking dinner for themselves or their family, a work meeting, a holiday season, going back to school and having a social life, getting together with friends, putting children to bed, a dinner party elsewhere or in their own home, a business conference, or a rough day with family—all without using substances to "help" them. Each time a woman gets through one of these situations substance-free, it sets up a kind of success that can be built on the next time. Through this process of building upon successes, it gradually gets easier to navigate these situations and feelings. At the beginning, though, it often takes a lot of support, and it is therefore very important to make room in your life for that support, whether it be group therapy, individual therapy, AA, NA, meditation, meetings with sponsors, or other recovery activities. Carving out time to engage in these activities early on in recovery optimizes your chance of success in the long term.

Achieving a Balance in Your Life

Many women find that over time, certain situations they felt they could not face substance-free become easier. Eventually many women report that, much to their surprise, they do not even think of using substances in those circumstances anymore. They have gotten to this point usually by working through each difficult situation, moment by moment, and learning a different way to manage it than to use substances. Slowly but surely, they can feel life moving into a *new type of balance*. This balance has at its center *recovery* and *sobriety*. No longer do these women feel they must invest so much internal energy in "just managing" things without using drugs or alcohol. New patterns have been created that eventually feel natural. Old patterns feel more distant. It can become easier to find the time and energy for other pursuits, whatever they may be.

Women achieve this balance by (1) setting priorities; (2) not using substances to manage internal and external triggers; (3) dealing with ambivalence and not using substances or dropping out of treatment when ambivalence arises; (4) learning new ways to manage triggers, urges, and cravings; (5) finding or resuming activities that are enjoyable and do not include substance use; and (6) practicing these new ways until they feel like a routine part of life.

Therapist Overview

Goals of This Session

- To learn about setting priorities.
- To learn about not using substances to manage internal and external triggers.
- To deal with ambivalence and not use substances or drop out of treatment when ambivalence arises.

- To learn new ways to manage triggers, urges, and cravings.
- To find or resume activities that are enjoyable and do not include substance use.
- To practice these new ways until they feel more natural.

Session 14 Outline

- **Introduction (*If Needed*)** (5 minutes).
- **Check-In** (15 minutes).
- **Review of Last Week's Skill Practice and Topic** (5 minutes).
- **Presentation of This Week's Topic and Distribution of Topic Overview** (25 minutes): Provide Participant Sheet 14.1.
- **Open Discussion** (30 minutes).
- **Wrap-Up and Reading of Take-Home Messages** (2 minutes): Provide Participant Sheet 14.2.
- **Distribution and Description of This Week's Skill Practice** (3 minutes): Provide Participant Sheet 14.3.
- **Check-Out** (5 minutes).

Session-Specific Materials Needed

- Bulletin Board Outline and Take-Home Messages for Session 14.
- Participant Sheet 14.1: Achieving a Balance in Your Life.
- Participant Sheet 14.2: Take-Home Messages.
- Participant Sheet 14.3: Skill Practice: Achieving a Balance in Your Life.

Introduction (If Needed)

As in the previous session, the therapist should provide an introduction to the group if there are new members.

Check-In

Pass around the Check-In Sheet and have each member respond orally to the three check-in questions.

Review of Last Week's Skill Practice and Distribution of Topic Overview

From the check-in, the therapist should have a sense of who has done the skill practice and commented on whether or not it was helpful. The therapist can build on the check-in by asking if anyone would like to comment on the skill practice and what she learned. The therapist can also comment on the main highlights from last week's topic. The therapist can then transition to presentation of this week's topic.

Presentation of This Week's Topic and Distribution of Topic Overview

The therapist should distribute Participant Sheet 14.1 at this time, which provides an overview of this topic. She should then try to highlight particular themes from the day's check-in relating to balance in one's life. If there were no related comments from participants on this particular day, the therapist can summarize themes from previous weeks that relate to the topic of balancing treatment or recovery-related activities with other parts of participants' lives. For example, this may include trying to balance taking care of everyone else and taking care of themselves and their recovery, or it may relate to wanting to have fun but also recognizing the need to avoid certain social events or people in order to preserve recovery. The therapist can begin the session by summarizing the take-home messages and then framing the session topic by saying something like, "In discussing balance, we will talk about the course of recovery, dealing with ambivalence, setting priorities, finding new activities to enjoy, and ultimately achieving a balance in your life."

The Course of Recovery

The therapist can then go on to discuss that two critical tasks of early recovery for a woman are learning about herself, including her internal and external triggers to use substances, and learning positive coping strategies to manage those triggers and not use substances. Early in recovery, it is important to have enough treatment supports, but sometimes these can seem like they make life feel out of balance, which can in turn lead to ambivalence about treatment and sobriety. Sometimes, ambivalent feelings about sobriety can highlight this feeling of "lack of balance." This can lead people to drop out of their recovery activities and can be the road back to using again. It is sometimes hard to remember that substance use and substance disorders also lead to life being "out of balance," with many activities and relationships given up or impaired or damaged due to addiction. Engaging in the necessary recovery work is the way to stay sober. One of the most important parts of *early recovery* is learning to recognize triggers, resist urges and cravings, and use other coping strategies, all of which take time and practice. As such, women need to prioritize recovery activities and treatment, and sometimes this means cutting back on some other activities or commitments for a while. Over time, some of the things that were difficult may become easier, which will likely make it possible for a woman to put other activities back into her life without jeopardizing recovery.

Dealing with Ambivalence

The therapist should outline the theme of dealing with ambivalence. She might ask something like, "Has anyone felt ambivalent about her recovery? What I mean by this is, has anyone felt like she both wants to recover and wants to use drugs at the same time?" The therapist may ask participants to name a few examples of ambivalent thinking, saying for example, "What types of thoughts do you have that you know are ambivalent thoughts?" After participants have a chance to relate their thoughts, the therapist can confirm that those are indeed ambivalent thoughts and then add others, such as "It really isn't that bad," or "I can do it on my own," or "I don't really need this group or that AA meeting."

The therapist can then ask the group what women can do when they have ambivalent thoughts or feelings. After group members share their own ideas on this topic, the therapist can suggest that another useful strategy for dealing with ambivalence is to communicate these thoughts to someone else and take action to make sure they stay in treatment and don't use substances. The therapist can remind participants that they should not make changes in their treatment or recovery work without first thinking it through with others. The pros and cons of dropping a treatment activity should be discussed thoroughly with a therapist, other clinician, or sponsor. Engaging in this type of conversation is a way for members to check themselves and *not* to act on ambivalent thinking in ways that will jeopardize their recovery.

Setting Priorities

The therapist can then discuss "setting priorities." Setting priorities is an important part of achieving balance at each phase of recovery. Early in recovery, recovery activities need to be high on the priority list so that women can learn how to manage situations and feelings substance-free. For some women it will be the first time they are facing situations, events, or feelings without using. It may be the first holiday period or birthday a woman experiences without using, or the first time handling extreme anger or frustration without using substances to try to cope with these feelings. It may be going back to school for the first time without using, traveling for work or leisure, or attending a family event. Each time a woman gets through an experience substance-free she can build on this success and over time it feels more natural to manage without substances. In order to gain these experiences of success, though, it is extremely important to make the necessary time for recovery activities early in her recovery.

Achieving a Balance in Your Life

The therapist can then relate that achieving a balance becomes easier over time. Many women report that they could not face situations or feelings substance-free in early recovery but over time are surprised to find that in those same circumstances, they no longer think of using. So, while early in recovery a woman may have found it difficult to go to a social event and not use, later in recovery she may find that using is not even on her mind. Similarly, a woman who used in the evening through the dinner hour to "relax" may find that during early recovery evenings were filled with cravings, but that later in recovery this time of day is no longer associated with using substances. The same is true for women who may have used alcohol or drugs at school, or may always have used them during family events or other activities. As many of these events are managed without using substances, new ways to have these experiences without substances become more routine. Over time, increased comfort will come with working through each difficult moment and learning different ways to manage them. Slowly but surely a woman may begin to feel that a new type of balance begins to characterize her life. She may then feel that she does not need to invest so much energy into "just managing" and that the new patterns she has created have begun to feel natural. At this point, the therapist can ask if women have faced challenges of setting priorities and prioritizing recovery in their own lives. After some discussion, she can point out the six ways that balance is achieved:

- Setting priorities.
- Not using substances to manage internal and external triggers.
- Dealing with ambivalence and not using substances or dropping out of treatment when ambivalence arises.

- Learning new ways to manage triggers, urges, and cravings.
- Finding or resuming activities that are enjoyable and do not include substance use.
- Practicing these new ways until they feel more natural.

Open Discussion

During open discussion, women may continue to pursue any aspect of today's topic. As always, the open discussion time may also focus on other recovery issues, including any issues that were raised during the check-in.

Wrap-Up and Reading of Take-Home Messages

As always, the therapist should summarize any themes regarding achieving a balance that have come up in the course of the session. She will want to highlight (1) setting priorities to achieve a balance; (2) not using substances to manage internal and external triggers; (3) dealing with ambivalence and not using substances or dropping out of treatment when ambivalence arises; (4) learning new ways to manage triggers, urges, and cravings; (5) finding or resuming activities that are enjoyable and do not include substance use; and (6) practicing these new ways until they feel more natural. Also, the therapist can point out that priorities may differ depending on the stage of recovery. As in previous sessions, distribute Participant Sheet 14.2. Then the Take-Home Messages can be reviewed by having members each read one of the messages in turn.

Distribution and Description of This Week's Skill Practice

The therapist should now distribute this week's Skill Practice Sheet (Participant Sheet 14.3). In this skill practice, participants will be asked to (1) write three examples of ways that they feel ambivalent about recovery or behaviors that have shown their ambivalence; (2) list the responsibilities and activities that are currently in their lives; (3) examine the list they wrote in question 2 and consider whether these can all fit comfortably in their lives right now; (4) rank the different activities and responsibilities according to priority—notice where they are listing treatment and recovery in this ranking; (5) write down how many of the things mentioned in the list in #2 they can "fit in" their lives now along with treatment and recovery activities—which of the things do they think they would need to defer or delay right now so that they can take care of their top priorities?; and (6) write down how they will set priorities for the coming week—What activities will they take care of, and which ones will they delay or defer for another time?

Check-Out

Pass around the Check-Out Sheet and ask participants each to answer orally the one-question check-out. Thank members and tell them you will see them next time.

Reproducible Participant Materials

This section includes all of the participant materials. The first three documents—the Pre-group Meeting Information, the List of Sessions and Topics, and the Readings and Resources for Recovery—are to be given to participants at the pre-group meeting. Then for each of the 14 sessions, there are three participant sheets: an outline of the session's topic, a list of take-home messages, and a skill practice. Purchasers of this book can download and print the materials in this appendix at *www.guilford.com/greenfield-forms* for personal use or use with clients.

Materials for Participants for the Pre-Group Meeting

Session-Specific Participant Materials

Pre-Group Meeting Information:
What You Need to Know to Help Yourself in Your Recovery

Please read this sheet. Your therapist will review it with you during your pre-group meeting. You and the therapist will sign this sheet. The therapist will keep a copy and will give you a copy to keep for yourself.

Show up to the group, no matter how you feel. It is hard to get better without making use of the help and support that is available to you. There are times you may be tempted to quit the group. This may happen because you are not doing well and think that the group won't help you. Or it may happen because you are doing well and think you no longer need the group. There may be other reasons as well. It is important, however, that no matter how you are feeling, you come to group. It is important for your own recovery. Also, as a part of a group, your absence will definitely affect others (even if you don't think so). You are needed for the group to work both for you and for the other group members.

Participate. There are four levels of participation. Participation includes (1) weekly attendance at group; (2) active listening to others in the group; (3) sharing, responding to others, and asking questions; and (4) doing the skill practices between groups. The Women's Recovery Group asks that you participate in each of these ways that you find comfortable. The more effort and participation you put in, the greater the potential gains you will make. Ideally, you will be able to participate at all four levels, but it is important that you participate within your zone of comfort.

Be honest. Your honesty in reporting your substance use and other life circumstances is essential for getting better. Also, please be honest with the group leader if you have a negative reaction to the group or to a particular session.

Stay focused on your own recovery, not that of others. Do not compare yourself to others. Comparisons at this stage will not help. Remember that everyone in the group shares a number of experiences and symptoms of substance use problems and substance use disorders or she would not be in the group. However, the path to recovery may be different for each person. Just keep trying to do *your* best. Also, remember to respect the confidentiality and privacy of other group members. What is said in the group, stays in the group.

Be aware that others in the group may be in a better or worse situation than you. The value of a group, in terms of symptoms, is that people who are still using substances or struggling to remain abstinent can learn from those who are already abstinent. If you are further along, you can reinforce your recovery by participating in discussion with people who are at an earlier stage than you.

(continued)

Be aware that the philosophy of this group is abstinence from substances of all types. Any substance can impair your judgment and ability to remain abstinent from other substances, as well as block your general growth and emotional development. While at first you may have mixed feelings about giving up substances entirely, it is necessary to be open to this idea and work on attaining this goal.

Complete the skill practices between sessions. Skill practice exercises are an important way to learn. Not completing your skill practices may be a sign of self-neglect; working on them is a way of taking care of yourself.

Patient Signature: _____ Date: _____

Therapist Signature: _____ Date: _____

List of Sessions and Topics

Session 1. The Effect of Drugs and Alcohol on Women's Health

Session 2. How to Manage Triggers and High-Risk Situations

Session 3. Overcoming the Obstacles to Recovery

Session 4. Managing Mood, Anxiety, and Eating Problems without Using Substances

Session 5. Women and Their Partners: The Effect on Recovery

Session 6. Coping with Stress

Session 7. Women as Caretakers: Can You Take Care of Yourself While You Are Taking Care of Others?

Session 8. Using Self-Help Groups to Help Yourself

Session 9. Women's Use of Substances through the Life Cycle

Session 10. Violence and Abuse: Getting Help

Session 11. The Issue of Disclosure: To Tell or Not to Tell?

Session 12. Substance Use and Women's Reproductive Health

Session 13. Can You Have Fun without Using Drugs or Alcohol?

Session 14. Achieving a Balance in Your Life

Your therapist is: _____   **Contact:** _____

Other important contacts: _____

_____

_____

_____

_____

_____

_____

_____

_____

_____

_____

_____

_____

_____

Readings and Resources for Recovery

Informational Websites

- National Institute on Drug Abuse (NIDA): *www.nida.nih.gov*
- National Institute on Alcohol Abuse and Alcoholism (NIAAA): *www.niaaa.nih.gov*
- Substance Abuse and Mental Health Services Administration (SAMHSA): *www.samhsa.gov*
- National Institute of Mental Health (NIMH): *www.nimh.nih.gov/health/topics/index.shtml*
- National Center on Domestic Violence, Trauma, and Mental Health: *www.nationalcenterdvtraumamh.org*
- National Women's Health Information Center (NWHIC): *www.4woman.gov*
- Centers for Disease Control and Prevention. (2013). Binge drinking: A serious, underrecognized problem among women and girls. *CDC Vital Signs.* Retrieved July 16, 2013, from *www.cdc.gov/VitalSigns/BingeDrinkingFemale/index.html.*
- NIDA: Medical Consequences of Drug Abuse. *http://nida.nih.gov/consequences*
- Helping Women Quit Smoking: *http://women.smokefree.gov*
- Safer Sex Skills Building (SSSB): *http://ctndisseminationlibrary.org/display/398.htm*
- Prescription Painkiller Overdoses: A Growing Epidemic, Especially among Women: *http://www.cdc.gov/vitalsigns/prescriptionpainkilleroverdoses/*

Self-Help Group Websites

- Alcoholics Anonymous (AA): *www.aa.org*
- Cocaine Anonymous (CA): *www.ca.org*
- Narcotics Anonymous (NA): *www.na.org*
- SMART Recovery: *www.smartrecovery.org*
- Al-Anon/Alateen: *www.al-anon.alateen.org*

Publications of Interest

Benderly, B. L. (1997). *In her own right: The Institute of Medicine's guide to women's health issues.* Washington, DC: National Academy Press.

Davis, M., Eshelman, E. R., & McKay, M. (2008). *The relaxation and stress reduction workbook* (6th ed.). Oakland, CA: New Harbinger.

Knapp, C. (1997). *Drinking: A love story.* New York: Random House.

National Center on Addiction and Substance Abuse at Columbia University (NCASA). (2013). *Women under the influence.* Baltimore: Johns Hopkins University Press.

NIAAA: Alcohol: A Women's Health Issue: *http://pubs.niaaa.nih.gov/publications/brochurewomen/women.htm.*

NIAAA: Are Women More Vulnerable to Alcohol's Effects?: *http://pubs.niaaa.nih.gov/publications/aa46.htm.*

NIAAA: Women and Alcohol: An Update: *http://pubs.niaaa.nih.gov/publications/arh26-4/toc26-4.htm.*

NIDA Notes: A Collection of Articles that Address Women's Health and Gender Differences: *www.drugabuse.gov/NIDA_Notes/NN0013.html.*

Scott, L. (2003). *The sober kitchen: Recipes and advice for a lifetime of sobriety.* Boston: Harvard Common Press.

Session 1 Overview:
The Effect of Drugs and Alcohol on Women's Health

Common Symptoms of Substance Problems and Substance Use Disorders

- Increasing the amount of the substance(s) used over time.
- Trying repeatedly but unsuccessfully to cut down or stop using substances.
- Spending an increasing amount of time using substances, often leading to decreasing time spent in other activities related to work, school, relationships, or recreation.
- Craving the substance(s) when you are not using.
- Continuing to use substances despite knowing they cause or worsen problems with work, family, school, relationships, or other activities.
- Using substances despite knowing they cause physical or mental health problems or when they may be physically dangerous to use.
- Developing tolerance to the substance over time (i.e., developing a need for more of the substance in order to achieve the desired or usual effect).
- Experiencing withdrawal symptoms when substance use stops or is reduced.

Telescoping Course of Illness

- Women's substance use disorders progress more rapidly from first using to first having problems with substances.
- Women get sicker faster using less alcohol or drugs.
- This telescoping course is true for both alcohol and other substances (e.g., cocaine and opioids).
- Women can have more severe health effects from substance problems than men.

Alcohol

- Major problem of binge drinking in women in the United States (ages 18–34 especially).
- Metabolized differently by men and women.
- Women have less enzyme in stomach lining to metabolize (break down) alcohol—more is absorbed as pure alcohol (i.e., ethanol) into bloodstream than in men.
- Women have less total body water than men; alcohol is distributed in total body water; ounce per ounce of alcohol consumed, women's blood alcohol concentration is higher than men's.
- May account for some of the telescoping course and adverse health consequences for women (including effects on heart, liver, lungs, and brain) as well as reproductive health effects and increased breast cancer risk.

(continued)

Cocaine

- Women using cocaine are more likely to smoke cigarettes than men.
- Women are more likely to have physical problems such as headaches, visit the emergency department.
- May have problems with menstrual cycle function, infertility.
- Other physical effects include increased heart rate and blood pressure.

Opioids

- Women become more rapidly addicted than men.
- Greater risk of death from heroin dependence than men.
- Injection drug users have greater mortality overall; women greater than men.
- Negative effects: overdose deaths, HIV/AIDS, hepatitis C, other physical consequences.
- Women have greater medical consequences but are less likely to access any medical care.

Marijuana

- Anxiety, panic attacks, paranoia most common reported health consequences, as well as memory impairment.
- Longer term effects on cognitive abilities including memory problems.
- Women who are frequent users may have greater impaired memory than men who use.
- Prolonged exposure to tar and other irritants in marijuana cigarettes can lead to lung issues.
- Possible increased risk of all these effects in women who smoke marijuana compared with men.

Neglected Self-Care

- While using, women often neglect themselves emotionally and physically.
- Emotional neglect can mean not doing the things necessary to nurture yourself.
- Women may neglect regular checkups, preventive care, or neglect other healthful activities, such as exercise or eating well.
- Neglecting your own needs can lead to unintended and unprotected sexual encounters.

Session 1 Take-Home Messages

1. Each drug has specific types of direct, negative effects on women's health.

2. For alcohol and drugs, women can experience a telescoping effect on the progress of their illness and the rapid advancement of these negative health effects and medical consequences.

3. Women's health, both physical and psychological, is also negatively affected by self-neglect.

4. This may lead to women neglecting to get routine physical health care.

5. It may also lead women to have sexual encounters that were unintended, unprotected, or done in order to obtain more drugs. These sexual encounters pose additional risks for women's health.

6. What you can do to be as healthy as possible:
   - **Be abstinent from drugs and alcohol.** Be on the road to recovery, and abstain from drugs. Many health effects are reversible, and others will stop worsening if you stop using.
   - **Get healthy.** See your primary care doctor or other clinician and sign up for routine physical checkups. Consult with your doctor about any adverse health conditions and what you can do to help care for yourself.
   - **Decrease self-neglect and increase self-care.** You can start by getting a physical exam. But don't let it stop there. What other things can you do to stay healthy? Exercise? Eat right? All of these things can help you be healthier and feel better, which in turn can help you continue your recovery and not use drugs and alcohol.

Session 1 Skill Practice:
The Effect of Drugs and Alcohol on Women's Health

(Please do this Skill Practice before the next group and bring it with you to the next session for the discussion at the beginning of group.)

1. List the symptoms of substance use problems that you recognize in your own experience: __

_____

_____

_____

_____

2. List any direct effects on your health that you think substances have had: _____

_____

_____

_____

_____

3. List any ways that you think substance use has led to neglect of self-care in your experience: _____

_____

_____

_____

_____

4. What have you done in the past to contribute to your own self-care and promote your own health? _____

_____

_____

_____

_____

5. List at least two ways you will contribute to self-care and your own health this week: _____

_____

_____

_____

_____

Session 2 Overview:
How to Manage Triggers and High-Risk Situations

What Is a Trigger?

- Any person, place, or thing that increases your urge to use drugs or alcohol.
  - **Internal:** thoughts and feelings.
  - **External:** people, places, situations, or things.

High-Risk Situations

Internal

- Feelings: loneliness, anger, anxiety, exhaustion, among others.
- Thoughts: "What difference does it matter if I use just once?" or "No one cares about me."
- Physical discomfort: acute or chronic pain.

External

- People: seeing dealer, hanging around friends who use, seeing friend/relative who always criticizes.
- Places: passing bar or liquor store, or place where you often used or bought drugs and alcohol.
- Things: money, cigarettes, liquor bottle, or drug paraphernalia.

Other High-Risk Situations

- Interpersonal conflict: arguments with family/partner/siblings/friends, or difficulties with employer/coworkers/other students.
- Social pressure: family/partner/friends putting pressure on you to use.

Gender Differences in Facing Triggers

- Women tend to relapse in negative mood states (e.g., depression).
- Women often use drugs or alcohol with a significant other.
- Negative mood states associated with premenstrual cycle also may be triggers.

Drug or Alcohol Availability

- Conditioned cues: alcohol or drugs, or internal or external experiences associated with alcohol or drug use.
- Conditioned responses: reactions to these cues, based on prior experiences.

(continued)

Avoiding High-Risk Situations

• Identify high-risk situations.
• Develop plan to avoid these situations.

Facing Unavoidable High-Risk Situations

• Don't face the situation alone.
• Do self-nurturing activities.
• Create structure in your day by scheduling tasks and activities.
• Distract yourself to manage internal triggers.

What to Do to Avoid or Manage High-Risk Situations

• Make a list of current and past high-risk situations.
• Which are internal?
• Which are external situations?
• Divide the list into avoidable and unavoidable situations.
• Develop a list of ways to avoid the ones that you can.
• Develop a list of ways to manage the unavoidable ones.

Examples of Some Triggers and Coping Strategies Identified by Women in Recovery

Use these lists when you do your skill practice for this session. (Circle any of these that are triggers for you. Add your own triggers to this list.)

Triggers

• Being in restaurants.
• Anxiety.
• Making dinner.
• Relationships or a particular relationship.
• Anger.
• Writing a letter that is difficult to write.
• Anniversary of a death.
• Watching a partner drink or use.
• Hurtful action by someone else (such as forgetting your birthday).
• Feeling sorry for yourself.
• Anger from relatives directed at you.
• Powerful strong difficult feelings (such as hatred).
• Guilt.
• Feeling imperfect.
• Drugs and alcohol being used by people in the household.

(continued)

- Separation.
- Doing paperwork (want to use to get through it).
- Family/children's/parent's/sibling's/partner's demands/needs.
- Dreaming about using.
- Nightmares.
- Depression.

Ways to Cope with Triggers

(Circle any of these that might be good ways for you to cope with your triggers.)

- Take care of others (but not at the expense of taking care of yourself).
- Exercise (unless this is not good for you due to another health condition).
- Make lists.
- Go to the gym (unless this is not good for you due to another health condition).
- Read.
- Take a bath.
- Get a massage if you can.
- Go to the movies.
- Be with people you like (who don't use).
- Get additional treatment if needed for substance use disorders or other psychiatric disorders (can include individual therapy, the WRG, self-help, etc.).
- Take care of responsibilities (will give you a feeling of accomplishment).
- Get rid of that bottle of wine for cooking in the refrigerator.
- Get rid of other substances that are around you.
- Start a journal or, if you have one, write in your journal.
- Do something positive to commemorate a loved one who is gone.
- Go to work or school.
- Write a goodbye note to someone you need to separate from.
- Talk with your significant other about what is going on or what you are feeling.
- Sleep a lot if you need to get rest.
- Rent movies or watch a favorite TV program.
- Find/go to an AA or other self-help meeting you really like.
- Altruism: do something for others to take your mind off yourself.
- Take time for yourself to do something you like.
- Garden.
- Go to church, synagogue, or other house of worship or service.
- Do yoga.
- Practice meditation or mindfulness.
- Take a walk.
- Listen to music you enjoy.
- Use your sponsor if you have one.
- Limit your access to money that you would spend on alcohol or drugs.
- Get rid of any drug paraphernalia.

Session 2 Take-Home Messages

1. **Avoid** high-risk situations whenever you can.

2. **If you can't avoid** the situation, don't face the situation alone. Get an ally who knows you are in recovery to accompany you.

3. Develop a way to "escape" or **leave early** from a high-risk event.

4. For triggers that are internal, such as feelings or negative thoughts, find ways to **distract yourself** with other activities or positive thoughts.

5. **Plan ahead** and think through situations in advance. Identify high-risk people, places, or things that you will come across, and plan how to avoid or manage them.

6. Learn to **tolerate the feelings** associated with triggers and know they will pass.

Session 2 Skill Practice:
How to Manage Triggers and High-Risk Situations

(Please do this Skill Practice before the next group and bring it with you to the next session for the discussion at the beginning of group.)

1. Using the Session-Specific Information Sheet (Participant Sheet 2.1), circle any of the triggers on that list that are relevant for you and any of the ways to cope that might be useful for you.

2. Using the template below, create your wallet-sized card that you can carry with you or photograph this card to carry on your smartphone, if you have one, stating: "I take care of myself because . . ."

```
I take care of myself because . . .




```

You can cut out this card and carry it with you. You can photograph it with your smartphone and refer to it on your phone. Refer to the card (hard copy or on your phone) when you need to remind yourself of the most important reasons you have to take good care of yourself.

3. Write down two of your avoidable high-risk situations: _____

_____

_____

4. Write down two ways you can avoid these situations: _____

_____

_____

(continued)

5. Write down two of your unavoidable high-risk situations: _____

    _____

    _____

6. Write down two ways you can manage these situations: _____

    _____

    _____

7. During this week, notice one or two triggers and write down the positive way you managed it or avoided it:

    Trigger: _____

    What I did to manage or avoid it: _____

    _____

    Trigger: _____

    What I did to manage or avoid it: _____

    _____

Session 3 Overview:
Overcoming Obstacles to Recovery

Stigma

- Substance problems may compromise women's life roles (as parents, partners, family members, students, workers, etc.).
- Fear of being labeled as "neglectful."
- Personal sense of shame, guilt, or embarrassment.
- May lead to keeping things secret from others and make it difficult to get the help and support you need.

Feeling That Other Problems Come First

- Women may think of their substance use as a *consequence* of other problems.
  For example: "My substance use is because of:
  - Relationships: partners, family, children, parents, friends.
  - Stressful life events: loss of job, spouse, marriage, parents, friend, or other loss.
  - Mood or anxiety symptoms.

This may lead to thoughts such as:

- "If these problems get fixed, I will be able to stop using. . . ."
- Defining the "problem" as other things, women minimize the *extent* and *negative consequences* of substance use and do not get the help they need.

Mood or Anxiety Symptoms

- Women don't always share information about substance problems with clinicians because they think the substance problem isn't really the issue and it will be resolved by treating the other illnesses or other life issues.

Role Conflicts

- Difficulty of balancing roles: as workers, students, caretakers of children and/or elder relatives.
- Stress of multiple roles can lead to feelings of being overwhelmed or "out of control."

(continued)

Other Barriers

- Lack of child or elder care.
- Lack of financial resources.
- Lack of partner or family support.
- Lack of stable housing.
- Lack of reliable transportation.
- Lack of information about the effectiveness of treatment and range of treatment options.

How Can You Overcome Recovery Obstacles?

- Make a personal inventory about your use of substances and their impact on your life (e.g., relationships, mood, health, and work or school).
- Make an inventory of the *feelings, ideas, and circumstances* that may be obstacles in recovery.
- Make a list of the ways substances affect your mood or feelings of anxiety.
- Learn about available treatment for substance disorders. Investigate what resources are available in your community, such as child care, services at school, medical care, housing, health insurance, transportation, or employment.
- Ask for help.

Session 3 Take-Home Messages

1. Women often have powerful obstacles to their recovery and these can include:
   - Stigma about getting help for drugs and alcohol: Feeling ashamed.
   - Thinking the problem is only about depression and anxiety.
   - Feeling that you must take care of others before taking care of yourself.
   - Having an unsupportive partner or family.
   - Lacking financial or child care resources.
   - Lacking information about the fact that treatment works.

2. These obstacles can be overcome by asking for help, getting treatment, and helping to create your own network of support for your recovery.

3. Do a **personal inventory** about the use of substances in your life and the effects drugs and alcohol have had and are having on all the areas of your life, including relationships, mood, health, mental health, and work or school.

4. Make an **inventory of the ideas, feelings, and circumstances** that may be barriers or obstacles to your recovery.

5. Write a **list** of the ways substances affect your mood, feelings of anxiety, or eating problems. Write another list of how feelings such as depression, anxiety, or other difficult emotional states may affect your use of substances.

6. **Learn** as much as you can about available treatments for substance disorders.

7. **Learn** about other community supports for child care, medical care, employment, school, housing, transportation, insurance, or any other area that you have identified as a barrier for you to get help yourself and move forward in recovery.

Session 3 Skill Practice:
Overcoming the Obstacles to Recovery

(Please do this Skill Practice before the next group and bring it with you to the next session for the discussion at the beginning of group.)

1. Write down two obstacles or barriers that you have experienced that are significant in making it difficult for your recovery: _____

   _____

   _____

   _____

   _____

   _____

   _____

   _____

   _____

2. Write down one thing that you plan to do differently that will help you overcome either of these obstacles (or any other current obstacle or barrier) to your recovery: _____

   _____

   _____

   _____

   _____

   _____

   _____

   _____

   _____

3. Write down any obstacle or barrier to your recovery that you encountered this week and what you did to help yourself: _____

   _____

   _____

   _____

   _____

   _____

   _____

   _____

Session 4 Overview:
Managing Mood, Anxiety, and Eating Problems
without Using Substances

Overview

- Women with drug and alcohol disorders often have other psychiatric symptoms/illnesses, such as depression, anxiety, and eating disorders.
- These disorders are much more common in women with substance use problems and substance use disorders than in men.
- Treatment is important for both substance use and these other psychiatric problems.

Depression

- Depressed mood most of the time.
- Feeling guilty, worthless, or helpless.
- Irritability, restlessness.
- Loss of interest in activities or hobbies once pleasurable.
- Fatigue and decreased energy.
- Difficulty concentrating, remembering details, and making decisions.
- Insomnia, early morning wakefulness, or excessive sleeping.
- Overeating, or appetite loss.
- Thoughts about death or suicide, suicide attempts.

People with depression usually experience a number of these types of symptoms most of the day nearly every day for weeks at a time, or longer. People can also have more minor depression where some of these symptoms are present continuously for much longer periods of time.

Depression can change the way you think through:

- Irrational beliefs.
- Pessimistic thinking.
- Hopelessness.
- Self-criticism and hearing criticism in what others say, even when it is not there.

Depressive thinking can lead to:

- "Self-fulfilling" prophecies: that is, you think that you can't succeed so you don't even try, thereby confirming your lack of success.
- Difficulty setting priorities and following through on tasks.
- Avoidance of other people, work situations, school, or other tasks.
- Problems taking care of yourself and your own recovery.

(continued)

Anxiety

- There are several types of anxiety disorders.
- Most common are social anxiety disorder (social phobia) and generalized anxiety disorder (GAD).

Social anxiety disorder (or social phobia) can be characterized by:

- Having extreme anxiety and fear of being judged by others.
- Being very self-conscious in front of other people.
- Feeling embarrassed, especially in social situations where you will be observed.
- Being afraid that other people will judge you and you will feel humiliated.
- Having excessive fear and worry before an event or social situation.
- Avoiding places or situations that will cause this anxiety.
- This fear can be so strong that it interferes with going to work or school or doing other everyday activities.

Generalized anxiety disorder (GAD) can be characterized by having an extreme amount of anxiety that is difficult to control, is more extreme than is warranted by the situation, and is focused on routine activities. Some common symptoms include:

- Difficulty relaxing or concentrating.
- Startling easily.
- Trouble falling or staying asleep.
- Physical symptoms such as fatigue, headaches, muscle tension, muscle aches, difficulty swallowing, trembling, twitching, irritability, nausea, sweating, lightheadedness, needing to use the bathroom frequently, breathlessness, and hot flashes.

Anxiety problems

- Often begin early in life, frequently in adolescence.
- Women often learn to "manage" their anxiety by using substances in situations that provoke anxiety.
- Anxiety problems can trigger substance use. Substance use → more anxiety → more substance use.

Eating Problems and Eating Disorders

- Unhealthy eating behaviors (e.g., overeating, undereating) can sometimes be used by women to manage stress.
- Common eating disorders in women with substance use disorders and substance problems are anorexia nervosa, bulimia nervosa, and binge eating disorder.

(continued)

Anorexia nervosa can be characterized by:

- Low body weight due to restricting calorie intake.
- Extreme fear of gaining weight or getting fat.
- Distorted perception of own body weight or shape.
- Weight loss occurring by food restriction with or without binge-eating or purging.

Bulimia nervosa can be characterized by the following symptoms:

- Having frequent episodes of eating unusually large amounts of food (i.e., binge-eating episodes).
- Feeling a lack of control over these episodes.
- Engaging in behaviors following these binge-eating episodes like forced vomiting (e.g., purging), taking laxatives or diuretics, fasting, exercising excessively, or a combination of these behaviors.
- Since these behaviors interfere with weight gain, individuals may maintain a normal body weight.
- Having excessive fear of gaining weight, wanting to lose weight, and feeling unhappy with body size and shape.

Bulimia can be accompanied by:

- Feelings of guilt and shame so that binging and purging often occur secretly.
- Other negative physical consequences including:
  - Chronically inflamed and sore throat.
  - Swollen salivary glands.
  - Damaged tooth enamel, increasingly sensitive and decaying teeth from exposure to stomach acid.
  - Acid reflux disorder and other gastrointestinal problems.
  - Intestinal irritation from laxative abuse.
  - Severe dehydration from purging of fluids.

Binge-eating disorder: People with binge-eating disorder can:

- Lose control over their eating.
- Have periods of binge eating that are not followed by purging, excessive exercising, or laxative use.
- Become overweight or obese.
- Often experience guilt, shame, and distress about these behaviors, and that can lead to more binge eating.

Craving, loss of control, and preoccupation with substance (drug, alcohol, or food) are hallmarks of both substance and eating disorders.

(continued)

Among women without an eating disorder:

- Urges and cravings for certain foods are common, especially in early recovery.
- Women may substitute foods for substances.
- One coping strategy that can be helpful is to focus on good nutrition and establishing healthy eating.
- Healthy eating can be helpful in all phases of recovery.

Coping Strategies

- Understand and accept that the substance use and other disorders are both/all important.
- Get treatment for both/all disorders.
- Help mood and anxiety and eating problems: learn to recognize early symptoms so you can report them and get help before they progress.
- Don't use substances to manage these other problems.
- Don't let these other disorders/problems stop your recovery from substance problems.
- Develop positive coping strategies for both/all disorders.

Session 4 Take-Home Messages

1. Mood, anxiety, and eating problems are common in women with drug and alcohol problems.

2. These problems can make it difficult to get well from your substance problem.

3. The substance problem can also make it hard to get well from your mood, anxiety, or eating problem.

4. Understand and accept that the substance use and these other disorders and problems are important.

5. Get treatment for both/all disorders.

6. Taking care of yourself is getting the help you need for your recovery from your substance use disorder and your co-occurring depression, anxiety, and/or eating disorders.

Session 4 Skill Practice: Managing Mood, Anxiety, and Eating Problems without Using Substances

(Please do this Skill Practice before the next group and bring it with you to the next session for the discussion at the beginning of group.)

1. Have you been diagnosed with another illness such as depression, anxiety, or an eating disorder? If so, write down the name of the illness(es): _____

   _____

   _____

   (If you have other illnesses, answer questions 2–4. If not, go on to question 5.)

2. If you have been diagnosed with another illness, please list symptoms or behaviors of the illness(es) that you have experienced: _____

   _____

   _____

3. For the symptoms and behaviors you listed in question 2, circle the ones that you think have interfered or do interfere in your recovery from substance use problems and substance use disorders.

4. List three ways (alternative behaviors or strategies) you can use to help yourself with the symptoms or behaviors associated with the other illness(es): _____

   _____

   _____

   _____

5. List any mood or anxiety symptoms or feelings or thoughts about food/eating that you think trigger your use of substances: _____

   _____

   _____

   _____

6. List three ways (alternative behaviors or strategies) you can use to help yourself with the symptoms, feelings, or behaviors that you listed in question 5 rather than have them interfere with your recovery: _____

   _____

   _____

   _____

Session 5 Overview:
Women and Their Partners: The Effect on Recovery

What Is a Partner?

- An individual with whom a woman is intimately involved (e.g., spouse, boyfriend, girlfriend, and/or father/mother of child[ren]).
  Relationships are strongly connected with women's addiction and recovery.

Partners' Influence on Substance Problems, Addiction, and Recovery

Having a Partner: Influence on Substance Problems and Recovery

Negative Influences

INITIATION OF SUBSTANCE USE

- Introduction to using substances by male partner is common among heterosexual women
- Less is known about lesbian couples, but prevalence of substance problems is estimated to be 28–35% in lesbian couples.
- Women with addiction are more likely to have a male partner who uses drugs or alcohol than men are to have a woman partner who uses.

CONTINUING SUBSTANCE USE

- Partners may supply women's drugs.
- Women may rely on male partners to maintain addiction.
- Male partners may supply drug/supervise or coerce illegal activities.
- Partners may continue to drink/keep alcohol or use drugs in the home while women try to be in recovery.

SUBSTANCE USE MAY BE MAIN FOCUS OF THE RELATIONSHIP

- Women may fear losing partner if she stops using.
- Sexual activity may have always been in context of drug/alcohol use.
- Use seen as way to maintain relationship.

SETTING UP OBSTACLES FOR GETTING TREATMENT

- Partners may have negative attitude toward women getting treatment.
- Women may fear loss of relationship.
- Sexual activity in context of drug/alcohol use.
- Women dependent on partners—may fear abandonment—may fear loss of financial resources.
- Physical threats by partners if women seek treatment.

(continued)

ROLE IN RELAPSE

- Relapse more likely when using with a partner.
- Use substances as a way to reconnect with a partner who uses.
- Women tend to relapse after difficult emotional/interpersonal experiences, often with partners.
- Some difficulties within a couple may have started before substances were a problem.
- Some difficulties within a couple may be a consequence of the substances themselves.
- If living with an addicted partner, may relapse because substances freely available.

Positive Influences

- Partners who do not use can help women enter treatment and remain in recovery.
- Partners can help maintain an alcohol- and drug-free home.
- Partners can support women's recovery through companionship without drugs or alcohol.
- Partners can provide support through high-risk situations.
- Partners can engage in treatment:
  - Individual treatment.
  - Couple counseling.
  - If using themselves, their own substance use disorder treatment.
  - Self-help groups such as Al-Anon, etc.

The Absence of a Partner: Influence on Substance Problems and Recovery

Negative Influences

- Feelings of loneliness or abandonment.
- Feeling more isolated or lack of social or other types of support.
- Common places to find a partner can involve use of drugs/alcohol.
- These can pose a high risk for relapse.

Positive Influences

- More flexible for recovery activities.
- Can make home a drug-free zone.
- Can "start from the beginning" and enter a new relationship without drugs or alcohol where there are no expectations/history of drug use.

What can you do?

- Examine past/present intimate relationships.
- Examine positive/negative roles that intimate partner plays in your recovery.

What are some things you could do that might be helpful?

- If your partner uses, is he or she willing to give up his or her own substance use?
- Is your partner willing to make home a substance-free zone?
- Is your partner willing to engage in treatment, either with you or on his or her own?

Session 5 Take-Home Messages

1. The first rule of recovery is: do **not use drugs and alcohol**.

2. Partners are people with whom a woman is intimately involved (e.g., spouse, boyfriend, girlfriend, and/or father/mother of child[ren]).

3. Partners can be **critically important** in supporting or getting in the way of your recovery.

4. The **absence of a partner** relationship can also influence your substance disorder and process of recovery in positive or negative ways.

5. It is important that you **think about what role** having or not having a partner plays in your recovery.

6. This is the **first step** to understanding and deciding the best way to help yourself be **abstinent from drugs and alcohol** and have the **healthiest possible relationships**.

Session 5 Skill Practice:
Women and Their Partners: The Effect on Recovery

(Please do this Skill Practice before the next group and bring it with you to the next session for the discussion at the beginning of group.)

1. Do you have an intimate partner now?   Yes _____ (please answer questions 5–8)

                                                     No _____ (please answer questions 2–4)

2. Write if you think lack of an intimate partner currently helps or hurts your recovery. Please explain how this happens: _____

   _____

   _____

   _____

   _____

3. Think about a past intimate partner that you have had and write ways you think that partner helped or hurt your recovery: _____

   _____

   _____

   _____

   _____

4. Write two things you will do this week to improve your relationships, seek out healthier relationships, or decrease loneliness: _____

   _____

   _____

   _____

   _____

5. Write the ways that you think your current partner helps you in your recovery: _____

   _____

   _____

   _____

   _____

(continued)

6. Write the ways that you think your current partner hurts you in your recovery: _____

_____

_____

_____

_____

7. Write ways that you have tried to make your relationship with your partner healthier in the past: _____

_____

_____

_____

_____

8. Write at least two things you will do this week to help make your relationship with your partner healthier and not use drugs or alcohol: _____

_____

_____

_____

_____

Session 6 Overview:
Coping with Stress

There are Different Causes of Stress, Including

- External Stressors.
- Internal Stressors.

External Stressors

- *Ordinary Stressors:* common and daily stressors (e.g., minor illnesses, traffic, work problems, minor conflicts with family or friends, among others).
- *Extraordinary Stressors:* less common and more extreme stressors (e.g., death in family, job loss, homelessness, severe illness, exposure to violence).

Internal Stressors

Negative feelings/attitudes that arise from experience of outside world

For example:

- Perfectionism.
- Pessimism.
- Negativism.
- Concern about others' opinions.
- Need for control.

Stressors Associated with Women's Roles

- Being the primary caregiver.
  - For your own family and/or elders.
  - Managing the household.
  - Providing primary/secondary income for self and family.
- Financial constraints.
- Limited access to child/elder care.
  - Single motherhood.
  - Other.
- Minimal or no support from partner/family member for household responsibilities.
- Own problems not given top priority.

Emotional Consequences of Stress

- Depression.
- Low self-esteem.
- Anxiety.
- Shame.

(continued)

- Guilt.
- Anger.

Which can lead to:

- Initiation of substance use.
- Rationale for continued use.
- Relapse.

Coping with Stressful Situations

- Best response to stressful situations is to develop and have healthy *coping skills*.

Unhealthy Coping

- Provides temporary escape from stressors (substance use can be one of these).
- Situation still exists or worsens.
- Does not provide model for resolving/ managing stressor.
- Smoking or using tobacco products is common unhealthy coping.
- Examples of unhealthy coping:
  ○ Smoking cigarettes.
  ○ Increasing unhealthy food consumption.
  ○ Keeping feelings to yourself.
  ○ Complaining about a problem but doing nothing.
  ○ Criticizing yourself/others.
  ○ Punishing yourself (e.g., over/undereating, excessive exercise).
  ○ Striving for perfection.
  ○ Developing harmful relationships.
  ○ Isolating yourself from others.
  ○ Being passive.

Healthy Coping Skills

- Help resolve/manage current stressor.
- Provides a model for managing future stressors.
- Examples:
  ○ Sharing feelings with others.
  ○ Making a plan to handle problem.
  ○ Seeing humor in situation.
  ○ Engaging in pleasurable activities (e.g., reading, hobbies).
  ○ Accepting your limitations.
- Developing positive relationships.
- Being assertive.
- Helping others.
- Meditating.
- Practicing yoga or exercise.
- Doing other self-care activities.

(continued)

Examples of unhealthy coping and suggested healthy coping:

Unhealthy Coping.	Healthy Coping Skills.
Setting unrealistic goals for yourself.	Setting realistic goals.
Complaining about a problem but doing nothing.	Making a plan to handle the problem.
Criticizing yourself/others for the situation.	Seeing humor in the situation.
Punishing yourself (e.g., over/undereating, excessive exercise).	Engaging in pleasurable, healthy activities (e.g., reading, hobbies).
Striving for perfection.	Accepting your limitations.
Developing harmful relationships or isolating yourself from others.	Developing positive relationships.
Passivity.	Assertiveness.
Selfishness.	Helping others.
Having high expectations of yourself in every situation.	Change expectations to be realistic in each situation.
Smoking cigarettes.	Quit smoking cigarettes.

What Can You Do to Cope With Stress?

- List current/past stressful situations/relationships that led to unhealthy coping skills (e.g., substance use).
- Divide list into stressors you can change and stressors you cannot.
- Develop alternative coping skills for different situations.
- Quit smoking cigarettes (resource: *http://women.smokefree.gov*).
- Practice meditation exercise daily.
- Practice yoga or exercise or other self-care activities.
- Use a telephone app if you can to help you with meditation, mindfulness, or other stress-relieving daily activities.

Session 6 Take-Home Messages

1. Stress can be caused by **routine life circumstances**, such as bad weather, deadlines, or traffic.

2. Stress can be caused by **more serious life events**, such as loss of a job, death a family member, serious illness, or exposure to violence.

3. Stress can also be caused by **internal states** such as feelings, thoughts, and attitudes such as perfectionism, negative thoughts, etc.

4. Stress can lead to feelings of depression, low self-esteem, anxiety, shame, guilt, and anger.

5. These feelings can lead to starting to use, continuing to use, or relapsing to using substances.

6. There are many ways to **cope with stress**. Some of these, like using drugs and alcohol, or smoking cigarettes, are **unhealthy**.

7. There are many **healthy** ways of coping with stress.

8. You can help your recovery by learning and practicing as many healthy ways to cope with stress as you can think of.

Session 6 Skill Practice: Coping with Stress

(Please do this Skill Practice before the next group and bring it with you at the next session for the discussion at the beginning of group.)

1. Write down two stressful situations you can change: _____

_____

_____

_____

_____

2. Write down two healthy coping strategies you can use to change the situations listed above:

_____

_____

_____

_____

3. Write down two stressful situations you cannot change: _____

_____

_____

_____

_____

4. Write down two healthy coping strategies you can use to manage the situations listed above:

_____

_____

_____

_____

5. If you are a current smoker, write down whether you use cigarettes to manage feeling stressed. Have you tried to quit in the past? If you currently smoke, please visit this site to help women quit smoking *http://women.smokefree.gov* and write whether it is/could be useful: _____

_____

_____

_____

_____

Session 7 Overview:
Women as Caretakers: Can You Take Care of Yourself While You Are Taking Care of Others?

Women's Role as Caretakers (or Caregivers)

- Women need to be able to take care of themselves (i.e., self-care) in order to be able to take care of others.
- Relationships are generally valued strongly by women.
- Caretaking (or caregiver) role can give self-esteem and fulfillment.
- Women's caretaking role can also interfere with self-care including treatment and recovery.

What Are Some Caretaking Roles?

On the home front:

- Children.
- Elders.
- Partners.
- Families.
- Friends.
- Siblings.
- Pets.

On the work or school front:

- Coworkers.
- Other students.
- People you supervise.
- Other people within a work or school organization.

In communities:

- Neighbors/neighborhoods.
- Schools.
- Religious groups.
- Other community groups.

Social Connectedness: Often a source of strength and value for women.

Lack of Social Connectedness: Can lead to feelings of isolation and lack of support.

The role of caretaker (or caregiver) can be a source of value, self-esteem, and motivation, but it can also interfere with the ability to take care of yourself (e.g., to get into treatment and recover from substance problems).

(continued)

How Do Caretaking Roles Interfere with the Ability to Get into Treatment and Recovery?

1. The Belief of Having No Time
    - Putting needs of others first.
    - Need to minimize the time spent at treatment/recovery to care for others.
    - Drugs and alcohol as coping with caretaking demands—may deter women from treatment.

2. The Role of Guilt and Shame
    - Actual or perceived neglect of others.
    - Neglecting others because of substance use.
    - Not available physically/emotionally because of substance use.
    - *Avoiding* these feelings may deter women from seeking treatment.

3. Fear of Losing Custody
    - Fear if enter treatment will lose custody of children.
    - Critically delays getting treatment.
    - May worsen substance problems.
    - Can lead to intervention from others (e.g., child welfare services).

How Can You Be a Caretaker (or Caregiver) and Take Care of Yourself?

Learn, acknowledge, accept, and *apply* these to your life:

- You cannot do the best job you'd like to do as a caretaker (e.g., parent, friend, daughter, sibling, sister, neighbor) when using drugs/alcohol.
- To be the caretaker you most want to be is dependent on *not* using drugs/alcohol.
- Using drugs/alcohol can take time and attention away from significant relationships.
- Waiting until you have time doesn't work; it only delays help and worsens substance problems.
- You *do* have time to get help and work toward recovery.
- Recovery = self-care.

Session 7 Take-Home Messages

1. You do have time to take care of yourself.

2. Use the strength of your role as a caretaker (or caregiver) and your desire to be the best you can as a motivation to seek the help you need for treatment and for your ongoing recovery.

3. Women sometimes avoid taking care of themselves and their recovery because they feel guilty that they might not be taking care of others.

4. Sometimes women convince themselves they have no time to take care of their recovery because of their other responsibilities. This is the "Belief of Having No Time."

5. It is important to take care of yourself so that you can take care of any others who are important to you.

6. Recovery is a major part of self-care and necessary to be able to take care of any others who are important to you.

Session 7 Skill Practice: Women as Caretakers: Can You Take Care of Yourself While You Are Taking Care of Others?

(Please do this Skill Practice before the next group and bring it with you to the next session for the discussion at the beginning of group.)

1. Name the roles in which you see yourself as a caretaker or caregiver (e.g., friend, partner, parent, spouse, sibling, child, neighbor, other): _____

   _____

   _____

   _____

2. Name as many ways as you can think of that you value your role as "caretaker" or "caregiver": _____

   _____

   _____

   _____

3. Name as many ways as you can think of when being a caretaker got in the way of your seeking treatment or being in recovery in *the past:* _____

   _____

   _____

   _____

4. Name as many ways as you can think of when being a caretaker gets in the way of your treatment and/or your recovery *currently:* _____

   _____

   _____

   _____

5. Name two things you did in the past to help yourself take care of yourself and your recovery:

   _____

   _____

   _____

6. Name two things you will do this week to help yourself take care of yourself and your recovery: _____

   _____

   _____

   _____

Session 8 Overview:
Using Self-Help Groups to Help Yourself

Self-Help Groups

- Alcoholics Anonymous (AA).
  - International fellowship of men/women with drinking problems.
  - Abstinence-based 12-step program.
  - Different types and formats for AA:
    - *Open:* open to individuals with or without a drinking or drug problem.
    - *Closed:* open only to individuals with a substance use problem.
    - *Speaker meeting:* members speak about how alcohol and/or drugs have affected their lives and how their lives have changed since stopping using.
    - *Discussion meetings:* led by one individual who briefly speaks about her/his experience with alcohol and/or drugs followed by a discussion.
    - *Step meeting:* A step meeting discusses one of the 12 steps of AA, NA, or CA.
    - *Women only:* There are meetings for women only.
    - *Other:* Other meetings identify themselves for men only, teenagers/young adults, LGBTQ, nonsmoking or smoking, or a combination of these characteristics.

- Narcotics Anonymous, Cocaine Anonymous, Gamblers Anonymous.
  - Same principles as AA.
  - Address problems with opioids, benzodiazepines, amphetamines, prescription drugs, marijuana (NA), cocaine (CA), or gambling (GA).

- SMART Recovery.
  - Self-Management and Recovery Training (SMART).
  - Treatment based on cognitive-behavioral (CB) model of addiction, viewing addiction as complex maladaptive behavior.
  - Smaller groups/less available than 12 step groups, such as AA.

Pros and Cons of 12-Step Groups

Pros/Advantages

- Education—learn more about recovery from others.
- Hope—experiences of others in recovery can inspire hope.
- Support—gain support from other members including sponsors.
- Availability—usually available 24/7/365 days each year.
- Spirituality—appeals to a Higher Power—consistent with your beliefs.
- Effectiveness—some studies show involvement associated with long-term recovery.

(continued)

Cons/Disadvantages

- Isolation—can feel isolated within the group.
- Spirituality—appeals to a Higher Power—not consistent with your beliefs.
- Unwarranted familiarity: may make you feel uncomfortable. Women may especially feel uncomfortable if approached and not sure of intentions.
- Language—members use language that others feel is offensive.
- "War stories"—members' recovery stories may be depressing rather than inspiring.

Pros and Cons of SMART Recovery

Pros/Advantages

- Group size—generally small group.
- CB approach—uses cognitive-behavioral approach to change cognitions and behaviors.
- Spirituality—does not appeal to a Higher Power—consistent with your beliefs.

Cons/Disadvantages

- Not always abstinence-focused—sometimes focused on moderation.
- Support—may feel that you should manage with CB approach and not reach out for other members' support.
- Effectiveness—no studies of effectiveness.
- Availability—not available 24/7/365 days and not available in all regions of United States and the world.
- Spirituality—does not appeal to a Higher Power—not consistent with your beliefs.

How to Use Self-Help Groups to Help Yourself

- Review list of groups and identify which ones to attend.
- After each meeting, write down what you liked/disliked about it.
- Keep track of groups attended and how much you participated.
- Consider women-only AA/NA.
- If you cannot attend specific groups, try visiting websites or calling different organizations to find other groups you can attend.

Session 8 Take-Home Messages

1. Involvement in self-help groups can help you achieve and maintain long-term recovery.

2. There are different kinds of self-help groups, including some for women only.

3. Sample a number of different types of self-help groups before deciding if they are for you.

4. Work on finding groups that best suit your recovery needs in terms of the type of meeting, location and timing of the meetings, and a membership with which you feel comfortable.

Session 8 Skill Practice: Using Self-Help Groups to Help Yourself

(Please do this Skill Practice before the next group and bring it with you to the next session for the discussion at the beginning of group.)

This week, find two self-help groups that you can attend this week. After attending each group, do the following skill practice:

1. Write down two self-help groups you attended this week: _____

   _____

   _____

   _____

2. Write down two things you liked about the meeting(s): _____

   _____

   _____

   _____

3. Write down two things you did not like about the meeting(s): _____

   _____

   _____

   _____

4. Name two ways you can make self-help groups a part of your life: _____

   _____

   _____

   _____

5. List for yourself pros and cons of attending self-help groups:

   Pros   Cons

   _____   _____

   _____   _____

   _____   _____

   _____   _____

6. If you were not able to attend self-help group meetings this week, you can do this skill practice any week that you are able to attend one or two self-help groups.

Session 9 Overview:
Women's Use of Substances through the Life Cycle

Substance Use Disorders

- Can occur or reoccur anytime in lifespan.
- Usually have early onset in adolescence or early 20s.
- Pressures, triggers, and risk factors vary at different times in women's lives.
- A risk factor is something that increases chance of developing substance problems.

Life Stages and Risk Factors

Adolescence

- Social context—influenced by peers and group exposure may be especially significant for girls.
- Depression.
- Alienation or isolation—especially among girls who are sexual minorities, girls who are bullied, or other girls who otherwise feel discrimination or marginalization.
- Earlier age of first use of substances increases risk for substance problems.
- Smoking cigarettes.
- Sexual trauma is a risk for onset of substance problems.
- Prescription drug use may become a risk for problem use or addiction.

Young Adulthood

- Partner with alcohol or drug problems.
- Depression—presence of depression, which can have onset in adolescence, is a risk for substance problems.
- Role-related issues leading to maladaptive coping strategies.
- Problem use of any substance increases risk of other substance problems.
- Sexual trauma is a risk for onset of substance problems.
- Prescription drug use may become a risk for problem use or addiction.

Middle Years

- Partner with alcohol or drug problems.
- Depression.
- Losses common to this stage of life: changes in physical selves or appearance, loss of marriage through death or divorce, children leave home.
- Feelings of unlikelihood/pessimism about acquiring new life roles.
- Substance problems: Any substance use problem predisposes to other use including prescription drugs, marijuana, alcohol, tobacco, other drugs.
- Prescription drug use may become a risk for problem use or addiction.

(continued)

Older Age

- Partner with alcohol or drug problems.
- Depression.
- Prescription drug use: women in this age group may have greater exposure and risk of problem use or addiction through increased likelihood of being prescribed drugs.
- Retirement: can be a welcome change or perceived as loss; retirement of spouse can be welcome or perceived as disruption from established routines.
- Widowhood/loss of a partner: grief and loneliness can lead to use of substances.
- Changes in metabolism: Older individuals have slower metabolism of drugs and alcohol, and same amount of alcohol consumed, for example, results in higher blood alcohol than in younger years.
- Retirement communities where alcohol can be prominent part of social life.

How to Help Yourself

- Understand that use of substances and risk for substance problems change throughout a woman's life cycle.
- Be aware of specific risks associated with your current life stage.
- Understand these risks and find and practice ways to manage them without using drugs or alcohol.

Session 9 Take-Home Messages

1. Women's life stages include adolescence, young adulthood, middle years, and older age.

2. Each stage of women's lives has different rewards and challenges.

3. The use of substances can change throughout women's life cycle, and the risks for substance problems can change over time.

4. Specific risks for substance use can be associated with each person's current stage of life.

5. Find and practice ways to manage these situations that do not include using drugs or alcohol.

6. Different stages in a woman's life cycle may also bring vulnerability to substances.

7. Identify the specific risks of this time in your life and think of opportunities now that can help in the recovery process.

Session 9 Skill Practice:
Women's Use of Substances through the Life Cycle

(Please do this Skill Practice before the next group and bring it with you to the next session for the discussion at the beginning of group.)

1. How do you identify your current life stage (e.g., adolescent, young adult, middle age, older age)? _____

   _____

   _____

   _____

   _____

2. What are the main risks/triggers for your substance use? _____

   _____

   _____

   _____

   _____

   _____

   _____

3. Which, if any, of these do you think may be related to your current stage of life? _____

   _____

   _____

   _____

   _____

   _____

   _____

4. List three things you can do to help yourself manage these triggers: _____

   _____

   _____

   _____

   _____

   _____

   _____

Session 10 Overview:
Violence and Abuse: Getting Help

Substance Use Disorders and Violence

- Many women in treatment for substance use disorders have experienced violence or other abuse such as sexual or physical abuse or intimate partner violence (IPV).
- Women who have had these experiences may use drugs/alcohol to "numb" or "mask" the pain of past (or current) abuse.
- Past abuse may lead to risk in adulthood of further violence or abuse.
- These experiences in childhood or adulthood can contribute to feelings of shame and to social isolation.

Experiences Associated with History of Violence

- Psychiatric disorders (that can co-occur with substance use disorders) such as depression, anxiety, or posttraumatic stress disorder (PTSD).
- Shame and guilt.
- Avoidant coping.
- Feelings of stigmatization.
- Inhibit trust in relationships.

These experiences of violence can:

- Predispose women to using substances to mask or numb the painful feelings.
- Contribute to feelings of low self-worth—lead to feeling socially disconnected.

All of these can serve as triggers to relapse and obstacles to recovery from substance problems.

Emotional, Psychological, and Verbal Abuse

- Partner controls woman's choices.
- Difference in power within relationship.
- **Childhood abuse** (including emotional abuse) makes women more vulnerable to substance use problems later in life.
- **Adulthood** emotional or psychological abuse can predispose women to using substances and acts as an obstacle to getting treatment and being in recovery.

Domestic Violence or Intimate Partner Violence (IPV)

- More common than is generally thought.
- Risk of domestic violence greater in setting of substance use and substance use disorders.
- Three-quarters of all incidents involve alcohol.

(continued)

- Another factor may be perceived inequality between partners (such as in unemployment, income, finances, family roles).
- One member of couple can feel less powerful or powerless and may, in fact, have fewer resources to express her autonomy.
- IPV occurs in both heterosexual and gay and lesbian couples.
- Drug and alcohol problems increase risk for IPV.
- **Vicious cycle:** *violence and abuse* → more substance *use and substance problems* → more *violence and abuse*.
- These patterns inhibit seeking treatment for substance problems and getting help to get physically safe and stop the violence.

Relationship of abuse and violence to problems with substances:

- Women who experience violence may use substances to try to cope with the trauma of abuse or violence.
- Women who use substances may be more vulnerable to violence through impaired judgment, vigilance, ability to react, etc.
- Women who are intoxicated may be less able to defend themselves against violence.
- Women who use substances can feel guilt and shame about their substance use, as well as about the abuse and violence; this can lead to decreased feelings of self-worth and the idea that they are less deserving of getting the help they need.
- Women (whether they use substances or not) who are with substance-using partners are at greater risk for abuse and IPV.

How to Get Help to Help Yourself

- Assess for yourself and communicate with your clinicians your own experience of violence and abuse: (1) before recovery; (2) during treatment and recovery; (3) while maintaining abstinence.

Before Treatment and Recovery

- Have you experienced abuse before your substance use/treatment for substance use?
- Do you think this may have contributed to use of substances and/or difficulty seeking treatment?

During Treatment and Recovery

- Are you currently being exposed to violence or other abuse?
- If you are not physically safe, it is important to seek a safe place.
- If you are not physically threatened or in danger, but have ongoing problems with your partner, consider counseling for you with or without your partner.
- Consider questions such as:
  - How often does your partner show disapproval toward you?
  - When was the last time you felt threatened by or controlled by or afraid of your partner?
  - How often does someone hurt you?
  - How often does your partner use words that put you down and make you feel bad about yourself?

(continued)

In Recovery and Maintaining Abstinence

- Are there any ongoing abusive relationships in your life?
- Do you need to find a place to be physically safe?
- What would be the best way to take care of yourself?
- If there are no current abusive relationships, were there past relationships that may be affecting how you feel now?
- What are the effects of past violence on you now?
- How do these play a role in your recovery?

If you are not physically safe, ask for HELP to get to a SAFE PLACE.

Safety is a priority. The self-assessments above and communications with clinicians are important and can lead to important next steps:

- Taking care of yourself physically and emotionally.
- Getting yourself physically safe if you are not physically safe now.
- Addressing emotional consequences of past abuse and violence.
- Getting treatment for other co-occurring disorders (e.g., PTSD, depression, anxiety).
- Grieving losses from abuse and violence.
- Learning to manage feelings from past abuse or violence *without using substances*.

Session 10 Take-Home Messages

1. Many women in treatment for substance use disorders have experienced violence or other abuse.

2. Sometimes women use substances to "numb" or "mask" the pain of past or current abuse.

3. In order to recover from substance problems you must be **SAFE,** both physically and emotionally.

4. The first step is to get yourself physically safe if physical safety is not part of your life now.

5. If you are not physically threatened, but you have ongoing problems with your partner, consider counseling for yourself and/or your partner.

6. If you have a history of past abuse and/or violence, addressing the emotional consequences (including PTSD, depression, or anxiety) and grieving the losses can be helpful in recovery.

7. **Most important is to learn to manage these feelings without using substances and to be physically and emotionally safe.**

Session 10 Skill Practice: Violence and Abuse: Getting Help

(Please do this Skill Practice before the next group and bring it with you to the next session for the discussion at the beginning of group.)

1. Have you experienced violence or abuse? _____

_____

2. If you have experienced violence or abuse, please write down if it is past or present: _____

_____

3. If in the past, write down whether it was violence from a person known to you, a partner, a family member, or a stranger, or other: _____

4. Write down any negative consequences you feel you have suffered as a result: _____

_____

_____

_____

5. Write down any ways that you feel this has been related to your substance problem: _____

_____

_____

_____

6. If the violence or abuse is current, write down whether it is from a person known to you, a partner, a family member, or a stranger, or other: _____

_____

7. If it is current, write down if you are in physical danger: _____

_____

8. If you are in physical danger, let your group leader know and discuss options and alternatives so you can get to a place of physical and emotional safety. Please list any options you are considering now to get yourself safe: _____

_____

_____

_____

_____

9. List three ways you will support your recovery this week: _____

_____

_____

_____

Session 11 Overview:
The Issue of Disclosure: To Tell or Not to Tell?

Disclosure means:

Revealing thoughts and feelings while stating crucial facts about yourself.

 —Can be a choice or necessity.
 —Can happen intentionally or unintentionally.
 —Dilemma: *secrecy and control versus getting it out in the open; to tell or not to tell?*

The issue of disclosure is <u>personal</u>, *requires* <u>careful thought</u>, *and can be made best with* <u>prudence</u>, <u>restraint</u> *and* <u>safety</u>.

Barriers and Potential Disadvantages to Disclosure

- Fear of discrimination/discrimination.
- Fear of stigma.
- Feelings of shame.
- Giving up feeling of privacy/giving up privacy.
- Fear of rejection/rejection.

Potential Benefits of Disclosure

- Recognition and acceptance of existing supports that enhance recovery.
- Gaining new supports and building new relationships.
- Decreasing isolation.
- Beginning and/or continuing the healing and recovery process.
- Sharing new perspectives/helping others.
- Obtaining reasonable accommodations in the workplace, school, and at home to support your recovery, access treatment.

Issues Surrounding Disclosure

- How much do you want to disclose?
- To whom will you disclose? *(Choose someone you trust.)*
- To whom is it important that you *not* disclose?
- In what form will disclosure be made?
- When will you disclose?
- Why are you disclosing? What do you hope to gain?
- Where will you disclose? *(Choose a safe environment.)*

(continued)

Dos and Don'ts of Disclosure

- Think about your own readiness and comfort with disclosure.
- It is important to feel a secure sense that you are ready.
- Choose carefully to whom you might disclose. Emphasize feelings of safety and comfort.
- Make sure the environment is right. Choose people (colleagues, friends, partners, family members, etc.) whom you think will be open and willing to listen and accept.
- Think carefully and discuss the pros and cons with someone. Consider "what if" situations. ("What if I disclose and this happens?"; "How will I feel?" etc.).
- Remember, that once you have disclosed personal information, you cannot take it back.
- Disclose carefully and wisely, not impulsively and generally.

Session 11 Take-Home Messages

1. There can be pros and cons to disclosing that you are in recovery.

2. Think about your own readiness and comfort with disclosure.

3. If you choose to disclose, it is important to disclose wisely and carefully.

4. Choose the time, people, and place to disclose so that your disclosure will help support your recovery.

Session 11 Skill Practice:
The Issue of Disclosure: To Tell or Not to Tell?

(Please do this Skill Practice before the next group and bring it with you to the next session for the discussion at the beginning of group.)

If you have disclosed your substance problem to family, friends, employer/coworkers, or important others, answer questions 1–3. If you have not disclosed your substance problem to close family, friends, employer/coworkers, or important others, but you have considered doing so and are unsure what to do, answer questions 4–7. If you have disclosed to some and are considering disclosing to others, you can answer all questions 1–7.

1. List any benefits you feel you have experienced from disclosing your substance problem: ___

   _____

   _____

   _____

   _____

   _____

2. List any negative consequences you feel you have experienced from disclosing your substance problem: _____

   _____

   _____

   _____

   _____

3. Please describe what (if any) circumstances made the disclosure a positive and/or negative experience for you: _____

   _____

   _____

   _____

   _____

4. To whom would you consider disclosing your substance problem? (e.g., your spouse, friend, partner, employer, coworker): _____

   _____

   _____

   _____

(continued)

5. List any possible benefits you might experience if you chose to disclose your substance problem: _____

_____

_____

_____

_____

6. List any negative consequences you are worried you might experience if you disclose your substance problem: _____

_____

_____

_____

_____

7. Write about any specific circumstances that you feel might make it either harder or easier for you to feel comfortable disclosing your substance problem: _____

_____

_____

_____

_____

_____

_____

_____

Session 12 Overview:
Substance Use and Women's Reproductive Health

Introduction

- Substance problems are most common during the reproductive years.
- Mood problems and stress can accompany reproductive events, which can change patterns of substance use and substance problems.
- Hormonal changes may influence substance use and the effects of substances on women.

Review of Hormonal Changes

- Menstrual cycles.
- Birth control medications.
- Pregnancy and postpartum.
- Menopause transition.

Relationship of Substances to Reproductive Events

Menstrual Cycle and Substance Use

- Follicular phase occurs between first day of period and day of ovulation (usual day 14); luteal phase is phase between ovulation and onset of period (menstrual bleeding).
- Premenstrual phase is the 7 days before onset of period.
- Menstrual cycles can be irregular for many reasons.
- Alcohol use may increase premenstrually.
  - may be caused by either:
    1. Increased stress.
    2. Alcohol may be processed (metabolized) differently in this phase.
- Quit rates for smoking may be more successful in follicular (first 14 days) than luteal (second 14 days) of menstrual cycle.

Substances' Effects on Menstrual Cycle

- Severe alcohol problems may lead to irregular cycles or amenorrhea (no periods).
- Can disrupt hormones required for a normal cycle.
- Cocaine, marijuana, opioids, and benzodiazepines can also cause menstrual irregularities.

Risks to Pregnant Woman and Fetus

- Many substances interfere with a woman's ability to get pregnant.
- Continued use during pregnancy can increase the likelihood of miscarriage.
- Most substances (including alcohol and nicotine) cross the placenta and can cause problems for the developing fetus.

(continued)

- Most substances (including alcohol and nicotine) put the fetus at risk for negative effects (including severe, permanent, and sometimes fatal conditions).
- Drinking alcohol during pregnancy puts the fetus at risk for a number of significant problems, including fetal alcohol syndrome (FAS).
- Smoking cigarettes during pregnancy puts the fetus at risk for a number of significant problems, including low birthweight.

Breastfeeding and the Effect on Infants

- Most drugs and alcohol can be passed onto the infant through breast milk and therefore potentially affect the developing infant.
- Infant exposure to substances can affect development.

Oral Contraceptive Medications

- Can alter how substances are processed or metabolized.
- Women on OCP (oral contraceptive pill) can metabolize alcohol and benzodiazepines more slowly.

Perimenopause/Menopause

- Menopause is reached when women have no periods for 12 months or more and the hormonal changes of menopause occur.
- These hormonal changes are experienced by the entire body including the brain.
- Vasomotor symptoms such as hot flashes are commonly experienced by two-thirds of U.S. women; hot flashes can persist after menopause.
- Alcohol use disorders may lead to earlier menopause.

Alcohol Use Increases the Risk of Breast Cancer

- High estradiol levels are a risk for breast cancer and alcohol increases estradiol.
- Alcohol use, especially heavy drinking, can increase a woman's risk for developing breast cancer.
- Low to moderate drinking can also increase a woman's risk for developing breast and other cancers.

Safer Sex and Protection for Prevention of STDs, Including HIV

- Regardless of hormonal status or intentions about pregnancy, women need to learn about safer sex and protection and to use protection (e.g., condoms) for intimate sexual behavior.
- Condom use during heterosexual intercourse is important for protection for prevention of HIV, hepatitis C, and other sexually transmitted diseases.
- Women who are sexually active need to learn how to discuss condom use with male partners, and feel empowered to learn how to use condoms, why to use condoms, and how to discuss this with male partners.
- Safer Sex Skills Building for Women is a program that can be downloaded without cost from the National Institute on Drug Abuse (see *http://ctndisseminationlibrary.org/display/398.htm*) to assist women in learning these skills.

(continued)

What Can You Do?

- *Know your body.* Keep track of your own cycle and symptoms. This can provide insight into how your body works and its relationship with substance use and substance problems.
- *Seek professional help.* Gynecologists, primary care clinicians, and others can help you regulate abnormal menstrual cycles and provide treatment for perimenopausal and menopausal symptoms. If you are considering pregnancy or are pregnant, regular prenatal care and getting substance use treatment is important for your health and for the pregnancy and the developing fetus.
- *Use contraception.* Avoiding unplanned pregnancies is important for establishing a stable environment for recovery.
- *Practice safer sex.* Use protection when having intimate sexual relations with male partners to protect yourself from HIV, hepatitis C, and other sexually transmitted diseases.
- *Learn.* Seek information about your reproductive health and how that can be affected by alcohol and drugs.

Session 12 Take-Home Messages

1. Substances can affect women's hormones and health.

2. Changes in hormones over the life cycle can also affect women's substance use.

3. If you are of childbearing age, avoiding unplanned pregnancies is important to maintaining sobriety and having a stable situation for continued recovery.

4. Use protection and practice safer sex to avoid sexually transmitted diseases, including HIV and hepatitis C.

5. Knowing your body, learning more about hormones and health, and seeking professional help can be useful in managing hormonal changes at all stages of life.

6. Good self-care includes taking care of yourself, protecting your health, and not using substances to stay as well and healthy as possible.

Session 12 Skill Practice:
Substance Use and Women's Reproductive Health

(Please do this Skill Practice before the next group and bring it with you to the next session for the discussion at the beginning of group.)

1. Write down two reproductive-health issues you have had that have affected your patterns of using substances: _____

_____

_____

_____

_____

_____

_____

2. Write down any concerns you have had regarding substance use and your reproductive health: _____

_____

_____

_____

_____

_____

_____

_____

_____

3. Write down one thing that you plan to do differently in your recovery with regard to your reproductive health: _____

_____

_____

_____

_____

_____

_____

_____

(continued)

4. Below is a weekly chart. Write down your mood, cravings, substance use, and any reproductive health events (e.g., OCP use, menstrual periods, PMS, hot flashes) associated with each day. You can reproduce this weekly calendar each week or substitute a monthly calendar:

Sunday: _____

_____

_____

Monday: _____

_____

_____

Tuesday: _____

_____

_____

Wednesday: _____

_____

_____

Thursday: _____

_____

_____

Friday: _____

_____

_____

Saturday: _____

_____

_____

Session 13 Overview:
Can You Have Fun without Using Drugs or Alcohol?

Introduction

- Many women experience recovery as effortful/requiring a great deal of time.
- Feeling of loss—both of substances and things related to substances (e.g., partners, jobs, friends, health).
- Importance of balancing the work of recovery with having fun in one's life.

Recovery Work Includes Relapse Prevention and Repair Work

Relapse Prevention Includes:

- Identifying triggers and high-risk situations.
- Planning to avoid such situations or develop coping strategies.
- Making your environment as trigger-free as possible.
- Getting treatment.

Repair Work Includes:

- Repairing damage to self and relationships due to substances.
- Learning to enjoy life substance-free.

Enjoying Your Life In Recovery

Areas of concern (among many others) such as:

- Can I ever entertain people in my own home?
- What should I do at the holidays?
- Can I attend a ballgame or other sporting event?
- Can I attend a music festival?
- What should I do on winter holidays? New Year's Eve?
- Can I attend the July 4th or Memorial Day barbeque or event?
- How can I see my friends when they always get together at a bar?
- I have to attend a lot of work events where alcohol is served. What can I do?
- I liked to go to jazz clubs/music venues/other to relax, but there was always a lot of alcohol and other substances around.
- Everyone in my book group drinks. Can I go?
- All my friends use. What do I do? They say they don't mind if I don't use, but I am not confident I can be with them and not use.
- We always watch the Super Bowl at my house and serve beer. Now what?
- My nephew's/friend's/daughter's wedding is coming up, what should I do when it is time to toast?
- How can I celebrate the holidays with my family? They always drink.

(continued)

- Everyone in my school drinks or uses drugs. How can I have a social life and not use? How can I have friends and not use alcohol or drugs?
- There is a lot of drug use where I live. How can I avoid that and not be completely isolated?

Useful Strategies

- Identify high-risk situations you feel are impossible for you to participate in and avoid them. (*Keep in mind that avoidance of these situations may only be temporary.*)
- If you must participate in a high-risk situation, you can:
  ○ Bring someone supportive with you.
  ○ Limit the amount of time you spend in the situation (e.g., attend wedding ceremony and skip reception).
  ○ Learn to manage the situation without substances (use nonalcoholic beverages, turn over the wine glass).
- There may be some activities that need to be given up temporarily or even for the long-term.
  ○ In this case, it is important to *think of other ways to spend your leisure time* or connect with friends or make new friends.
  ○ You may *discover/rediscover interests* given up due to using.
- Some situations and/or people may have only been enjoyable while intoxicated.
- Find other activities you enjoy to substitute for these activities or events.
- Some strategies that may be useful include:
  ○ At a dinner party or restaurant, turn your wine glass over; the waiter will not ask if you want alcohol.
  ○ When you go to a reception, immediately get a nonalcoholic drink, so others will not try to give you a drink.
  ○ Attend events with a friend supportive of your recovery.
  ○ **Practice "substance refusal lines,"** such as "I am taking a medicine I can't use with alcohol." Try your own substance refusal lines.
  ○ Make your own home a "substance-free zone." This way frequent visitors will know there will be no substances in your home.
  ○ Many colleges have dormitories that are alcohol- and drug-free and students living in them make a commitment not to use.

Conclusions

- *Remember to think through situations and plan ahead.*
- *Remember that slowly but surely it is possible to find yourself having fun and feeling satisfied with life in recovery.*
- *It may take some time, but it can happen.*

Session 13 Take-Home Messages

1. Having fun when you are in recovery takes some advance planning.

2. There may be some activities that need to be avoided because they are too high risk.

3. Look for other things you like to do that don't include substances.

4. Find friends and relationships with whom you are comfortable not drinking or using drugs.

5. Practice drink and drug refusal lines to find the ones you are most comfortable using.

6. You can be substance-free, have fun, and feel satisfied with life in recovery.

Session 13 Skill Practice:
Can You Have Fun without Using Drugs or Alcohol?

(Please do this Skill Practice before the next group and bring it with you to the next session for the discussion at the beginning of group.)

1. Make a list of fun or satisfying events and activities that you enjoyed before recovery: _____

    _____

    _____

    _____

    _____

    _____

    _____

    _____

2. Make a list of fun or satisfying events and activities that are too high risk to include in your recovery life: _____

    _____

    _____

    _____

    _____

    _____

    _____

    _____

3. Make a list of fun or satisfying events and activities that you think you can enjoy in your recovery life that do not include drugs or alcohol: _____

    _____

    _____

    _____

    _____

    _____

    _____

    _____

(continued)

4. For any events or activities listed previously, are there special strategies you would use so that you could enjoy yourself and protect your recovery? _____

_____

_____

_____

_____

_____

5. Write down activities (new or old) that can be enjoyed without substances: _____

_____

_____

_____

6. Write in your own words three substance refusal lines that you know you would be comfortable using. Say them out loud. Bring these with you to share at the next group.

   1. _____

   _____

   2. _____

   _____

   3. _____

   _____

Session 14 Overview: Achieving a Balance in Your Life

Introduction

- Early recovery can be a time that feels "out of balance."
- Can feel that life is filled with treatment.
- Getting treatment can lead to excluding some other important activities.

Course of Recovery

- Tasks of early recovery include:
  - Learning about yourself.
  - Identifying internal and external triggers to use substances.
  - Determining positive coping strategies to manage triggers.
- Early in recovery, it is important to have enough treatment support for these tasks.
- Treatment supports can include:
  - Self-help groups.
  - Group treatment.
  - Individual treatment.
- Important to deal with ambivalence, set priorities, and achieve balance.

Dealing with Ambivalence

- Almost everyone experiences ambivalence some time in recovery.
- What are examples of ambivalent thinking?
  - Wondering whether you really have a substance problem or if it is as serious as others' substance problems.
  - Leads to thoughts such as:
      "It really isn't that bad."
      "I can do it on my own."
- What do you do when you experience ambivalent thoughts or behaviors?
  - Share the thoughts with someone else.
  - Stay in treatment, and don't use substances.
  - Anytime you consider changing your treatment, don't do it on your own.
- *Be sure to discuss pros and cons with your therapist, clinician, or sponsor, and reach an agreement before making changes to your treatment.*

Setting Priorities

- Early in recovery, recovery activities need to be high on the priority list.
- Learning to manage situations without substances takes a lot of support and practice.

(continued)

Achieving Balance in Your Life

- Over time, many women find managing situations substance-free to be easier.
- Slowly, life moves back into a new type of balance.
- This balance has at its center recovery and sobriety.

How to Achieve Balance

- Setting priorities.
- Not using substances to manage internal and external triggers.
- Dealing with ambivalence and not using substances or dropping out of treatment when ambivalence arises.
- Learning new ways to manage cravings and triggers and urges.
- Finding or resuming activities that are enjoyable and do not include substance use.
- Practicing these new behaviors and patterns until they feel more natural.

Session 14 Take-Home Messages

1. In early recovery it is important to deal with ambivalence.

2. At all stages of recovery, learn to know when you are having ambivalent thinking.

3. Setting priorities and valuing self-care is very important.

4. This can mean putting your recovery before other commitments.

5. Dealing with ambivalence and setting priorities can help you achieve a new kind of balance in your life.

Session 14 Skill Practice: Achieving a Balance in Your Life

(Please do this Skill Practice before the next group and bring it with you at the next session for the discussion at the beginning of group.)

1. Write three examples of ways that you feel ambivalent about recovery or behaviors you have had that show your ambivalence: _____

    _____

    _____

    _____

    _____

    _____

2. List the responsibilities and activities that you have right now in your life: _____

    _____

    _____

    _____

    _____

    _____

    _____

3. Look at the list you wrote in question 2. Do you think all of the things you wrote down can fit comfortably in your life right now? _____

    _____

    _____

    _____

    _____

4. Rank the different activities and responsibilities you listed in question 2 in order of priority for you. Notice where you are listing treatment and recovery in this ranking. _____

    _____

    _____

    _____

    _____

    _____

    _____

(continued)

5. Write how many of the things you mentioned in question 2 you can "fit in" your life now along with treatment and recovery activities. Which of the things do you think you would need to defer or delay right now so that you can take care of your top priorities? _____

_____

_____

_____

_____

_____

6. Write how you will set priorities for the coming week. What activities will you take care of, and which ones will you delay or defer for another time? Where does self-help fit? _____

_____

_____

_____

_____

_____

Reproducible Therapist Materials

This section includes all of the materials needed for each group session. There is a Check-In Sheet and Check-Out Sheet that should be reproduced and laminated if possible for durability. It is possible to create a two-sided laminated page with one side consisting of the check-in questions and the other side the check-out question. During the check-in and check-out portions of the session, the "Check-In" and "Check-Out" Sheets are passed from one group member to the next, as each participant orally answers the questions on the sheet. The three bulletin board posters that are present at every session (i.e., the Group Theme, the Central Recovery Rule, and the Common Symptoms of Substance Problems) are then followed by the session outline and take-home messages for each of the 14 sessions and these are posted for the specific topic of the week. Enlarged versions of the general and session-specific bulletin board materials for posting are available online. Purchasers of this book can download and print the materials in this appendix at *www.guilford.com/greenfield-forms* for personal use or use with clients. A therapist self-assessment for adherence to the treatment protocol can also be found here, as well as additional informational resources.

Check-In and Check-Out Sheets

Bulletin Board Posters

Bulletin Board Outlines and Take-Home Messages

Therapist Self-Assessment and Resources

Each group member will have 2–3 minutes to share the following with the group:

1. **Did you have any cravings or urges to use?**

2. **Did you use? If not, how were you able to remain sober?**

3. **Did you do the skill practice? If so, what did you do or find helpful?**

Check-Out Sheet

Each group member will have 1–2 minutes to share the following with the group:

What will you do in the coming week to support your recovery?

RECOVERY MEANS TAKING CARE OF YOURSELF

RECOVERY

=

RELAPSE PREVENTION

+

REPAIR WORK

Common Symptoms of Substance Problems

(Note: The word "substance" includes drugs and alcohol.)

- Increasing the amount of the substance(s) used over time.

- Trying unsuccessfully to cut down or stop using substances.

- Spending an increasing amount of time using substances, often leading to decreasing time spent in other activities related to work, school, relationships, or recreation.

- Having craving for the substance(s) when you are not using.

- Continuing to use substances even when knowing they cause or worsen problems with work, family, school, relationships, or other activities.

- Using substances even when knowing they cause physical or mental health problems or when they may be physically dangerous to use.

- Developing tolerance to the substance over time (i.e., developing a need for more of the substance in order to achieve the desired or usual effect).

- Experiencing withdrawal symptoms when substance use stops or is reduced.

Bulletin Board Outline for Session 1:
The Effect of Drugs and Alcohol on Women's Health

Common Symptoms of Substance Problems

(Please note that the word "substance" includes drugs and alcohol.)

- Increasing the amount of the substance(s) used over time.
- Trying unsuccessfully to cut down or stop using substances.
- Spending an increasing amount of time using substances, often leading to decreasing time spent in other activities related to work, school, relationships, or recreation.
- Craving the substance(s) when you are not using.
- Continuing to use substances despite knowing they cause or worsen problems with work, family, school, relationships, or other activities.
- Using substances despite knowing they cause physical or mental health problems or when they may be physically dangerous to use.
- Developing tolerance to the substance over time (i.e., developing a need for more of the substance in order to achieve the desired or usual effect).
- Experiencing withdrawal symptoms when substance use stops or is reduced.

Telescoping Course of Illness

- Women's substance use progress more rapidly from first using to first having problems with substances.
- Women get sicker faster using smaller quantities of alcohol or drugs than men.
- This telescoping course is true for both alcohol and other substances.
- Women can have more severe health effects from substance problems than men.

Neglected Self-Care

- While using, women often neglect themselves emotionally and physically.
- Emotional neglect can mean not doing the things necessary to nurture yourself.
- Women who use often neglect regular checkups or preventive care (i.e., mammograms, PAP smears, routine lab work) or neglect other healthful activities, such as exercise or eating well.
- Substance use may also lead to unintended and unprotected sexual encounters.

Take-Home Messages for Session 1:
The Effect of Drugs and Alcohol on Women's Health

1. Each drug has specific types of direct, negative effects on women's health.

2. For alcohol and drugs, women can experience a telescoping effect on the progress of their illness and the rapid advancement of these negative health effects and medical consequences.

3. Women's health, both physical and psychological, is also negatively affected by self-neglect.

4. This may lead to women neglecting to get routine physical health care.

5. It may also lead women to have sexual encounters that were unintended, unprotected, or done in order to obtain more drugs. These sexual encounters pose additional risks for women's health.

6. What you can do to be as healthy as possible:
   - *Be abstinent from drugs and alcohol.* Be on the road to recovery, and abstain from drugs. Many health effects are reversible, and others will stop worsening if you stop using.
   - *Get healthy.* See your primary care doctor or other clinician and sign up for routine physical checkups. Consult with your doctor about any adverse health conditions and what you can do to help care for yourself.
   - *Decrease self-neglect and increase self-care.* You can start by getting a physical exam. But don't let it stop there. What other things can you do to stay healthy? Exercise? Eat right? All of these things can help you be healthier and feel better, which in turn can help you continue your recovery and not use drugs and alcohol.

Bulletin Board Outline for Session 2:
How to Manage Triggers and High-Risk Situations

What Is a Trigger?

- Any person, place, or thing that increases your urge to use drugs or alcohol.
    Internal: thoughts and feelings.
    External: people, places, situations, or things.

High-Risk Situations

Internal

- Feelings: loneliness, anger, anxiety, or exhaustion.
- Thoughts: "What difference does it matter if I use just once?" or "No one cares about me."
- Physical discomfort: acute or chronic pain.

External

- People: seeing dealer, hanging around friends who use, seeing friend/relative who always criticizes.
- Places: passing bar or liquor store, or place where you often used or bought drugs.
- Things: money, cigarettes, liquor bottle, or drug paraphernalia.

Other High-Risk Situations

- Interpersonal conflict: arguments with family/partner/friends, difficulties with employer/coworkers/other students.
- Social pressure: family/partner/friends putting pressure on you to use.

Gender Differences in Facing Triggers

- Women tend to relapse in negative mood states (e.g., depression).
- Women often use with significant other.
- Negative mood states associated with premenstrual cycle also may be triggers.

Drug or Alcohol Availability

- Conditioned cues: alcohol or drugs, or internal or external experiences associated with their use.
- Conditioned responses: reactions to these cues, based on prior experiences.

(continued)

Avoiding High-Risk Situations

- Identify high-risk situations.
- Develop plans to avoid these situations.

Facing Unavoidable High-Risk Situations

- Don't face the situation alone.
- Do self-nurturing activities.
- Create structure in your day by cheduling tasks and activities.

What to Do to Avoid or Manage High-Risk Situations

- Make a list of current and past high-risk situations.
- Which are internal?
- Which are external situations?
- Divide the list into avoidable and unavoidable situations.
- Develop a list of ways to avoid the ones that you can.
- Develop a list of ways to manage the unavoidable ones.

Take-Home Messages for Session 2:
How to Manage Triggers and High-Risk Situations

1. **Avoid** high-risk situations whenever you can.

2. **If you can't avoid** the situation, don't face the situation alone. Get an ally who knows you are in recovery to accompany you.

3. Develop a way to "escape," or **leave early,** from a high-risk event.

4. For triggers that are internal, such as feelings or negative thoughts, find ways to **distract yourself** with other activities or positive thoughts.

5. **Plan ahead** and think through situations in advance. Identify high-risk people, places, or things that you will come across, and plan how to avoid or manage them.

6. Learn to **tolerate the feelings** associated with triggers and know they will pass.

Bulletin Board Outline for Session 3:
Overcoming Obstacles to Recovery

Stigma

- Substance problems may compromise women's life roles (as parents, partners, family members, students, workers, etc.).
- Fear of being labeled as "neglectful."
- Personal sense of shame, guilt, or embarrassment.
- May lead to keeping things secret from others and make it difficult to get the help and support you need.

Feeling That Other Problems Come First

- Women may think of their substance use as a *consequence* of other problems.

For example: *My substance use is because of . . .*

- Relationships: partners, family, children.
- Stressful life events: loss of job, spouse, marriage, parent, or friend.
- Mood or anxiety symptoms.

This may lead to thoughts such as

- "If these problems get fixed, I will be able to stop using . . ."
- Defining the "problem" as other things, women minimize the *extent* and *negative consequences* of substance use and do not get the help they need.

Mood or Anxiety Symptoms

- Women don't always share information about substance problems with clinicians because they think the substance problem isn't really the issue and it will be resolved by treating the other illnesses or other life issues.

Role Conflicts

- Difficulty of balancing roles: as workers, caretakers, children, and/or elder relatives.
- Stress of multiple roles can lead to feelings of being overwhelmed or "out of control."

(continued)

Other Barriers

- Lack of child or elder care.
- Lack of financial resources.
- Lack of partner or family support.
- Lack of information about the effectiveness of treatment and range of treatment options.
- Lack of stable housing or reliable transportation.

How Can You Overcome Recovery Obstacles?

- Make a personal inventory about your use of substances and their impact on your life (e.g., relationships, mood, health, work, or school).
- Make an inventory of the *feelings, ideas, and circumstances* that may be obstacles in recovery.
- Make a list of the ways substances affect your mood or feelings of anxiety.
- Learn about available treatment for substance disorders. Investigate resources that are available in your community, such as child care, medical care, employment, school, housing, health insurance.
- Ask for help.

Take-Home Messages for Session 3:
Overcoming the Obstacles to Recovery

1. Women often have powerful obstacles to their recovery. these can include:

   - Stigma about getting help for drugs and alcohol: Feeling ashamed.
   - Thinking the problem is only about depression and anxiety.
   - Feeling that they must take care of others before taking care of themselves.
   - Having an unsupportive partner or family.
   - Lacking financial or child care resources.
   - Lacking information about the fact that treatment works.

2. These obstacles can be overcome by asking for help, getting treatment, and helping to create your own network of support for your recovery.

3. Do a **personal inventory** about the use of substances in your life and the effects drugs and alcohol have had and are having on all the areas of your life, including relationships, mood, health, mental health, and work or school.

4. Make an **inventory of the ideas, feelings, and circumstances** that may be barriers or obstacles to your recovery.

5. Write a **list** of the ways substances affect your mood, feelings of anxiety, or eating problems. Write another list of how feelings such as depression, anxiety, or other difficult emotional states may affect your use of substances.

6. **Learn** as much as you can about available treatments for substance disorders.

7. **Learn** about other community supports for child care, medical care, employment, school, housing, transportation, insurance, or any other area that you have identified as a barrier for you to get help yourself and move forward in recovery.

Bulletin Board Outline for Session 4:
Managing Mood, Anxiety, and Eating Problems without Using Substances

Overview

- Women with drug and alcohol disorders often have other psychiatric symptoms/illnesses, such as depression, anxiety, and eating disorders.
- These disorders are much more common in women with substance use problems and substance use disorders than in men.
- Treatment is important for both substance use and these other psychiatric problems.

Depression

- Depressed mood most of the time.
- Feeling guilty, worthless, or helpless.
- Irritability, restlessness.
- Loss of interest in activities or hobbies once pleasurable, including sex.
- Fatigue and decreased energy.
- Difficulty concentrating, remembering details, and making decisions.
- Insomnia, early morning wakefulness, or excessive sleeping.
- Overeating or appetite loss.
- Thoughts about death or suicide.

People with depression usually experience a number of these types of symptoms most of the day nearly every day for at least 2 weeks. People can also have more "minor" depressions where some of these symptoms are present continuously for much longer periods of time.

Depression can change the way you think through:
- Irrational beliefs.
- Pessimistic thinking.
- Sense of hopelessness.
- Self-criticism and hearing criticism in what others say, even when it is not there.

Depressive thinking can lead to:
- "Self-fulfilling" prophecies: that is, you think that you can't succeed so you don't even try, thereby confirming your lack of success.
- Difficulty setting priorities and following through on tasks.
- Avoidance of other people, work situations, school, or other tasks.
- Problems taking care of yourself and your own recovery.

Anxiety

- There are several types of anxiety disorders.
- Most common are social anxiety disorder (social phobia) and generalized anxiety disorder (GAD).

(continued)

Social anxiety disorder (or social phobia) can be characterized by:

- Having an extreme amount of anxiety and fear of being judged by others and being embarrassed when observed by other people.
- Being very self-conscious in front of other people and feeling embarrassed especially in social situations or situations where you will be observed.
- Being afraid that other people will judge you and you will feel humiliated.
- Having excessive fear and worry before an event or social situation.
- Avoiding places or situations that will cause this anxiety.
- This fear can be so strong that it interferes with going to work or school or doing other everyday activities, as well as in social situations or settings such as performing, speaking.

Generalized anxiety disorder (GAD) can be characterized by:
Having an extreme amount of anxiety that is difficult to control, is more extreme than is warranted by the situation, and is focused on routine activities. Some common symptoms include:

- Difficulty relaxing or concentrating.
- Startling easily.
- Trouble falling or staying asleep.
- Physical symptoms such as fatigue, headaches, muscle tension, muscle aches, difficulty swallowing, trembling, twitching, irritability, nausea, sweating, lightheadedness, needing to use the bathroom frequently, breathlessness, and hot flashes.

Anxiety problems

- Often begin early in life, frequently in adolescence.
- Women often learn to "manage" their anxiety by using substances in situations that provoke anxiety.
- Anxiety problems → can trigger substance use. Substance use → more anxiety → more substance use.

Eating Problems and Eating Disorders

- Unhealthy eating behaviors (e.g., overeating, undereating) can sometimes be used by women to manage stress.
- Common eating disorders in women with substance use disorders and substance problems are anorexia nervosa, bulimia nervosa, and binge-eating disorder.

Anorexia nervosa can be characterized by:

- Low body weight due to restriction of calorie intake.
- Extreme fear of gaining weight or becoming fat.
- Distorted perception of own body weight or shape.
- Weight loss occurs by food restriction with or without binge eating or purging.

Bulimia nervosa can be characterized by the following symptoms:

- Having recurrent and frequent episodes of eating unusually large amounts of food (i.e., binge-eating episodes).
- Feeling a lack of control over these episodes.

(continued)

- After binge eating, doing things like forced vomiting (e.g., purging), taking laxatives or diuretics, fasting, or exercising excessively.
- Since these behaviors interfere with weight gain; individuals may maintain a normal body weight.
- Having excessive fear of gaining weight, wanting to lose weight, and feeling unhappy with body size and shape.

Bulimia can be accompanied by:

- Feelings of guilt and shame so that binging and purging often occur secretly.
- Other negative physical consequences including:
  o Chronically inflamed and sore throat.
  o Swollen salivary glands in the neck and jaw area.
  o Damaged tooth enamel, increasingly sensitive and decaying teeth as a result of exposure to stomach acid.
  o Acid reflux disorder and other gastrointestinal problems.
  o Intestinal distress and irritation from laxative abuse.
  o Severe dehydration from purging of fluids.

Binge-eating disorder: People with binge-eating disorder can:

- Lose control over their eating.
- Have periods of binge eating that are not followed by purging, excessive exercising, or laxative use.
- Become overweight or obese.
- Often experience guilt, shame and distress about these behaviors and that can lead to more binge eating.

Craving, loss of control, and preoccupation with substances (drug, alcohol, or food) are hallmarks of both substance and eating disorders.

Among women without an eating disorder:

- Urges and cravings for certain foods are common, especially in early recovery.
- Women may substitute unhealthy foods for substances.
- One coping strategy that can be helpful is to focus on good nutrition and establishing healthy eating.
- Healthy eating can be helpful in all phases of recovery.

Coping Strategies

- Understand and accept that the substance use and other disorders are both/all important.
- Get treatment for both/all disorders.
- Help mood and anxiety and eating problems: learn to recognize early symptoms so you can report them and get help before they progress.
- Don't use substances to manage these other problems.
- Don't let these other disorders/problems stop your recovery from substance problems.
- Develop positive coping strategies for both/all disorders.

Take-Home Messages for Session 4:
Managing Mood, Anxiety, and Eating Problems without Using Substances

1. Mood, anxiety, and eating problems are common in women with drug and alcohol problems.

2. These other problems can make it difficult to get well from your substance problem.

3. The substance problem can also make it hard to get well from your mood, anxiety, or eating problem.

4. Understand and accept that the substance use and these other disorders and problems are important.

5. Get treatment for both/all disorders.

6. Taking care of yourself is getting the help you need for your recovery from your substance use disorder and your co-occurring depression, anxiety, and/or eating disorders.

Bulletin Board Outline for Session 5:
Women and Their Partners: The Effect on Recovery

What Is a Partner?

- An individual with whom a woman is intimately involved (e.g., spouse, boyfriend, girlfriend, and/or father/mother of child[ren]).
- Relationships are strongly connected with women's addiction and recovery.

Partners' Influence on Substance Problems, Addiction, and Recovery

Having a Partner: Influence on Substance Problems and Recovery

Negative Influences

INITIATION OF SUBSTANCE USE

- Introduction to using substances by male partner is common among heterosexual women.
- Less is known about lesbian couples regarding partner influence on initiation but their prevalence of substance problems in lesbian couples is estimated to be 28–35%.
- Women with addiction are more likely to have a male partner who uses drugs and alcohol than men are to have a woman partner who uses.

CONTINUING SUBSTANCE USE

- Partners may supply women's drugs.
- Women may rely on male partners to maintain addiction.
- Male partner may supply drug/supervise or coerce illegal activities.
- Partner may continue to drink/keep alcohol or use drugs in the home while woman tries to be in recovery.

SUBSTANCE USE MAY BE MAIN FOCUS OF THE RELATIONSHIP

- Women may fear losing partner if she stops using.
- Sexual activity may have always been in context of drug/alcohol use.
- Use seen as way to maintain relationship.

SETTING UP OBSTACLES FOR GETTING TREATMENT

- Partners may have negative attitude toward women getting treatment.
- Women may fear loss of relationship.
- Sexual activity in context of drug/alcohol use.
- Women dependent on partners, fear abandonment, fear loss of financial resources.
- Physical threats by partners if woman seek treatment.

(continued)

ROLE IN RELAPSE

- Relapse more likely when using with a partner.
- Use substances as a way to reconnect with a partner who uses.
- Women tend to relapse after difficult emotional/interpersonal experiences, often with partner.
- Some difficulties within a couple may have started before substances were a problem.
- Some difficulties within a couple may be a consequences of the substances themselves.
- If living with an addicted partner, may relapse because substances freely available.

Positive Influences

- Partners who do not use can help women enter treatment and remain in recovery.
- Partners can help maintain an alcohol- and drug-free home.
- Partners can support a woman's recovery through companionship without drugs or alcohol.
- Partners can provide support through high-risk situations.
- Partners can engage in treatment.
  - Individual treatment.
  - Couple counseling.
  - If using themselves, their own substance use disorder treatment.
  - Self-help groups such as Al-Anon, etc.

The Absence of a Partner: Influence on Substance Problems and Recovery

Negative Influences

- Feelings of loneliness or abandonment.
- Feeling more isolated or lack of social or other types of support.
- Common places to find a partner can involve use of drugs/alcohol.
- *These can pose a high risk for relapse.*

Positive Influences

- More flexible for recovery activities.
- Can make home a drug-free zone.
- Can "start from the beginning" and enter a new relationship without drugs or alcohol where there are no expectations/history of drug use.

What Can You Do?

- Examine past/present intimate relationships.
- Examine positive/negative roles that an intimate partner plays in your recovery.

What Are Some Things You Could Do That Might Be Helpful?

- If your partner uses, is he/she willing to give up his/her own substance use?
- Is your partner willing to make home a substance-free zone?
- Is your partner willing to engage in treatment, either with you or on his/her own?

Take-Home Messages for Session 5:
Women and Their Partners: The Effect on Recovery

1. The first rule of recovery is: **do not use drugs and alcohol**.

2. Partners are people with whom a woman is intimately involved (e.g., spouse, boyfriend, girlfriend, and/or father/mother of child[ren]).

3. Partners can be **critically important** in supporting or getting in the way of your recovery.

4. The **absence of a partner** relationship can also influence your substance disorder and process of recovery in positive or negative ways.

5. It is important that you **think about what role** having or not having a partner plays in your recovery.

6. This is the **first step** to understanding and deciding the best way to help yourself be **abstinent from drugs and alcohol** and have the **healthiest possible relationships**.

There Are Different Causes of Stress, Including:

- External stressors.
- Internal stressors.

External Stressors

- *Ordinary stressors:* common and daily stressors (e.g., minor illnesses, traffic, work problems, minor conflicts with family/friends).
- *Extraordinary stressors:* less common and more extreme (e.g., death in family, job loss, homelessness, severe illness).

Internal Stressors

Negative feelings/attitudes that arise from experience of outside world. For example:
- Perfectionism.
- Pessimism.
- Negativism.
- Concern about others' opinions.
- Need for control.

Stressors Associated with Women's Roles

- Being the primary caregiver.
  - For one's own family and/or elders.
  - Managing the household.
  - Providing primary/secondary income for self and family.
- Financial constraints.
- Limited access to child/elder care.
  - Single motherhood.
  - Other.
- Minimal or no support from partner/family member for household responsibilities.
- Own problems not given top priority.

Emotional Consequences of Stress

- Depression.
- Low self-esteem.
- Anxiety.
- Shame.
- Guilt.
- Anger.

Which can lead to:
- Initiation of substance use.
- Rationale for continued use.
- Relapse.

(continued)

Coping with Stressful Situations

- Best response to stressful situations is to develop and have **healthy coping skills.**

Unhealthy Coping

- Provides temporary escape from stressors (substance use can be one of these).
- Situation still exists or worsens.
- Does not provide model for resolving/managing stressor.
- Examples:
  - Smoking cigarettes.
  - Increasing unhealthy food consumption.
  - Keeping feelings to yourself.
  - Complaining about a problem but doing nothing.
  - Criticizing yourself/others.
  - Punishing yourself (e.g., overeating/undereating, excessive exercise).
  - Striving for perfection.
  - Developing harmful relationships.
  - Isolating yourself from others.
  - Being passive.

Healthy Coping Skills

- Help resolve/manage current stressor.
- Provides a model for managing future stressors.
- Examples:
  - Sharing feelings with others.
  - Making a plan to handle problem.
  - Seeing humor in situation.
  - Engaging in pleasurable activities (e.g., reading, hobbies).
  - Accepting your limitations.
  - Developing positive relationships.
  - Being assertive.
  - Helping others.
  - Meditating.
  - Practicing yoga or exercising.
  - Doing other self-care activities.

What Can You Do to Cope with Stress?

- List current/past stressful situations/relationships that led to unhealthy coping skills (e.g., substance use).
- Divide list into stressors you can change and stressors you cannot change.
- Develop alternative coping skills for different situations.
- Quit smoking cigarettes (resource: *http://women.smokefree.gov*).
- Practice meditation daily.
- Practice yoga or exercise or do other self-care activities.
- Use a telephone app if you can to help with meditation, mindfulness, or other stress-relieving daily activities.

Take-Home Messages for Session 6:
Coping with Stress

1. Stress can be caused by **routine life circumstances**, such as bad weather, deadlines, or traffic.

2. Stress can be caused by **more serious life events**, such as loss of a job, death of a family member, serious illness, or exposure to violence.

3. Stress can also be caused by **internal states** such as feelings, thoughts, and attitudes such as perfectionism, negative thoughts, etc.

4. Stress can lead to feelings of depression, low self-esteem, anxiety, shame, guilt, and anger.

5. These feelings can lead to starting to use, continuing to use, or relapsing to using substances.

6. There are many ways to **cope with stress**. Some of these, like using drugs and alcohol, or smoking cigarettes, are **unhealthy**.

7. There are many **healthy** ways of coping with stress.

8. You can help your recovery by learning and practicing as many healthy ways to cope with stress as you can think of.

Bulletin Board Outline for Session 7:
Women as Caretakers: Can You Take Care of Yourself While You Are Taking Care of Others?

Women's Role as Caretakers (or Caregivers):

- Women need to be able to take care of themselves (self-care) in order to be able to take care of others.
- Relationships are generally valued strongly by women.
- Caretaking role can give self-esteem and fulfillment.
- Women's caretaking role can also interfere with self-care, including treatment and recovery.

What Are Some Caretaking Roles?

On the home front:

- Children.
- Elders.
- Partners.
- Families.
- Friends.
- Siblings.
- Pets.

On the work or school front:

- Coworkers.
  - Other students.
  - People you supervise.
- People within work or school organization.

In communities:

- Neighbors/neighborhoods.
- Schools.
- Religious groups.
- Other community groups.

Social Connectedness: often a source of strength and value for women.

Lack of Social Connectedness: can lead to feelings of isolation and lack of support.

The role of caretaker can be a source of value, self-esteem, and motivation, but it can also interfere with the ability to take care of self (e.g., to get into treatment and recover from substance problems).

(continued)

How Do Caretaking Roles Interfere with the Ability to Get into Treatment and Recovery?

1. The Belief of Having No Time
   - Putting needs of others first.
   - Need to minimize the time spent at treatment/recovery to care for others.
   - Drugs and alcohol as coping with caretaking demands—may deter women from seeking treatment.
2. The Role of Guilt and Shame
   - Actual or perceived neglect of others.
   - Neglecting others because of substance use.
   - Not available physically/emotionally because of substance use.
   - *Avoiding* these feelings may deter women from seeking treatment.
3. Fear of Losing Custody
   - Fear if enter treatment will lose custody of children.
   - Critically delays getting treatment.
   - May worsen substance problems.
   - Can lead to intervention from others (e.g., child welfare services).

How Can You Be a Caretaker and Take Care of Yourself?

Learn, acknowledge, accept, and *apply* these to your life:

- You cannot do the best job you'd like to do as a caretaker when using drugs/alcohol.
- To be the caretaker you most want to be is dependent on *not* using drugs/alcohol.
- Using drugs/alcohol can take time and attention away from significant relationships.
- Waiting until you have time doesn't work; it only delays help and worsens substance problems.
- You *do* have time to get help and work toward recovery.
- Recovery = Self-Care.

Take-Home Messages for Session 7:
Women as Caretakers: Can You Take Care of Yourself While You Are Taking Care of Others?

1. You do have time to take care of yourself.

2. Use the strength of your role as a caretaker (or caregiver) and your desire to be the best you can be as a motivation to seek the help you need for treatment and for your ongoing recovery.

3. Women sometimes avoid taking care of themselves and their recovery because they feel guilty that they might not be taking care of others.

4. Sometimes women convince themselves they have no time to take care of their recovery because of their other responsibilities. This is the "Belief of Having No Time."

5. It is important to take care of yourself so that you can take care of any others who are important to you.

6. Recovery is a major part of self-care and necessary to be able to take care of any others who are important to you.

Bulletin Board Outline for Session 8:
Using Self-Help Groups to Help Yourself

Self-Help Groups

- Alcoholics Anonymous (AA)
  - International fellowship of men/women with drinking problems.
  - Abstinence-based 12-step program.
  - Different types and formats for AA (open, closed, speaker meeting, discussion meetings, step meetings, women-only, and others such as men-only, non-smoking, teenagers/young adults/LGBTQ, or combination of these).
- Narcotics Anonymous, Cocaine Anonymous, Gamblers Anonymous
  - Same principles as AA.
  - Address problems with opioids, benzodiazepines, marijuana, amphetamines, prescription drugs (NA), cocaine (CA), or gambling (GA).
- SMART Recovery
  - Self-Management and Recovery Training (SMART).
  - Treatment based on CBT model of addiction.
  - Smaller than groups/less available 12-step groups, such as AA.

Pros and Cons of 12-Step Groups

Pros/Advantages

- Education—learn about recovery from others.
- Hope—others' experiences can inspire hope.
- Support—gain support from other members or sponsor.
- Availability—usually available 24/7/365 worldwide.
- Spirituality—appeals to a Higher Power consistent with your beliefs.
- Effectiveness—some evidence that involvement associated with long-term recovery.

Cons/Disadvantages

- Isolation—can feel isolated within the group.
- Spirituality—not consistent with your beliefs.
- Language—language used can be offensive.
- "War stories"—members' stories are depressing and not inspiring.
- Unwanted familiarity—makes you uncomfortable.

Pros and Cons of SMART Recovery

Pros/Advantages

- Group size—generally small group.
- CB approach—change cognitions and behaviors.
- No spirituality—consistent with your beliefs.

(continued)

Cons/Disadvantages

- Abstinence—not always abstinence-focused.
- Support—may feel you should use CB approach and not reach for member support.
- Effectiveness—no studies of effectiveness.
- Availability—not available 24/7/365 and not available in all regions of the United States.
- No spirituality—not consistent with your beliefs.

How to Use Self-Help Groups to Help Yourself

- Review list of groups and identify which ones to attend.
- After each meeting, write down what you liked/disliked about it.
- Consider women-only AA/NA meetings.
- Keep track of groups attended and how much you participated.
- If you cannot attend specific groups, try visiting websites or calling different organizations to identify groups and times you can attend.

Take-Home Messages for Session 8:
Using Self-Help Groups to Help Yourself

1. Involvement in self-help groups can help you achieve and maintain long-term recovery.

2. There are different kinds of self-help groups, including some for women only.

3. Sample a number of different types of self-help groups before deciding if they are for you.

4. Work on finding groups that best suit your recovery needs in terms of the type of meeting, location and timing of the meetings, and membership with which you feel comfortable.

Bulletin Board Outline for Session 9:
Women's Use of Substances through the Life Cycle

Substance Use Disorders

- Usually have early onset in adolescence or early 20s.
- However, onset can occur or reoccur at any time during the lifespan.
- Pressures, triggers, and risk factors vary at different times in women's lives.
- A risk factor is something that increases chance of developing substance problems.

Life Stages and Risk Factors

Adolescence

- Social context.
- Depression.
- Feelings of alienation or isolation, especially among sexual minority girls, girls who are bullied, or girls who otherwise feel discrimination or marginalization.
- Earlier age of first use of substances increases risk for abuse.
- Smoking cigarettes.
- Trauma.
- Prescription drug use carries risk for problems/addiction.

Young Adulthood

- Partner with alcohol or drug problem.
- Depression.
- Role-related issues leading to maladaptive coping strategies.
- Problems with any substance increases risk of other substance problems.
- Trauma.
- Prescription drug use carries risk for problems/addiction.

Middle Years

- Partner with alcohol or drug problem.
- Depression.
- Losses common to this stage of life.
- Feelings of unlikelihood about acquiring new life roles.
- Substance problems—any substance problem can predispose to problems with other substances.
- Prescription drug use carries risk for problems/addiction.

(continued)

Older Age

- Partner with alcohol or drug problem.
- Depression.
- Prescription drug use.
- Retirement.
- Widowhood/loss of a partner.
- Changes in metabolism.
- Retirement communities where alcohol is prominent part of social life.

How to Help Yourself

- Understand that use of substances and risk for substance problems changes throughout women's life cycle.
- Be aware of specific risks associated with your current life stage.
- Understand these risks and construct ways to manage them without using drugs or alcohol.

Take-Home Messages for Session 9:
Women's Use of Substances through the Life Cycle

1. Women's life stages include adolescence, young adulthood, the middle years, and older age.

2. Each stage of women's lives has different rewards and challenges.

3. The use of substances can change throughout women's life cycle, and the risks for substance problems can change over time.

4. Specific risks for substance use can be associated with each person's current stage of life.

5. Find ways to manage these situations that do not include using drugs or alcohol.

6. Different stages in a woman's life cycle may also bring vulnerability to substances.

7. Identify the specific risks of this time in your life and think of opportunities now that can help in the recovery process.

Bulletin Board Outline for Session 10:
Violence and Abuse: Getting Help

Substance Use Disorders and Violence

- Many women in treatment for substance use disorders have experienced violence or other abuse (e.g., sexual or physical abuse or intimate partner violence).
- They may use drugs/alcohol to "numb" or "mask" the pain of past (or current) abuse.
- Past abuse may lead to risk in adulthood for further violence or abuse.
- These experiences in childhood or adulthood can contribute to feelings of shame and social isolation.

Experiences Associated with History of Violence

- Co-occurring disorders with substance use disorders (e.g., depression, anxiety, PTSD).
- Shame and guilt.
- Avoidant coping.
- Feelings of stigmatization.
- Inhibit trust in relationships.

These feelings can:

- Predispose women to using substances to mask or numb the painful feelings.
- Contribute to feelings of low self-worth—lead to feeling socially disconnected.

All of these can serve as triggers to relapse and obstacles to recovery from substance problems.

Emotional, Psychological, and Verbal Abuse

- Partner controls woman's choices.
- Difference in power within relationship.
- Childhood abuse (including emotional abuse) makes women more vulnerable to substance use problems later.
- Adulthood abuse predisposes women to using substances and acts as an obstacle to getting treatment and being in recovery.

Domestic Violence/Interpersonal Violence (IPV)

- More common than is generally thought.
- Risk of domestic violence greater in setting of substance use and substance use disorders.
- Three-quarters of all incidents involve alcohol.
- Another factor may be perceived inequality between partners (such as in unemployment, income, finances, family roles).

(continued)

- One member of couple can feel less powerful or powerless and may, in fact, have fewer resources to express her autonomy.
- IPV occurs in both heterosexual and gay and lesbian couples.
- Drug and alcohol problems increase risk for IPV.
- **Vicious cycle:** → *violence and abuse* → *more substance abuse* → *more violence and abuse.*
- These patterns inhibit seeking treatment for substance problems and getting help to get safe and stop the violence.

Relationship of abuse and violence to problems with substances:

- Women who experience violence may use substances to try to cope with the trauma of abuse or violence.
- Women who use substances may be more vulnerable to violence.
- Women who are intoxicated may be less able to defend themselves against violence.
- Women who use substances can feel guilt and shame about their substance use, as well as about the abuse and violence; this can lead to decreased feelings of self-worth and the idea that they are less deserving of getting the help they need.
- Women (whether they use substances or not) who are with substance-using partners are at greater risk for abuse and IPV.

How to Get Help to Help Yourself

- Assess for yourself and communicate with your clinicians your own experience of violence and abuse.

Before Treatment and Recovery

- Have you experienced abuse before your substance use/treatment for substance use?
- Do you think this may have contributed to use of substances and/or difficulty seeking treatment?

During Treatment and Recovery

- Are you currently being exposed to violence or other abuse?
- If you are not physically safe, it is important to seek a safe place.
- If you are not physically threatened or in danger, but have ongoing problems with your partner, consider counseling for yourself and/or your partner.
- Consider questions such as:
  - How often does your partner show disapproval toward you?
  - When was the last time you felt threatened by or controlled by or afraid of your partner?
  - How often does someone hurt you?
  - How often does your partner use words that put you down and make you feel bad about yourself?

(continued)

In Recovery and Maintaining Abstinence

- Are there any ongoing abusive relationships in your life?
- Do you need to find a place to be physically safe?
- What would be the best way to take care of yourself?
- If there are no current abusive relationships, were there past relationships that may be affecting how you feel now?
- What are the effects of past violence on you now?
- How do these play a role in your recovery?

If you are not physically safe, ask for HELP to get to a SAFE PLACE.

Safety is a priority. The self-assessments above and communications with clinicians are important and can lead to important next steps:

- Taking care of yourself physically and emotionally.
- Getting yourself physically safe if you are not physically safe now.
- Addressing emotional consequences of past abuse and violence.
- Getting treatment for other co-occurring disorders (PTSD, depression, anxiety).
- Grieving losses from abuse and violence.
- Learning to manage feelings from past abuse or violence *without using substances*.

Take-Home Messages for Session 10:
Violence and Abuse: Getting Help

1. Many women in treatment for substance use disorders have experienced violence or other abuse.

2. Sometimes women use substances to "numb" or "mask" the pain of past or current abuse.

3. In order to recover from substance problems you must be **SAFE**, both physically and emotionally.

4. The first step is to get yourself physically safe if physical safety is not part of your life now.

5. If you are not physically threatened, but you have ongoing problems with your partner, consider counseling for yourself and/or your partner.

6. If you have a history of past abuse and/or violence, addressing the emotional consequences (including PTSD, depression, anxiety) and grieving the losses can be helpful in recovery.

7. **Most important is to learn to manage these feelings without using substances and to be physically and emotionally safe.**

Bulletin Board Outline for Session 11:
The Issue of Disclosure: To Tell or Not to Tell?

Disclosure means:

Revealing thoughts and feelings while stating crucial facts about yourself.

- Can be a choice or necessity.
- Can happen intentionally or unintentionally.
- Dilemma: *secrecy and control versus getting it out in the open*; to tell or not to tell?

The issue of disclosure is personal, requires careful thought, and can be made best with prudence, restraint, and safety.

Barriers and Potential Disadvantages to Disclosure

- Fear of discrimination/discrimination.
- Fear of stigma.
- Feelings of shame.
- Feelings of loss of privacy/loss of privacy.
- Fear of rejection/rejection.

Potential Benefits of Disclosure

- Recognition and acceptance of existing supports enhance recovery.
- Gaining new supports and building new relationships.
- Decreasing isolation.
- Beginning and/or continuing the healing and recovery process.
- Sharing new perspectives/helping others.
- Obtaining reasonable accommodations in the workplace, school, and at home.

Issues Surrounding Disclosure

- How much do you want to disclose?
- To whom will you disclose? *(Choose someone you trust.)*
- To whom is it important that you *not* disclose?
- In what form will disclosure be made?
- When will you disclose?
- Why are you disclosing? What do you hope to gain?
- Where will you disclose? *(Choose a safe environment.)*

Dos and Don'ts of Disclosure

- Think about your own readiness and comfort with disclosure.
- It is important to feel a secure sense that you are ready.

(continued)

From *Treating Women with Substance Use Disorders: The Women's Recovery Group Manual* by Shelly F. Greenfield. Copyright © 2016 The Guilford Press. Permission to photocopy this material is granted to purchasers of this book for personal use or use with individual clients (see copyright page for details). Purchasers can download additional copies of this material (see the box at the end of the table of contents).

- Choose carefully to whom you might disclose. Emphasize to yourself feelings of safety and comfort.
- Make sure the environment is right. Choose people whom you think will be open and willing to listen and accept.
- Think carefully and discuss the pros and cons with someone. Consider "what if" situations.
- Remember that once you have disclosed personal information, you cannot take it back.
- Disclose carefully and wisely, not impulsively and generally.

Take-Home Messages for Session 11:
The Issue of Disclosure: To Tell or Not to Tell?

1. There can be pros and cons of disclosing that you are in recovery.

2. Think about your own readiness and comfort with disclosure.

3. If you choose to disclose, it is important to disclose wisely and carefully.

4. Choose the time, people, and place to disclose so that your disclosure will help support your recovery.

Bulletin Board Outline for Session 12:
Substance Use and Women's Reproductive Health

Introduction

- Substance use problems are most common during the reproductive years.
- Mood problems and stress can accompany reproductive events, which can change patterns of use and substance problems.
- Hormonal changes may influence substance use and effects of substances on women.

Review of Hormonal Changes

- Menstrual cycles.
- Birth control medications.
- Pregnancy and postpartum.
- Menopause transition.

RELATIONSHIP OF SUBSTANCES TO REPRODUCTIVE EVENTS

Menstrual cycle and substance use

- Alcohol use may increase premenstrually.
- May be caused by either:
  1. Increased stress.
  2. Alcohol may be processed differently.
- Quit rates for smoking may be more successful in follicular (first 14 days) than luteal (second 14 days) of menstrual cycle.

Substances' effect on menstrual cycle

- Severe alcohol problems may lead to irregular cycles or amenorrhea (no periods).
- Can disrupt hormones required for a normal cycle.
- Cocaine, marijuana, opioids, and benzodiazepines can also cause irregularities.

Risks to pregnant woman and fetus

- Substances can interfere with a woman's ability to get pregnant.
- Continued use during pregnancy can increase the likelihood of miscarriage.
- Most substances (including alcohol and nicotine) cross placenta and can cause problems for the developing fetus.
- Most substances put the fetus at risk for negative effects (including severe, permanent, and sometimes fatal conditions).
- Drinking alcohol during pregnancy puts the fetus at risk for a number of significant problems.
- Smoking cigarettes during pregnancy puts the fetus at risk for a number of significant problems.

(continued)

Breastfeeding and the effect on infants

- Most alcohol and drugs can be passed on to the infant through breast milk and therefore possibly affect the developing infant.
- Infant exposure to substances can affect development.

Oral contraceptive medications

- Can alter how substances are metabolized or processed.
- Women on OCP (oral contraceptive pill) metabolize alcohol and benzodiazepines more slowly.

Perimenopause/Menopause

- Menopause is reached when women have no periods for 12 or more months and the hormonal changes of menopause occur.
- Alcohol use disorders may lead to earlier menopause.
- Alcohol use, especially heavy drinking, can increase a woman's risk of breast cancer.
- Low to moderate drinking can also increase a woman's risk for developing breast and other cancers.

Safer sex and protection for prevention of STDs including HIV

- Women need to learn about safer sex and protection and to use protection (e.g., condoms) for intimate sexual behavior.
- Condom use during heterosexual intercourse is important for protection for prevention of HIV, hepatitis C, and other sexually transmitted diseases.
- Women who are sexually active need to learn how to discuss condom use with male partners, and feel empowered to learn how to use condoms, why to use condoms, and how to discuss this use with male partners.
- "Safer Sex Skills Building" for women can be downloaded without cost from the National Institute on Drug Abuse (Safer Sex Skills Building [SSSB]: *http://ctndisseminationlibrary.org/display/398.htm*) to assist women with these skills.

What Can You Do?

- ***Know your body***. Keep track of your own cycle and symptoms. This can provide insight into how your body works and its relationship with substance use and substance problems.
- ***Seek professional help***. Gynecologists, primary care clinicians, and other clinicians can help you regulate abnormal menstrual cycles and provide treatment for perimenopausal and menopausal symptoms. If you are considering pregnancy or are pregnant, regular prenatal care and getting substance use treatment is important for your health and for the pregnancy and the developing fetus.
- ***Use contraception***. Avoiding unplanned pregnancies is important for establishing a stable environment for recovery.
- ***Practice safer sex***. Use protection when having intimate sexual relations to protect yourself from HIV, hepatitis C, and other sexually transmitted diseases.
- ***Learn***. Seek information about your reproductive health and how that can be affected by alcohol and drugs.

Take-Home Messages for Session 12:
Substance Use and Women's Reproductive Health

1. Substances can affect women's hormones and health.

2. Changes in hormones over the life cycle can also affect women's substance use.

3. If you are of childbearing age, avoiding unplanned pregnancies is important to maintaining sobriety and having a stable situation for continued recovery.

4. Use protection and practice safer sex to avoid sexually transmitted diseases including HIV and hepatitis C.

5. Knowing your body, learning more about hormones and health, and seeking professional help can be useful in managing hormonal changes at all stages of life.

6. Good self-care includes taking care of yourself, protecting your health, and not using substances in order to stay as well and healthy as possible.

Bulletin Board Outline for Session 13:
Can You Have Fun without Using Drugs or Alcohol?

Introduction

- Many women experience recovery as effortful/requiring a great deal of time.
- Feeling of loss—both of substances and things related to substances (e.g., partners, jobs, friends).
- Importance of balancing work of recovery with having fun in one's life.

Recovery Work Includes Relapse Prevention and Repair Work

Relapse Prevention includes:

- Identifying triggers and high-risk situations.
- Planning to avoid such situations or develop coping strategies.
- Making your environment as trigger-free as possible.
- Getting treatment.

Repair Work includes:

- Repairing damage to self and relationships due to substances.
- Learning to enjoy life substance-free.

Enjoying Your Life In Recovery

Areas of concern (among many others) such as:

- Can I ever entertain people in my own home?
- What should I do at the holidays?
- Can I attend a ballgame or other sporting event?
- Can I attend a music event?
- Can I attend the July 4th or Memorial Day barbecue or event?
- How can I see my friends when they always get together at a bar?
- I have to attend a lot of work events where alcohol is served. What can I do?
- I liked to go to jazz clubs/music venues/other places to relax, but there was always a lot of alcohol and other substances around.
- Everyone in my book group drinks. Can I go?
- All my friends use. What do I do? They say they don't mind if I don't use, but I am not confident that I can be with them and not use.
- We always watch the Super Bowl at my house and serve beer. Now what?
- My nephew's/friend's/daughter's wedding/birthday, etc. is coming up. What should I do when it is time to toast?
- How can I celebrate the holidays with my family? They always drink.
- Everyone in my school drinks or uses drugs. How can I have a social life and not use? How can I have friends and not use alcohol or drugs?
- There is a lot of drug use where I live. How can I avoid that and not be completely isolated?

(continued)

Useful Strategies

- **Identify high-risk situations you feel are impossible for you to participate in and avoid them. *(Keep in mind that avoidance of these situations may only be temporary.)***
- **If you must participate in a high-risk situation, you can:**
  - Bring someone supportive with you.
  - Limit the amount of time you spend in the situation (e.g., attend wedding ceremony and skip reception).
  - Learn to manage the situation without substances (use nonalcoholic beverages, turn over the wine glass).
- There may be some activities that need to be given up temporarily or even for the long term.
  - In this case, it is important to think *of other ways to spend your leisure* time or connect with friends or make new friends.
  - You may *discover/rediscover interests* given up due to using.
- Some situations and/or people may have only been enjoyable while you were intoxicated.
- Find other activities you enjoy to substitute for these activities.
- Some strategies that may be useful include:
  - At a dinner party, turn your wine glass over; the waiter will not ask if you want alcohol.
  - When you go to a reception, immediately get a nonalcoholic drink, so others will not try to give you a drink.
  - Attend events with a friend supportive of your recovery.
  - **Practice "substance refusal lines,"** such as "I am taking a medicine I can't use with alcohol," "I am not drinking right now," or "I don't use that anymore." Try your own substance refusal lines.
  - Make your own home a "substance-free zone." This way frequent visitors will know there will be no substances in your home.
  - Many colleges have dormitories that are alcohol- and drug-free and students living in them make a commitment not to use.

Conclusions

- *Remember to think through situations and plan ahead.*
- *Remember that slowly but surely it is possible to find yourself having fun and feeling satisfied with life in recovery.*
- *It may take some time, but it can happen.*

Take-Home Messages for Session 13:
Can You Have Fun without Using Drugs or Alcohol?

1. Having fun when you are in recovery takes some advance planning.

2. There may be some activities that need to be avoided because they are too high risk.

3. Look for other things you like to do that don't include substances.

4. Find friends and relationships with whom you are comfortable not drinking or using drugs.

5. Practice drink and drug refusal lines to find the ones you are most comfortable using.

6. You can be substance-free, have fun, and feel satisfied with life in recovery.

Bulletin Board Outline for Session 14:
Achieving a Balance in Your Life

Introduction

- Early recovery can be a time that feels "out of balance."
- Can feel that life is filled with "treatment."
- Getting treatment can lead to excluding some other important activities.

Course of Recovery

- Tasks of early recovery include:
  - Learning about yourself.
  - Identifying internal and external triggers to use substances.
  - Determining positive coping strategies to manage triggers.
- Early in recovery, it is important to have enough treatment support for these tasks.
- Treatment supports can include:
  - Self-help groups.
  - Group treatment.
  - Individual treatment.
- Important to deal with ambivalence, set priorities, and achieve balance.

Dealing with Ambivalence

- Almost everyone experiences ambivalence some time in recovery.
- What are examples of ambivalent thinking?
  - Wondering whether you really have a substance problem or if it is as serious as others' substance problems.
  - Leads to thoughts such as:
    "It really isn't that bad."
    "I can do it on my own."
- What do you do when you experience ambivalent thoughts or behaviors?
  - Share the thoughts with someone else.
  - Stay in treatment, and don't use substances.
  - Anytime you consider changing treatment, don't do it on your own.
  - *Be sure to discuss pros and cons with your therapist, clinician, or sponsor, and reach an agreement about making changes to your treatment.*

Setting Priorities

- Early in recovery, recovery activities need to be high on the priority list.
- Learning to manage situations without substances takes a lot of support and practice.

(continued)

Achieving Balance in Your Life

- Over time, many women find managing situations substance-free to be easier.
- Slowly, life moves back into a new type of balance.
- This balance has at its center recovery and sobriety.

How to Achieve Balance

- Setting priorities.
- Not using substances to manage triggers.
- Dealing with ambivalence and not using substances or dropping out of treatment when ambivalence arises.
- Learning new ways to manage cravings and triggers.
- Finding or resuming activities that are enjoyable and do not include substance use.
- Practicing these new behaviors and patterns until they feel more natural.

Take-Home Messages for Session 14:
Achieving a Balance in Your Life

1. In early recovery it is important to deal with ambivalence.

2. At all stages of recovery, learn to know when you are having ambivalent thinking.

3. Setting priorities that value self-care is very important.

4. This can mean putting your recovery before other commitments.

5. Dealing with ambivalence and setting priorities can help you achieve a new kind of balance in your life.

Therapist Self-Assessment
in Conducting the Women's Recovery Group

Complete the following self-assessment scale after each session. Recording these points will help you assess the extent to which you are following the basic guidelines of the WRG manual. For each question, rate how extensively you engaged in specific therapist behaviors as you conducted each session:

0	1	2	3	4
not at all	rarely	somewhat	frequently	extensively

_____ 1. Highlighted how session topic is relevant to women with substance use disorders.

_____ 2. Kept check-in brief and structured, focusing specifically on the three check-in questions: (1) Did you have any cravings or urges to use? (2) Did you use? If not, how were you able to remain sober? (3) Did you do the skill practice? If so, what was helpful? Helped members address these questions briefly (i.e., approximately 3 minutes each).

_____ 3. Briefly reviewed lapses and relapses with members who have used since previous session (when appropriate) to help members process the event and learn ways to reduce relapse risk.

_____ 4. Encouraged discussion of specific issues relevant to women with substance use disorders.

_____ 5. Enabled members to share personal details of their own lives relevant to relapse prevention and recovery.

_____ 6. Helped group members relate their discussion to issues of women's physical health, including effects of substance problems on women's health, life cycle issues, self-care, balancing recovery with relationships and caretaking roles, or other themes relevant to relapse prevention and recovery in women.

_____ 7. When presenting session topic, paused occasionally throughout presentation of information to encourage group members' brief discussion of, or questions about, the material and then returned to topic presentation after several minutes.

_____ 8. Stressed the theme of self-care as central to recovery. Can be referred to as "taking care of yourself," "not neglecting your own needs," etc.

_____ 9. Created an atmosphere of trust, respect, and confidentiality.

_____ 10. Made appropriate references to bulletin board materials, core themes of the group on the bulletin board, or skill practices when relevant to session topic and/or participants' open discussion.

_____ 11. Focused the session around a core theme and remained on a recovery or relapse prevention topic (can be multiple different recovery or relapse prevention topics).

_____ 12. Stressed the importance of group attendance.

(continued)

____ 13. Stressed the importance of the four levels of participation (attending group, reflective listening, sharing, and doing the skill practice), and helped members participate at the level with which they were comfortable.

____ 14. Provided open-discussion time for group members to discuss the day's topic or related recovery topics and experiences so that they could support one another.

____ 15. Encouraged members to identify triggers to relapse (can be internal or external triggers: thoughts, feelings, places where one used to use, people, etc.) and alternative strategies to managing these triggers rather than using substances.

____ 16. Encouraged participants to openly discuss experiences concerning addiction and recovery

____ 17. Stressed the importance of abstinence (may be referred to as sobriety, not using, staying clean, staying off, not using drugs or alcohol).

____ 18. Presentation, body language, or verbal feedback characterized by warmth, openness, acceptance, and attention to cues.

____ 19. Handed out skill practice and emphasized helpfulness of doing skill practice during the upcoming week.

____ 20. Ended the session with a wrap-up of highlights or basic themes of the group.

____ 21. Asked group members to each take a turn reading the take-home messages.

____ 22. Completed all parts of the group session (check-in and review of skill practice, topic presentation, discussion, skill practice for next week, take-home messages, and check-out).

____ 23. Completed all parts of group as in question 22 in specified order *and* held to time range for each part of group.

Additional Resources for Therapists

The Women's Recovery Group Study

Cummings, A., Gallop, R. J., & Greenfield, S. F. (2010). Self-efficacy and substance use outcomes for women in single-gender versus mixed-gender group treatment. *Journal of Groups in Addiction and Recovery, 5,* 4–16.

Greenfield, S. F., Crisafulli, M. A., Kaufman, J. S., Freid, C. M., Bailey, G. L., Connery, H. S., et al. (2014). Implementing substance abuse group therapy clinical trials in real-world settings: Challenges and strategies for participant recruitment and therapist training in the Women's Recovery Group Study. *American Journal on Addictions, 23*(3), 197–204.

Greenfield, S. F., Cummings, A. M., Kuper, L. E., Wigderson, S. B., & Koro-Ljungberg, M. (2013). A qualitative analysis of women's experiences in single-gender versus mixed-gender substance abuse group therapy. *Substance Use and Misuse, 48*(9), 772–782.

Greenfield, S. F., Kuper, L. E., Cummings, A. M., Robbins, M. S., & Gallop, R. J. (2013). Group process in the single-gender Women's Recovery Group compared with mixed-gender Group Drug Counseling. *Journal of Groups in Addiction and Recovery, 8*(4), 270–293.

Greenfield, S. F., Sugarman, D. E., Freid, C. M., Bailey, G. L., Crisafulli, M. A., Kaufman, J. S., et al. (2014). Group therapy for women with substance use disorders: Results from the Women's Recovery Group Study. *Drug and Alcohol Dependence, 142,* 245–253.

Greenfield, S. F., Trucco, E. M., McHugh, R. K., Lincoln, M., & Gallop, R. J. (2007). The Women's Recovery Group Study: A stage I trial of women-focused group therapy for substance use disorders versus mixed gender group drug counseling. *Drug and Alcohol Dependence, 90,* 39–47.

Kuper, L. E., Gallop, R. J., & Greenfield, S. F. (2010). Changes in coping moderate substance abuse outcomes differentially across behavioral treatment modality. *American Journal on Addictions, 19,* 543–549.

McHugh, R. K., & Greenfield, S. F. (2010). Psychiatric symptom improvement in women following group substance abuse treatment: Results from the Women's Recovery Group Study. *Journal of Cognitive Psychotherapy, 24,* 26–36.

SUDs in General and Additional Tools and Tips

National Clearinghouse for Alcohol and Drug Information (NCADI): *www.ncadi.samhsa.gov.*
National Institute on Alcohol Abuse and Alcoholism (NIAAA): *www.niaaa.nih.gov.*
National Institute on Drug Abuse (NIDA): *www.nida.nih.gov.*
Substance Abuse and Mental Health Services Administration (SAMHSA): *www.samhsa.gov.*

(continued)

Women and SUDs

Brady, K., Back, S., & Greenfield, S. F. (Eds.). (2009). *Women and addiction: A comprehensive textbook*. New York: Guilford Press.

Centers for Disease Control and Prevention. (2013). Binge drinking: A serious, under-recognized problem among women and girls. *CDC Vital Signs*. Retrieved July 16, 2013, from *www.cdc.gov/VitalSigns/BingeDrinkingFemale/index.html*.

Greenfield, S. F. (2002). Women and alcohol use disorders. *Harvard Review of Psychiatry, 10,* 76–85.

Greenfield, S. F., Back, S., & Brady, K. (2011). Women's issues. In P. Ruiz & E. Strain (Eds.), *Lowinson and Ruiz's substance abuse: A comprehensive textbook* (5th ed., pp. 847–870). Baltimore: Lippincott, Williams and Wilkins.

Greenfield, S. F., Back, S., Lawson, K., & Brady, K. (2010). Substance abuse in women. In S. Kornstein & A. Clayton (Eds.), Women's mental health. *Psychiatric Clinics of North America, 33,* 339–355.

Greenfield, S. F., Brooks, A. J., Gordon, S. M., Green, C. A., Kropp, F., McHugh, R. K., et al. (2007). Substance abuse treatment entry, retention, and outcome in women: A review of the literature. *Drug and Alcohol Dependence, 86,* 1–21.

Greenfield, S. F., & Grella, C. (2009). What is "women-focused" treatment for substance use disorders? *Psychiatric Services, 60,* 880–882.

McHugh, R. K., Wigderson, S., & Greenfield, S. F. (2014). Epidemiology of substance use in reproductive-age women. *Obstetrics and Gynecology Clinics of North America, 41*(2), 177–189.

National Center on Addiction and Substance Abuse at Columbia University (NCASA). (2013). *Women under the influence*. Baltimore: Johns Hopkins University Press.

National Women's Health Information Center (NWHIC): *www.4woman.gov*.

NIAAA: Alcohol: A Women's Health Issue: *http://pubs.niaaa.nih.gov/publications/brochurewomen/women.htm*.

NIAAA: Are Women More Vulnerable to Alcohol's Effects?: *http://pubs.niaaa.nih.gov/publications/aa46.htm*.

NIDA: Substance Use in Women: *www.drugabuse.gov/publications/research-reports/substance-use-in-women/sex-gender-differences-in-substance-use*.

NIDA: Women and Sex Gender Differences Research Group: *www.drugabuse.gov/about-nida/organization/workgroups-interest-groups-consortias/women-sex-gender-differences-research-group*.

SAMHSA Treatment Improvement Protocol: Substance Abuse Treatment: Addressing the Specific Needs of Women: *www.ncbi.nlm.nih.gov/books/NBK26013*.

Sugarman D. E., Brezing C., & Greenfield, S. F. (2013). Women and substance abuse. In A. H. Mack, K. T. Brady, & R. J. Frances (Eds.), *Clinical textbook of addictive disorders* (4th ed., pp. 481–506). New York: Guilford Press.

(continued)

Additional Reading for Specific WRG Topics

The Effect of Drugs and Alcohol on Women's Health

Cao, Y., Willett, W. C., Rimm, E. B., Stampfer, M. J., & Giovannucci, E. L. (2015). Light to moderate intake of alcohol, drinking patterns, and risk of cancer: Results from two prospective U.S. cohorts. *British Medical Journal, 315,* h4238.

Centers for Disease Control and Prevention (CDC): Binge drinking: A serious under-recognized problem among girls and women, 2013: *www.cdc.gov/vitalsigns/bingedrinkingfemale.*

NIAAA: Are Women More Vulnerable to Alcohol's Effects?: *http://pubs.niaaa.nih.gov/publications/aa46.htm.*

NIAAA: Women and Alcohol: An Update: *http://pubs.niaaa.nih.gov/publications/arh26-4/toc26-4.htm*

NIDA Medical Consequences of Drug Abuse: *http://nida.nih.gov/consequences.*

NIDA Notes: A Collection of Articles that Address Women's Health and Gender Differences: *http://archives.drugabuse.gov/NIDA-Notes/NN00013.htm.*

How to Manage Triggers and High-Risk Situations

NIAAA Publications: Relapse prevention: *http://pubs.niaaa.nih.gov/publications/arh23-2/151-160.pdf.*

NIDA Notes: Coping skills help patients recognize and resist the urge to use cocaine: *www.archives.drugabuse.gov/NIDA_Notes/NNVol13N6/Coping.html.*

NIDA Notes: Men and women in drug abuse treatment relapse at different rates and for different reasons: *http://archives.drugabuse.gov/NIDA_Notes/NNVol13N4/Relapse.html.*

Rubin, A., & Stout, R. L. (1996). Gender differences in relapse situations. *Addiction, 91*(Suppl.), S111–S120.

Veenstra, M. Y., Lemmens, P. H. H., Friesema, I. H. M., Tan, F. E. S., Garretsen, H. F. L., Knottnerus, J. A., et al. (2007). Coping style mediates impact of stress on alcohol use: A prospective population-based study. *Addiction, 102,* 1890–1898.

Overcoming Obstacles to Recovery

Greenfield, S. F., Brooks, A. J., Gordon, S. M., Green, C. A., Kropp, F., McHugh, R. K., et al. (2007). Substance abuse treatment entry, retention, and outcome in women: A review of the literature. *Drug and Alcohol Dependence, 86,* 1–21.

Kelly, J. F., & Westerhoff, C. M. (2010). Does it matter how we refer to individuals with substance-related conditions?: A randomized study of two commonly used terms. *International Journal of Drug Policy, 21,* 202–207.

Kessler, R. C., Aguilar-Gaxiola, S., Berglund, P. A., Caraveo-Anduago, J. J., DeWit, D. J., Greenfield, S. F., Kolody, B., et al. (2001). Patterns and predictors of treatment seeking after onset of a substance use disorder. *Archives of General Psychiatry, 58,* 1065–1071.

SAMHSA's Resource Center to Promote Acceptance, Dignity and Social Inclusion Associated with Mental Health (ADS Center): *www.stopstigma.samhsa.gov.*

SAMHSA Treatment Improvement Protocol: Addressing the Specific Needs of Women: Treatment Engagement, Placement, and Planning: *www.ncbi.nlm.nih.gov/books/NBK25634.*

(continued)

Managing Mood, Anxiety, and Eating Problems without Using Substances

Brownell, K. D., & Gold, M. S. (Eds.). (2012). *Food and addiction: A comprehensive handbook.* New York: Oxford University Press.

Magura, S. (2008). Effectiveness of dual focus mutual aid for co-occurring substance use and mental health disorders: A review and synthesis of the "double trouble" in recovery evaluation. *Substance Use and Misuse, 43,* 1904–1926. Also see *www.doubletroubleinrecovery.org.*

NIAAA Alcohol Research and Health: Alcohol and Comorbid Mental Health Disorders: *http://pubs.niaaa.nih.gov/publications/arh26-2/toc26-2.htm.*

NIDA Notes: Gender Affects Relationships between Drug Abuse and Psychiatric Disorders: *http://archives.drugabuse.gov/NIDA_Notes/NNVol12N4/gender.html.*

NIDA Research Report Series: Comorbidity: Addiction and Other Mental Illnesses: *www.drugabuse.gov/ResearchReports/comorbidity/.*

Rounsaville, B. J., Dolinsky, Z. S., Babor, T. F., & Meyer, R. E. (1987). Psychopathology as a predictor of treatment outcome in alcoholics. *Archives of General Psychiatry, 44,* 505–513.

SAMHSA's Co-Occurring Center for Excellence (COCE): *www.coce.samhsa.gov/products/overview_papers.aspx.*

SAMHSA Treatment Improvement Protocol: Substance Abuse Treatment for Persons With Co-Occurring Disorders: A Brief Overview of Specific Mental Disorders and Cross-Cutting Issues: *www.ncbi.nlm.nih.gov/books/NBK26283.*

Women and Their Partners: The Effect on Recovery

Brown, T. G., Kokin, M., Seraganian, P., & Shields, N. (1995). The role of spouses of substance abusers in treatment: Gender differences. *Journal of Psychoactive Drugs, 27,* 223–229.

Fals-Stewart, W., Lam, W., & Kelley, M. L. (2009). Learning sobriety together: Behavioural couples therapy for alcoholism and drug abuse. *Journal of Family Therapy, 31,* 115–125.

Fals-Stewart, W., O'Farrell, T. J., & Lam, W. K. K. (2009). Behavioral couple therapy for gay and lesbian couples with alcohol use disorders. *Journal of Substance Abuse Treatment, 37,* 379–387.

Room, R. (1996). Gender roles and interactions in drinking and drug use. *Journal of Substance Abuse, 8,* 227–239.

Winters, J., Fals-Stewart, W., O'Farrell, T. J., Birchler, G. R., & Kelley, M. L. (2002). Behavioral couples therapy for female substance-abusing patients: Effects on substance use and relationship adjustment. *Journal of Consulting and Clinical Psychology, 70,* 344–355.

Coping with Stress

Brady, K. T., & Sonne, S. C. (1999). The role of stress in alcohol use, alcoholism treatment, and relapse. *Alcohol Research and Health, 23,* 263–271. Also see *http://pubs.niaaa.nih.gov/publications/arh23-4/263-271.pdf.*

Holahan, C. J., Moos, R. H., Holahan, C. K., Cronkite, R. C., & Randall, P. K. (2001). Drinking to cope, emotional distress, and alcohol use and abuse: A ten-year model. *Journal of Studies on Alcohol, 62,* 190–198.

Weaver, G. D., Turner, N. H., & O'Dell, K. J. (2000). Depressive symptoms, stress and coping among women recovering from addiction. *Journal of Substance Abuse Treatment, 18,* 161–167.

(continued)

Women as Caretakers: Can You Take Care of Yourself While You Are Taking Care of Others?

McMahon, T. J., Winkel, J. D., Suchman, N. E., & Luthar, S. S. (2002). Drug dependence, parenting responsibilities, and treatment history: Why doesn't mom go for help? *Drug and Alcohol Dependence, 65,* 105–114.

National Alliance for Caregiving: *www.caregiving.org.*

NWHIC page on caregiver stress: *www.womenshealth.gov/publications/our-publications/ fact-sheet/caregiver-stress.html.*

Sher, K. J. (1997). Psychological characteristics of children of alcoholics. *Alcohol Health and Research World, 21,* 247–255.

Using Self-Help Groups to Help Yourself

Al-Anon/Alateen: *www.al-anon.alateen.org.*

Alcoholics Anonymous (AA): *www.aa.org.*

Cocaine Anonymous (CA): *www.ca.org.*

Fiorentine, R., & Hillhouse, M. P. (2000). Drug treatment and 12-step program participation: The additive effects of integrated recovery activities. *Journal of Substance Abuse Treatment, 18,* 65–74.

Kelly, J. F., & Yeterian, J. D. (2011). The role of mutual-help groups in extending the framework of treatment. *Alcohol Research and Health, 33*(4), 350–355.

Narcotics Anonymous (NA): *www.na.org.*

SMART Recovery: *www.smartrecovery.org.*

Women's Use of Substances through the Life Cycle

Blow, F. C., & Barry, K. L. (2002). Use and misuse of alcohol among older women. *Alcohol Research and Health, 26,* 308–315. Also see *http://pubs.niaaa.nih.gov/publications/ arh26-4/308-315.pdf.*

Centers for Disease Control and Prevention Compendium of Evidence-Based HIV Behavioral Interventions: *www.cdc.gov/hiv/prevention/research/compendium/rr/sssb.html.*

DASIS Report: Drug and Alcohol Services Information System: *www.dasis.samhsa.gov/dasis2/ index.htm.*

Gomberg, E. S. L. (1996). Women's drinking practices and problems from a lifespan perspective. In J. M. Howard, S. E. Matin, P. D. Mail, M. E. Hilton, & E. D. Taylor (Eds.). *Women and alcohol: Issues for prevention research.* Bethesda, MD: National Institute on Alcohol Abuse and Alcoholism.

Klatsky, A. L., Li, Y., Tran, N. H., et al. (2015). Alcohol intake, beverage choice, and cancer: A cohort study in a large Kaiser Permanente population. *The Permanente Journal, 19,* 28–34.

Risk and Protective Factors for Adolescent Drug Use: Findings from the 1999 National Household Survey on Drug Abuse: *www.oas.samhsa.gov/1999Prevention/toc.htm.*

Safer Sex Skills Building: Manual for HIV/STD Safer Sex Skills Groups for Women in Outpatient Substance Abuse Treatment. This treatment manual can be accessed and a PDF downloaded at the National Institute on Drug Abuse website: *http://ctndisseminationlibrary. org/display/398.htm.*

SAMHSA Treatment Improvement Protocol: Substance Abuse among Older Adults: *www.ncbi. nlm.nih.gov/books/NBK14467.*

(continued)

Violence and Abuse: Getting Help

National Center on Domestic Violence, Trauma, and Mental Health: *www. nationalcenterdvtraumamh.org.*

Rape, Abuse and Incest National Network: *www.rainn.org.*

SAMHSA Treatment Improvement Protocol: Substance Abuse Treatment and Domestic Violence: *www.ncbi.nlm.nih.gov/books/NBK14419.*

SAMHSA Treatment Improvement Protocol: Substance Abuse Treatment for Persons with Child Abuse and Neglect Issues: *www.ncbi.nlm.nih.gov/books/NBK14695.*

Study of Women with Co-Occurring Disorders and Lifetime Histories of Interpersonal Trauma: *http://home.fmhi.usf.edu/common/file/ahca/ahca2004/2004-Becker_co_disorders.pdf.*

U.S. Department of Justice Office on Violence against Women: *www.ovw.usdoj.gov.*

Substance Use and Women's Reproductive Health

Connery, H. C., & Rayburn, W. F. (Eds.). (2014). Substance abuse during pregnancy. *Obstetrics and Gynecology Clinics of North America, 41*(2), 1–342.

NIAAA: Alcohol's Effects of Female Reproductive Function: *http://pubs.niaaa.nih.gov/ publications/arh26-4/274-281.htm.*

NIAAA: Effects of Prenatal Alcohol Exposure on Child Development: *http://pubs.niaaa.nih.gov/ publications/arh26-4/282-286.htm.*

Safer Sex Skills Building (SSSB): *http://ctndisseminationlibrary.org/display/398.htm.*

SAMHSA Treatment Improvement Protocol: Pregnant, Substance-Using Women: Treatment Improvement Protocol (TIP) Series 2: *http://adaiclearinghouse.org/downloads/TIP-2-Pregnant-Substance-Using-Women-83.pdf.*

Can You Have Fun without Using Drugs or Alcohol?

Correia, C. J., Benson, T. A., & Carey, K. B. (2005). Decreased substance use following increases in alternative behaviors: A preliminary investigation. *Addictive Behaviors, 30,* 19–27.

Murphy, J. G., Barnett, N. P., Goldstein, A. L., & Colby, S. M. (2007). Gender moderates the relationship between substance-free activity enjoyment and alcohol use. *Psychology of Addictive Behaviors, 21,* 261–265.

Roozen, H. G., Wiersema, H., Strietman, M., Feji, J. A., Lewinsohn, P. M., Meyers, R. J., et al. (2008). Development and psychometric evaluation of the Pleasant Activities List. *American Journal on Addictions, 17,* 422–435.

References

American Psychiatric Association. (2000). *Diagnostic and statistical manual of mental disorders* (4th ed., text rev.). Washington, DC: Author.

American Psychiatric Association. (2013). *Diagnostic and statistical manual of mental disorders* (5th ed.). Arlington, VA: Author.

Anderson, G. L., Judd, H. L., Kaunitz, A. M., Barad, D. H., Beresford, S. A., Pettinger, M., et al. (2003). Effects of estrogen plus progestin on gynecologic cancers and associated diagnostic procedures: The Women's Health Initiative randomized trial. *Journal of the American Medical Association, 290,* 1739–1748.

Ashley, O. S., Marsden, M. E., & Brady, T. M. (2003). Effectiveness of substance abuse treatment programming for women: A review. *American Journal of Drug and Alcohol Abuse, 29*(1), 19–53.

Back, S. E., Killeen, T., Foa, E. B., Ana, E. J. S., Gros, D. F., & Brady, K. T. (2012). Use of an integrated therapy with prolonged exposure to treat PTSD and comorbid alcohol dependence in an Iraq veteran. *American Journal of Psychiatry, 169*(7), 688–691.

Beck, A. T., Brown, G., Epstein, N., & Steer, R. A. (1988). An inventory for measuring clinical anxiety: Psychometric properties. *Journal of Consulting and Clinical Psychology, 56,* 893–897.

Beck, A. T., & Steer, R. A. (1987). *Manual for the revised Beck Depression Inventory.* San Antonio, TX: Psychological Corporation.

Berry, R., & Sellman, J. (2001). Childhood adversity in alcohol- and drug-dependent women presenting to out-patient treatment. *Drug and Alcohol Review, 20*(4), 361–367.

Brady, K. T., Back, S. E., & Greenfield, S. F. (Eds.). (2009). *Women and addiction: A comprehensive handbook.* New York: Guilford Press.

Bride, B. E. (2001). Single-gender treatment of substance abuse: Effect on treatment retention and completion. *Social Work Research, 25,* 223–232.

Brown, P. J. (2000). Outcome in female patients with both substance use and post-traumatic stress disorders. *Alcoholism Treatment Quarterly, 18*(3), 127–135.

Cao, Y., Willett, W. C., Rimm, E. B., Stampfer, M. J., & Giovannucci, E. L. (2015). Light to moderate intake of alcohol, drinking patterns, and risk of cancer: Results from two prospective U.S. cohorts. *British Medical Journal, 315,* h4238.

Centers for Disease Control and Prevention. (2013). Binge drinking: A serious, under-recognized problem among women and girls. *CDC Vital Signs*. Retrieved July 16, 2013, from *www.cdc.gov/VitalSigns/BingeDrinkingFemale/index.html*.

Claus, R. E., Orwin, R. G., Kissin, W., Krupski, A., Campbell, K., & Stark, K. (2007). Does gender-specific substance abuse treatment for women promote continuity of care? *Journal of Substance Abuse Treatment, 32*, 27–39.

Cohen, L. R., Greenfield, S. F., Gordon, S., Killeen, T., Jiang, H., Zhang, Y., et al. (2010). Survey of eating disorder symptoms among women in treatment for substance abuse. *American Journal on Addictions, 19*(3), 245–251.

Comfort, M., Sockloff, A., Loverro, J., & Kaltenbach, K. (2003). Multiple predictors of substance-abusing women's treatment and life outcomes: A prospective longitudinal study. *Addictive Behaviors, 28*(2), 199–224.

Compton, W. M. III, Cottler, L. B., Jacobs, J. L., Ben-Abdallah, A., & Spitznagel, E. L. (2003). The role of psychiatric disorders in predicting drug dependence treatment outcomes. *American Journal of Psychiatry, 160*(5), 890–895.

Copeland, J., & Hall, W. (1992). A comparison of women seeking drug and alcohol treatment in a specialist women's and two traditional mixed-sex treatment services. *British Journal on Addictions, 87*(9), 1293–1302.

Covington, S. S. (2003). *Beyond trauma: A healing journey for women: Facilitator's guide*. Center City, MN: Hazelden.

Crean, R. D., Crane, N. A., & Mason, B. J. (2011). An evidence-based review of acute and long-term effects of cannabis use on executive cognitive functions. *Journal of Addiction Medicine, 5*(1), 1–8.

Cummings, A., Greenfield, S. F., & Gallop, R. (2010). Self-efficacy and substance use outcomes for women in single gender versus mixed-gender group treatment. *Journal of Groups in Addiction and Recovery, 5*, 4–16.

Dawson, D. A. (1996). Gender differences in the probability of alcohol treatment. *Journal of Substance Abuse, 8*(2), 211–225.

Drake, R. E., Mueser, K. T., Brunette, M. F., & McHugo, G. J. (2004). A review of treatments for people with severe mental illnesses and co-occurring substance use disorders. *Psychiatric Rehabilitation Journal, 27*(4), 360–374.

Fiorentine, R., & Hillhouse, M. P. (1999). Drug treatment effectiveness and client–counselor empathy. *Journal of Drug Issues, 29*(1), 59–74.

Franklin, T. R., Ehrman, R., Lynch, K. G., Harper, D., Sciortino, N., O'Brien, C. P., et al. (2008). Menstrual cycle phase at quit date predicts smoking status in an NRT treatment trial: A retrospective analysis. *Journal of Women's Health, 17*(2), 287–292.

Gjersing, L., & Brettville-Jensen, A. L. (2014). Gender differences in mortality and risk factors in a 13-year cohort study of street-recruited injecting drug users. Available at *www.drugabuse.gov/publications/research/reports/substance-use-in-women/sex-gender-differences-in-substance-use*.

Graham, H. L., Copello, A., Birchwood, M. J., Orford, J., McGovern, D., Maslin, J., et al. (2003). Cognitive-behavioral integrated treatment approach for psychosis and problem substance use. In H. L. Graham, A. Copello, M. J. Birchwood, & K. T. Mueser (Eds.), *Substance misuse in psychosis: Approaches to treatment and service delievery* (pp. 181–206). West Sussex UK: Wiley.

Graham, K., Bernards, S., Wilsnack, S. C., & Gmel, G. (2011). Alcohol may not cause partner violence but it seems to make it worse: A cross national comparison of the relationship between alcohol and severity of partner violence. *Journal of Interpersonal Violence, 26*(8), 1503–1523.

Green, C. A., Polen, M. R., Lynch, F. L., Dickinson, D. M., & Bennett, M. D. (2004). Gender differences in outcomes in an HMO-based substance abuse treatment program. *Journal of Addictive Diseases, 23*(2), 47–70.

Greenfield, S. F., Brooks, A. J., Gordon, S. M., Green, C. A., Kropp, F., McHugh, R. K., et al. (2007a). Substance abuse treatment entry, retention, and outcome in women: A review of the literature. *Drug and Alcohol Dependence, 86*(1), 1–21.

Greenfield, S. F., Crisafulli, M. A., Kaufman, J. S., Freid, C. M., Bailey, G. M., Connery, H. S., et al. (2014a). Implementing substance abuse group therapy clinical trials in real-world settings: Challenges and strategies for participant recruitment and therapist training in the Women's Recovery Group Study. *American Journal of Addiction, 23*(3), 197–204.

Greenfield, S. F., Cummings, A. M., Kuper, L. E., Wigderson, S. B., & Koro-Ljungberg, M. (2013a). A qualitative analysis of women's experiences in single-gender versus mixed-gender substance abuse group therapy. *Substance Use and Misuse, 48*(9), 772–782.

Greenfield, S. F., & Grella, C. E. (2009). What is "women-focused" treatment for substance use disorders? *Psychiatric Services, 60*(7), 880–882.

Greenfield, S. F., & Hennessy, G. (2008). Assessment of the patient. In M. Galanter & H. D. Kleber (Eds.), *The American Psychiatric Publishing textbook of substance abuse treatment* (4th ed., pp. 55–78). Arlington, VA: American Psychiatric Publishing.

Greenfield, S. F., & Hennessy, G. (2015). Assessment of the patient. In M. Galanter, H. D. Kleber, & K. Brady (Eds.), *The American Psychiatric Publishing textbook of substance abuse treatment* (5th ed., pp. 81–98). Arlington, VA: American Psychiatric Publishing.

Greenfield, S. F., Kolodziej, M. E., Sugarman, D. E., Muenz, L. R., Vagge, L. M., He, D. Y., et al. (2002). History of abuse and drinking outcomes following inpatient alcohol treatment: A prospective study. *Drug and Alcohol Dependence, 67*(3), 227–234.

Greenfield, S. F., Kuper, L. E., Cummings, A. M., Robbins, M. S., & Gallop, R. J. (2013b). Group process in the single-gender Women's Recovery Group compared with mixed-gender Group Drug Counseling. *Journal of Groups in Addiction and Recovery, 8*(4), 270–293.

Greenfield, S. F., Sugarman, D. E., Freid, C. M., Bailey, G. L., Crisafulli, M. A., Kaufman, J. S., et al. (2014b). Group therapy for women with substance use disorders: Results from the Women's Recovery Group Study. *Drug and Alcohol Dependence, 142*, 245–253.

Greenfield, S. F., Trucco, E. M., McHugh, R. K., Lincoln, M. F., & Gallop, R. (2007b). The Women's Recovery Group Study: A Stage I trial of women-focused group therapy for substance use disorders versus mixed-gender group drug counseling. *Drug and Alcohol Dependence, 90*, 39–47.

Greenfield, S. F., Weiss, R. D., Muenz, L. R., Vagge, L. M., Kelly, J. F., Bello, L. R., et al. (1998). The effect of depression on return to drinking: A prospective study. *Archives of General Psychiatry, 55*(3), 259–265.

Grella, C. E. (2008). From generic to gender-responsive treatment: Changes in social policies, treatment services, and outcomes of women in substance abuse treatment. *Journal of Psychoactive Drugs, Suppl. 5*, 327–343.

Grella, C. E., Scott, C. K., & Foss, M. A. (2005). Gender differences in long-term drug treatment outcomes in Chicago PETS. *Journal of Substance Abuse Treatment, 28*(Suppl. 1), S3–S12.

Grucza, R. A., Bucholz, K. K., Rice, J. P., & Bierut, L. J. (2008). Secular trends in the lifetime prevalence of alcohol dependence in the United States: A re-evaluation. *Alcoholism: Clinical and Experimental Research, 32*(5), 763–770.

Hernandez-Avila, C. A., Rounsaville, B. J., & Kranzler, H. R. (2004). Opioid-, cannabis- and alcohol-dependent women show more rapid progression to substance abuse treatment. *Drug and Alcohol Dependence, 74*(3), 265–272.

Hien, D. A., Cohen, L. R., & Campbell, A. (2005). Is traumatic stress a vulnerability factor for women with substance use disorders? *Clinical Psychology Review, 25*(6), 813–823.

Hien, D. A., Cohen, L. R., Miele, G. M., Litt, L. C., & Capstick, C. (2004). Promising treatments for women with comorbid PTSD and substance use disorders. *American Journal of Psychiatry, 161*(8), 1426–1432.

Huang, C., & Lee, C. (2013). Factors associated with mortality among heroin users after seeking treatment with methadone: A population-based cohort study in Taiwan. *Journal of Substance Abuse Treatment, 44*(3), 295–300.

Jones, C. M., Logan, J., Gladden, R. M., & Bohm, M. K., (2015). Vital signs: Demographic and substance use trends among heroin users—United States, 2002–2013. *Morbidity and Mortality Weekly Report, 64*, 719–725.

Kaskutas, L. A., Zhang, L., French, M. T., & Witbrodt, J. (2005). Women's programs versus mixed-gender day treatment: Results from a randomized study. *Addiction, 100*(1), 60–69.

Kauffman, E., Dore, M. M., & Nelson-Zlupko, L. (1995). The role of women's therapy groups in the treatment of chemical dependence. *American Journal of Orthopsychiatry, 65*(3), 355–363.

Klatsky, A. L., Li, Y., Tran, N. H., et al. (2015). Alcohol intake, beverage choice, and cancer: A cohort study in a large Kaiser Permanente population. *The Permanente Journal, 19*, 28–34.

Kranzler, H. R., & Tinsley, J. A. (2004). *Dual diagnosis and psychiatric treatment: Substance abuse and comorbid disorders* (2nd ed.). New York: Marcel Dekker.

Kuper, L. E., Gallop, R., & Greenfield, S. F. (2010). Changes in coping moderate substance abuse outcomes differentially across behavioral treatment modality. *American Journal on Addictions, 19*(6), 543–549.

Liebschutz, J., Savetsky, J. B., Saitz, R., Horton, N. J., Lloyd-Travaglini, C., & Samet, J. H. (2002). The relationship between sexual and physical abuse and substance abuse consequences. *Journal of Substance Abuse Treatment, 22*, 121–128.

Linehan, M. M., Schmidt, H. III, Dimeff, L. A., Craft, J. C., Kanter, J., & Comtois, K. A. (1999). Dialectical behavior therapy for patients with borderline personality disorder and drug-dependence. *American Journal on Addictions, 8*(4), 279–292.

Lopez-Quintero, C., de los Cobos, J. P., Hasin, D. S., Okuda, M., Wang, S., Grant, B. F., et al. (2011). Probability and predictors of transition from first use to dependence on nicotine, alcohol, cannabis, and cocaine: Results of the National Epidemiologic Survey on Alcohol and Related Conditions (NESARC). *Drug and Alcohol Dependence, 115*(1–2), 120–130.

Luthar, S. S., & Suchman, N. E. (2000). Relational Psychotherapy Mothers' Group: A developmentally informed intervention for at-risk mothers. *Development and Psychopathology, 12*(2), 235–253.

Mackie-Ramos, R. L., & Rice, J. M. (1988). Group psychotherapy with methadone-maintained pregnant women. *Journal of Substance Abuse Treatment, 5*(3), 151–161.

Mathers B. M., Degenhardt, L., Bucello, C., Lemon, J., Wiessing, L., & Hickman, M. (2013). Mortality among people who inject drugs: A systematic review and meta-analysis. *Bulletin of the World Health Organization, 91*(2), 81–156. Retrieved from *www.who.int/bulletin/volumes/91/2/12–108282/en*.

McHugh, R. K., & Greenfield, S. F. (2010). Psychiatric symptom improvement in women following group substance abuse treatment: Results from the Women's Recovery Group Study. *Journal of Cognitive Psychotherapy, 24*(1), 26–36.

McHugh, R. K., Wigderson, S., & Greenfield, S. F. (2014). Epidemiology of substance use in reproductive-age women. *Obstetrics and Gynecology Clinics of North America, 41*(2), 177–189.

McKay, J. R., Lynch, K. G., Pettinati, H. M., & Shepard, D. S. (2003). An examination of potential sex and race effects in a study of continuing care for alcohol- and cocaine-dependent patients. *Alcoholism: Clinical and Experimental Research, 27*(8), 1321–1323.

McLellan, A. T., Kushner, H., Metzger, D., Peters, R., Smith, I., Grissom, G., et al. (1992). The fifth edition of the Addiction Severity Index. *Journal of Substance Abuse Treatment, 9*, 199–213.

Mojtabai, R. (2005). Use of specialty substance abuse and mental health services in adults with substance use disorders in the community. *Drug and Alcohol Dependence, 78*(3), 345–354.

Morgan-Lopez, A. A., & Fals-Stewart, W. (2006). Analytic complexities associated with group therapy in substance abuse treatment research: Problems, recommendations, and future directions. *Experimental and Clinical Psychopharmacology, 14*(2), 265–273.

Murty, S. A., Peek-Asa, C., Zwerling, C., Stromquist, A. M., Burmeister, L. F., & Merchant, J. A. (2003). Physical and emotional partner abuse reported by men and women in a rural community. *American Journal of Public Health, 93*(7), 1073–1075.

Najavits, L., Weiss, R., Shaw, S., & Muenz, L. (1998). "Seeking safety": Outcome of a new cognitive-behavioral psychotherapy for women with postttraumatic stress disorder and substance dependence. *Journal of Traumatic Stress, 11*, 437–456.

National Institute of Mental Health. (n.d.-a). What are the signs and symptoms of depression? Retrieved April 25, 2015, from *www.nimh.nih.gov/health/publications/depression/index.shtml?ct=39994*.

National Institute of Mental Health. (n.d.-b). What is generalized anxiety disorder? Retrieved April 25, 2015, from *www.nimh.nih.gov/health/topics/generalized-anxiety-disorder-gad/index.shtml*.

National Institute of Mental Health. (n.d.-c). What is social phobia? Retrieved April 25, 2015, from *www.nimh.nih.gov/health/topics/social-phobia-social-anxiety-disorder/index.shtml*.

National Institute of Mental Health. (n.d.-d). Signs and symptoms of anorexia nervosa. Retrieved April 25, 2015, from *www.nimh.nih.gov/health/topics/eating-disorders/index.shtml*.

National Institute of Mental Health. (n.d.-e). Signs and symptoms of bulimia nervosa. Retrieved April 25, 2015, from *www.nimh.nih.gov/health/topics/eating-disorders/index.shtml*.

National Institute of Mental Health. (n.d.-f). Binge eating disorder. Retrieved April 25, 2015, from *www. nimh.nih.gov/health/topics/eating-disorders/index.shtml*.

Nelson-Zlupko, L., Dore, M., Kauffman, E., & Kaltenbach, K. (1996). Women in recovery: Their perceptions of treatment effectiveness. *Journal of Substance Abuse Treatment, 13*(1), 51–59.

Nguyen, T. D., Attkisson, C. C., & Stegner, B. L. (1983). Assessment of patient satisfaction: Development and refinement of a service evaluation questionnaire. *Evaluation and Program Planning, 6*, 299–314.

Orwin, R. G., Francisco, L., & Bernichon, T. (2001). *Effectiveness of women's substance abuse treatment programs: A meta-analysis.* Arlington, VA: Substance Abuse and Mental Health Services Administration.

Perucci, C. A., Davoli, M., Rapiti, E., Abeni, D. D., & Forastiere, E. (1991). Mortality of intravenous drug users in Rome: A cohort study. *American Journal of Public Health, 81*(10), 1307–1310.

Piazza, N. J., Vrbka, J. L., & Yeager, R. D. (1989). Telescoping of alcoholism in women alcoholics. *International Journal of the Addictions, 24*, 19–28.

Quaglio, G., Talamini, G., Lechi, A., Venturini, L., Lugoboni, F., & Mezzelani, P. (2001). Study of 2708 heroin-related deaths in north-eastern Italy 1985–98 to establish the main causes of death. *Addiction, 96*(8), 1127–1137.

Randall, C. L., Roberts, J. S., Del Boca, F. K., Carroll, K. M., Connors, G. J., & Mattson, M. E. (1999). Telescoping of landmark events associated with drinking: A gender comparison. *Journal of Studies on Alcohol, 60*(2), 252–260.

Robins, L. N., & Regier, D. A. (1991). *Psychiatric disorders in America: The Epidemiologic Catchment Area Study.* New York: Free Press.

Ruiz, P., & Strain, E. (Eds.). (2011). *Lowinson and Ruiz's substance abuse: A comprehensive textbook* (5th ed.). Philadelphia: Lippincott Williams & Wilkins.

Satre, D. D., Blow, F. C., Chi, F. W., & Weisner, C. (2007). Gender differences in seven-year alcohol and drug treatment outcomes among older adults. *American Journal on Addictions, 16*(3), 216–221.

Sinha, R., & Rounsaville, B. J. (2002). Sex differences in depressed substance abusers. *Journal of Clinical Psychiatry, 63*(7), 616–627.

Smith, B. D., & Marsh, J. C. (2002). Client–service matching in substance abuse treatment for women with children. *Journal of Substance Abuse Treatment, 22*(3), 161–168.

Sobell, L. C., & Sobell, M. B. (1992). Timeline follow-back: A technique for assessing self-reported alcohol consumption. In R. Z. Litten & J. P. Allen (Eds.), *Measuring alcohol consumption: Psychosocial and biochemical methods* (pp. 41–72). Totowa, NJ: Humana Press.

Sterling, R. C., Gottheil, E., Weinstein, S. P., & Serota, R. (1998). Therapist/patient race and sex matching: Treatment retention and 9–month follow-up outcome. *Addiction, 93*(7), 1043–1050.

Sterling, R. C., Gottheil, E., Weinstein, S. P., & Serota, R. (2001). The effect of therapist/patient race- and sex-matching in individual treatment. *Addiction, 96*(7), 1015–1022.

Stewart, D., Gossop, M., Marsden, J., Kidd, T., & Treacy, S. (2003). Similarities in outcomes for men and women after drug misuse treatment: Results from the National Treatment Outcome Research Study (NTORS). *Drug and Alcohol Review, 22*(1), 35–41.

Substance Abuse and Mental Health Services Administration. (2012). Results from the 2011 National Survey on Drug Use and Health: Summary of national findings. Retrieved from *www.samhsa.gov/data/nsduh/2k11results/NSDUHresultsAlts2011*.

Substance Abuse and Mental Health Services Administration. (2013). *Results from the 2012 National Survey on Drug Use and Health: Detailed tables.* Rockville, MD: Author.

Sugarman, D. E., Brezing, C., & Greenfield, S. F. (2013). Women and substance abuse. In A. H. Mack, K. T. Brady, S. I. Miller, & R. J. Frances (Eds.), *Clinical textbook of addictive disorders* (4th ed., pp. 481–506). New York: Guilford Press.

Sugarman, D. E., Kaufman, J. S., Trucco, E. M., Brown, J. C., & Greenfield, S. G. (2014). Predictors of drinking and functional outcomes in men and women following inpatient alcohol treatment. *American Journal on Addictions, 23*(3), 226–233.

Terner, J. M., & De Wit, H. (2006). Menstrual cycle phase and responses to drugs of abuse in humans. *Drug and Alcohol Dependence, 84*(1), 1–13.

Timko, C., DeBenedetti, A., Moos, B. S., & Moos, R. H. (2006). Predictors of 16–year mortality among individuals initiating help-seeking for an alcoholic use disorder. *Alcoholism: Clinical and Experimental Research, 30*(10), 1711–1720.

Tross, S., Campbell, A. N. C., Cohen, L. R., Calsyn, D., Pavlicova, M., Miele, G. M., et al. (2008). Effectiveness of HIV/STD sexual risk reduction groups for women in substance abuse treatment programs: Results of NIDA clinical trials network trial. *Journal of Acquired Immune Deficiency Syndromes, 48*(5), 581–589.

Trucco, E. M., Connery, H. S., Griffin, M., & Greenfield, S. F. (2007). The relationship of self-efficacy and self-esteem to treatment outcomes in alcohol dependent men and women. *American Journal on Addictions, 16*(2), 85–92.

Ullman, S. E., Najdowski, C. J., & Adams, E. B. (2012). Women, Alcoholics Anonymous, and related mutual aid groups: Review and recommendations for research. *Alcoholism Treatment Quarterly, 30*(4), 443–486.

Washton, A. M. (2005). Group therapy with outpatients. In J. H. Lowinson, P. Ruiz, R. B. Millman, & J. G. Langrod (Eds.), *Substance abuse: A comprehensive textbook* (4th ed., pp. 671–679). Philadelphia: Lippincott Williams & Wilkins.

Wechsberg, W. M., Craddock, S. G., & Hubbard, R. L. (1998). How are women who enter substance abuse treatment different than men?: A gender comparison from the Drug Abuse Treatment Outcome Study (DATOS). *Drugs and Society, 13*(1–2), 97–115.

Weisner, C. (1993). Toward an alcohol treatment entry model: A comparison of problem drinkers in the general population. *Alcoholism: Clinical and Experimental Research, 17*(4), 746–752.

Weisner, C., & Schmidt, L. (1992). Gender disparities in treatment for alcohol problems. *Journal of the American Medical Association, 268*, 1872–1876.

Weiss, R. D., & Connery, H. S. (2011). *Integrated group therapy for bipolar disorder and substance abuse.* New York: Guilford Press.

Wells, E. A., Donovan, D. M., Doyle, S. R., & Hatch-Maillette, M. A. (2014). Is level of exposure to a twelve step facilitation therapy associated with treatment outcome? *Journal of Substance Abuse Treatment, 47*(4), 265–274.

World Health Organization. (1992). *International classification of diseases* (version 10). Geneva, Switzerland: Author.

Wu, L.-T., & Ringwalt, C. L. (2004). Alcohol dependence and use of treatment services among women in the community. *American Journal of Psychiatry, 161*(10), 1790–1797.

Index

Note: *f* following a page number indicates a figure; *t* indicates a table.